Essential Hypertension

Essential Hypertension

John Malcolm Cruickshank, BM, BCH, MA,
DM(Oxford), FRCP(London)
Independent Cardiovascular Consultant
London, United Kingdom

2013
PEOPLE'S MEDICAL PUBLISHING HOUSE—USA
SHELTON, CONNECTICUT

People's Medical Publishing House-USA
2 Enterprise Drive, Suite 509
Shelton, CT 06484
Tel: 203-402-0646
Fax: 203-402-0854
E-mail: info@pmph-usa.com

PMPH-USA

13 14 15 16/SBI/9 8 7 6 5 4 3 2 1

ISBN-13 978-1-60795-168-1
ISBN-10 1-60795-168-1
eISBN-13 978-1-60795-253-4

Printed in the United States of America by Sheridan Books, Inc.
Editor: Jason Malley; Copyeditor/Typesetter: diacriTech; Cover designer: Allison Dibble

Library of Congress Cataloging-in-Publication Data

Cruickshank, J. M.
Essential hypertension / John Malcolm Cruickshank.
p. ; cm.
Includes bibliographical references and index.
ISBN-13: 978-1-60795-168-1
ISBN-10: 1-60795-168-1
ISBN-13: 978-1-60795-253-4 (eISBN)
1. Title.

[DNLM: 1. Hypertension. WG 340]
LC Classification not assigned
616.1 32—dc23

2012037763

Sales and Distribution

Canada
McGraw-Hill Ryerson Education
Customer Care
300 Water St
Whitby, Ontario L1N 9B6
Canada
Tel: 1-800-565-5758
Fax: 1-800-463-5885
www.mcgrawhill.ca

Foreign Rights
John Scott & Company
International Publisher's Agency
P.O. Box 878
Kimberton, PA 19442, USA
Tel: 610-827-1640
Fax: 610-827-1671

Japan
United Publishers Services Limited
1-32-5 Higashi-Shinagawa
Shinagawa-ku, Tokyo 140-0002
Japan
Tel: 03-5479-7251
Fax: 03-5479-7307
Email: kakimoto@ups.co.jp

United Kingdom, Europe, Middle East, Africa
McGraw Hill Education
Shoppenhangers Road
Maidenhead
Berkshire, SL6 2QL
England
Tel: 44-0-1628-502500
Fax: 44-0-1628-635895
www.mcgraw-hill.co.uk

Singapore, Thailand, Philippines, Indonesia, Vietnam, Pacific Rim, Korea
McGraw-Hill Education
60 Tuas Basin Link
Singapore 638775
Tel: 65-6863-1580
Fax: 65-6862-3354
www.mcgraw-hill.com.sg

Australia, New Zealand
Elsevier Australia
Locked Bag 7500
Chatswood DC NSW 2067
Australia
Tel: 161 (2) 9422-8500
Fax: 161 (2) 9422-8562
www.elsevier.com.au

Brazil
SuperPedido Tecmedd
Beatriz Alves, Foreign Trade Department
R. Sansao Alves dos Santos
102l7th floor
Brooklin Novo
Sao Paolo 04571-090
Brazil
Tel: 55-16-3512-5539
www.superpedidotecmedd.com.br

India, Bangladesh, Pakistan, Sri Lanka, Malaysia
CBS Publishers
4819/X1 Prahlad Street
24 Ansari Road, Darya Ganj
New Delhi-110002
India
Tel: 91-11-23266861/67
Fax: 91-11-23266818
Email: cbspubs@vsnl.com

People's Republic of China
People's Medical Publishing House
International Trade Department
No. 19, Pan Jia Yuan Nan Li
Chaoyang District
Beijing 100021
P.R. China
Tel: 8610-67653342
Fax: 8610-67691034
www.pmph.com/en/

Foreword

Essential Hypertension is a strange name for the most prevalent of the diseases of a westernized society. There is nothing essential about it. Very few areas of medicine of such apparent simplicity have been subject to so much research. Blood pressure is a characteristic; a physiological variable that is subject to large postural, emotional, and physiological changes, which is both closely monitored and stabilized by means of short-term reflexes and yet is subject to large increases over time in asymptomatic people who indulge in a modern "Western" diet and lifestyle. Chronically elevated blood pressure, defined as hypertension only on the basis of a numerical increase in blood pressure the precise cut-off of which is still uncertain, puts people at dramatically increased risk of vascular damage and consequent organ damage, including stroke, heart attack, dementia, renal failure, blindness, and death. The "essential" of the title merely means it is not due to any identifiable primary disease like an endocrine tumour, metabolic disorder, aortic coarctation, renal disease, or renal arterial stenosis.

The book by John Cruickshank, a veteran of early drug development in hypertension and an early champion of beta-blockers, is full of statistics that would surprise most non-medical people. The lifetime risk of developing hypertension once you reach the age of 60 years is 90%; over 7 million deaths per year are attributable to high blood pressure alone; and you, the reader, If an adult living in a modern Western country, will have has more than a one in three chance of having hypertension. Can it really be a disease if virtually all of us get it? Yet we believe that with traditional diets and lifestyles hypertension is uncommon; it is the disease of a developed society, with genetic factors playing a more minor role in causation and the environment—including salt intake—contributing the majority, around 70%, of causation. John is a pioneer, not just in the use of beta-blockers but also in the role of sympathetic overactivity in the genesis of hypertension and of the so-called "J-curve," wherein there is a point below which further reduction of blood pressure ceases to protect and may actually increase the risk of future cardiovascular events. He is a passionate advocate for the use of traditional drug classes (especially beta blockers and diuretics) in treating high blood pressure, arguing against recent attempts to relegate beta blockers to a second-, or third-, or even fourth-line therapy for hypertension. He argues instead for profiling patients based on age, co-morbidities, and heart rate (as a surrogate of sympathetic tone) into those more or less likely to respond to the wide array of drug classes we have today to manage high blood pressure.

This book is, in my opinion, an invaluable source of information and perspective on this most common and enigmatic of the conditions of modern life. Pickering won the argument over Platt: hypertension is not a disease we can diagnose, but a measurement we should make, yet we still treat hypertension as a disease one either has or does not have rather than as an aspect of risk we should manage. Pre-hypertension, "white coat" hypertension, masked hypertension, labile hypertension, and isolated systolic hypertension all are ways to describe a physiological variable outside of the healthy range that tells us something about the state of our blood vessels and our risk for vascular events in the future. What we need to know is, when is it on balance worthwhile doing something to change our blood pressure, whether through lifestyle changes or drug intervention? Even the measurement of blood pressure remains controversial, with guidelines beginning to recommend central aortic blood pressure measurement and ambulatory and/or home blood pressure monitoring rather than the 100-year-old clinic cuff method. This change has come only after decades of research showing that the cuff method in a clinic setting may be quite unreliable for making an accurate prediction of an individual's risk for cardiovascular disease! In hypertension, as in many other things, John Cruickshank's masterly book tells us nothing is as simple as it seems, and yet the old and traditional may still be very worthwhile.

—Andrew J. Stewart Coats
Melbourne, November 2012

Preface

The global burden of hypertension is extremely high, the prevalence in Europe being a staggering 44%. The Framingham Heart Study tells us that, from the age of 65, the lifetime risk of developing hypertension is about 90%!

Thus, not surprisingly, hypertension is the number one risk factor for premature death in the world, way ahead of cigarette smoking and high cholesterol. About 80% of this burden is in low- to middle-income populations.

Genetic factors are linked to about 30% of essential hypertensive cases. Of the remaining 70%, environmental factors are involved, and the world-wide epidemic of obesity is a key component in the young to middle-aged diastolic hypertensive person. In the elderly, aging and stiffening of the arteries play the vital role in the development of systolic hypertension. Thus, diastolic hypertension and isolated systolic hypertension are quite different disease entities, and each requires its own form of optimal treatment.

In the younger or middle-aged diastolic hypertensive, whether overweight/obese or normal weight, there is underlying increased sympathetic nerve activity. In this group (with sensitized beta receptors), it is the level of blood pressure that relates to stroke. By contrast, myocardial infarction is related to the degree of sympathetic nerve activity. Clearly, this will have an impact on the choice of antihypertensive agent in this younger to middle-aged group, where myocardial infarction is three times more common than stroke. Thus, antihypertensive agents that increase sympathetic nerve activity, that is, thiazide-type diuretics, dihydropyridine calcium blockers and ARBs, do not reduce (and may increase) the risk of myocardial infarction in the young to middle-aged diastolic hypertensive. Resting heart rate is a good surrogate for sympathetic nerve activity. Hence, among young to middle-aged hypertensives, resting heart rates greater than 80–85 bpm are strong predictors of premature coronary/cardiovascular deaths. It is this scenario that, unlike elderly systolic hypertension, is ideal for beta-1 blockade, where not only is stroke risk diminished, but also that of myocardial infarction. In elderly systolic hypertension (with desensitized beta-receptors), first-line diuretics or calcium blockers are appropriate.

There is much disagreement in the recommendations of guideline committees around the world. Thus, (a) the UK NICE committee recommends ACE/ARB for younger diastolic hypertensive subjects and calcium blockers for elderly systolic hypertensive subjects; beta-blockers and diuretics have been discarded as first-line choices for uncomplicated hypertension. (b) The US JNC-7 committee recommends diuretics as the first choice for all hypertensive cases. (c) The European guidelines recommend all classes of antihypertensive agents for both young and old.

This book seeks to throw a little light on a very confused, but vitally important, area termed essential hypertension.

I would like to thank Moira, my wife, for her sterling secretarial efforts, and Alan Thompson (retired head-master) for his stern attention to my spelling and grammatical errors.

—JMC
June 2012

Contents

Essential Hypertension

CHAPTER 1

A BRIEF HISTORY

1. Measurement

Descriptions from Egypt in the "Edwin Smith Papyrus," dating to 1600 BC, contain references to the examination of the pulse (1). It was Stephen Hales who first directly measured blood pressure, by inserting a brass tube into the crural artery of a horse and connecting it to a glass tube! (2). Clearly, Hales' methods are not applicable to humans.

It was Etienne Jules Marcy who, in 1860, was the first to measure blood pressure in humans (2). He designed the sphygmograph that measured the arterial pressure wave noninvasively (**Figure 1-1**). The radial pulse wave transmitted directly to a metal plate applied closely to the skin of the forearm, amplified closely to the skin of the forearm, and amplified and recorded on a smoked paper. It

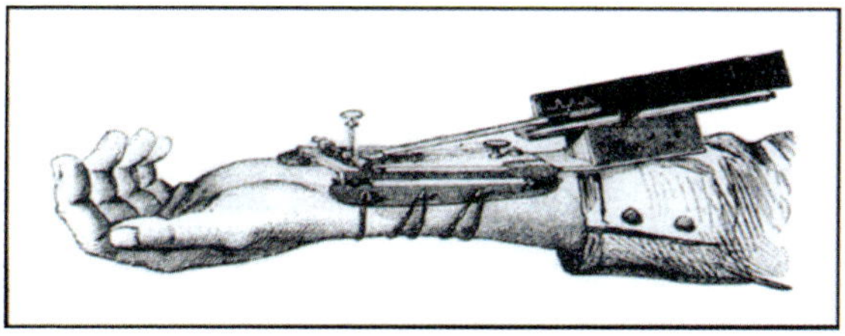

Fig. 1-1 Sphygmograph by Etienne Marie 1860.

was Frederick Mahomid who adapted Marey's sphygmograph for clinical practice (2). It was derived from the pressure with which the sphygmograph had to be applied to the forearm to secure a maximal pressure wave. When the applied pressure exceeded the blood pressure, it was hypothesized that progressive dampening of the waveform would occur (expressed in ounces). Thus, he was able to demonstrate the elevation of blood pressure in patients without renal disease, and he also predicted a long asymptomatic phase ending in breathlessness or apoplectic seizure. It was von Basch who was more successful in using a carefully positioned (against the head of radius) fluid-filled bulb connected to a manometer, recording the pressure needed to prevent oscillations in the radial artery (2). It was not until Riva-Rocci, in 1896, designed an air-filled rubber bag as an occlusive device, that measurement of systolic blood pressure became a routine part of the clinical examination (3). However, there was no measurement of diastolic pressure until Korotkoff described them in 1905 (**Figure 1-2**) (4). He became interested in the sounds created by changes in vascular lumen diameter, particularly the sounds created by arterial constriction resulting from application of the Riva-Rocci cuff to the upper arm. Phase 1 (appearance), phase 4 (muffling), and phase 5 (disappearance) of the Korotkoff sounds are still used in manual measurement of blood pressure.

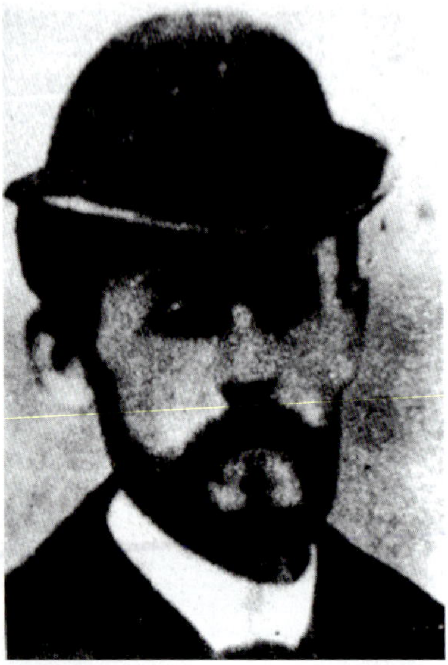

Fig. 1-2 Nikolai Korotkoff.

2. Laboratory aspects

It was in 1904 that high blood pressure was linked to renal disease and salt intake (5). Even earlier, in 1889, Tigerstedt and Bergman (6) had noted a renal hormone with a prolonged pressor action. It was much later that, in 1934, Goldblatt et al. identified this pressor substance as renin (7). The components of the renin–angiotensin system were identified in 1940s, the amino acid sequences of the peptides angiotensin I and II were identified in 1950s, and the gene-coding for renin, angiotensinogen, and converting enzymes were identified in the 1980s.

3. Growth of epidemiology and the controlled clinical trial

It was the second half of the 20th century that the rapidly developing science of epidemiology occurred. The universal assumption that hypertension was a discrete, largely inherited disorder, championed by Platt, was challenged by George Pickering. He introduced the concept that high blood pressure was a quantitative deviation from the population mean (8). Pickering's views prevailed, and hypertension was regarded as a multifactorial condition arising from the interaction of an unknown number of genetic and environmental influences.

Since the early 1950s, the clinical trial has become progressively more sophisticated, culminating in the double-blind, randomized, crossover/parallel group design. Thus, therapeutic interventions can be precisely assessed and, with the advent of large "hard end-point" trials, drug effects on death, stroke, myocardial infarction, heart failure, and so forth, can be measured. Meta-analysis techniques can prove powerful tools in bringing together the results of many (possibly underpowered) studies.

4. Modern methods of measuring blood pressure

During the first half of the 20th century, mercury, aneroid, and oscillometric manometers came into regular use. However, the universal mercury sphygmomanometer was replaced by other devices for safety reasons (mercury is poisonous).

It is now recognized that the so-called "office," or clinical blood pressures, are somewhat unreliable and inaccurate, and are prone to "white-coat" hypertension. Automated devices used at home can remove observer error, avoid white-coat hypertension, and provide printouts of blood pressure over time (9). The ultimate home blood pressure assessment is through 24-hour ambulatory blood pressure monitoring, which gives information of nocturnal as well as daytime blood pressure (10).

Central (aortic) blood pressure is now recognized as the "ultimate" pressure that vital organs such as the heart, brain, and kidney are exposed to. The central pressures can be assessed either invasively (research tool) or indirectly through arterial (usually radial) tonometry. Applanation tonometry can assess aortic waveforms from the radial artery; waveform analysis can indicate central pressures (11).

REFERENCES

1. Breasted JH. *The Edwin Smith Surgical Papyrus*, Vol 1. Chicago, IL: University of Chicago Press; 1930:105.
2. Swales JD. *Text Book of Hypertension*. Oxford: Blackwell Scientific Publications; 1994:1–7.
3. Riva-Rocci S. Un stigmmomanometro nuovo. *Gaz Med Torino* 1896;47:981–96, 1001–17.
4. Korotkoff NS. K voprosu o metodoach eezldovania Krovyanovo davlenia. *ISV Imperatoor Vorenno Med Akad* 1905;11:365–7.
5. Ambard L, Beaujard E. Causes de l'hypertension arterielle. *Arch Gen Med* 1904;1:520–33.
6. Tigerstedt R, Bergman PG. Niere und Kreislauf. *Skand Archiv Physiol* 1898;7–8:223–71.
7. Goldblatt H, Lynch J, Hanzal RF, et al. Studies on experimental hypertension. Part 1. The production of persistent elevation of systolic blood pressure by means of renal ischaemia. *J Exp Med* 1934;59:347–78.
8. Swales JD. *Platt Versus Pickering*. London: Keynes Press; 1985:156.
9. Jones DW, Appel LJ, Sheps SG, et al. Measuring blood pressure accurately. *JAMA* 2003;289:1027–30.
10. Prasad N, Isles C. Ambulatory blood pressure monitoring: a guide for general practitioners. *BMJ* 1996;313:1535–41.
11. Nelson MR, Stepanek J, Cevette M, et al. Noninvasive measurement of central vascular pressures with arterial tonometry: clinical revival of the pulse pressure wave form. *Mayo Clin Proc* 2010;85:460–72.

What Is High Blood Pressure?

CHAPTER 2

BRACHIAL BLOOD PRESSURE IN CLINIC

1. Defining hypertension

It is important to differentiate brachial blood pressure (BP) from central BP. Historically, the term "high blood pressure" is related to brachial BP assessed in the clinic. Central (aortic) BPs are a more recent development and can be measured either directly or indirectly in only specialized units.

The definition of hypertension, as pointed out by Pickering (1), is arbitrary. Looking at the frequency/distribution curves of arterial BP in populations, there is no dividing line, although there have been several suggested divisions of normotension and hypertension over the years (**Table 2-1**) (1). The dividing line is in fact nothing but an artifact. Having said that, most modern physicians regard a rested clinic blood pressure greater than 140/90 mm Hg as hypertensive. On that basis, about 40% of the middle-aged population of westernized countries has a diastolic BP (DBP) greater than 90 mm Hg, with 35% being mild to moderate and 5% severe (**Figure 2-1**) (2).

To come back to Pickering's "artifact" of an arbitrary dividing line between hypertension and normal BP, there is now a recognized group of patients with so-called prehypertension (3).

TABLE 2-1 Suggested dividing lines between "normotension" and "hypertension"

Division (pressure, mm Hg)	Source
120/80	Robinson and Brucer 1939 (1)
130/70	Browne until 1947 (2)
140/80	Ayman 1934 (3)
140/90	Perera 1948 (4)
150/90	Thomas 1952 (5)
160/100	Bechgaard 1946 (6)
180/100	Burgees 1948 (7)
180/110	Evans 1956 (8)

From Pickering G. Hypertension: definitions, natural history and consequences. In: Laragh JH, Brenner BM, editors. *Hypertension*. Vol. 1. New York: Raven Press; 1995, pp 3–16.

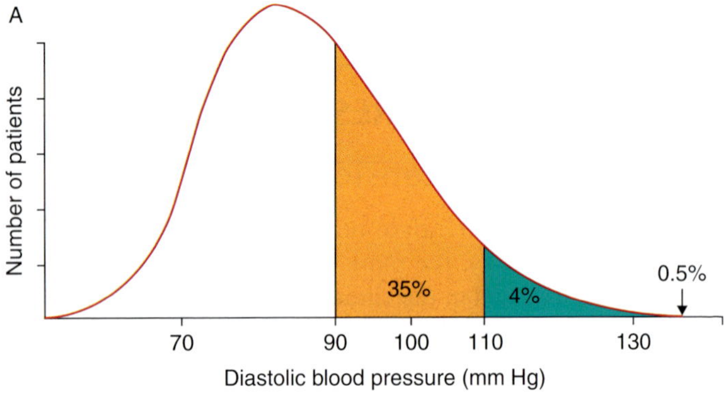

Fig. 2-1 About 4–5% of the middle-aged population Western of countries have a DBP > 110 mm Hg with a further 35% > 90 mm Hg. (From Fox KM, Shapiro LM. *Hypertension*. London: Wolfe Medical Publications Ltd.; 1986, p 13.)

Prehypertension is related to a clinic BP of 130–139/80–89 mm Hg and linked to increased risk. Indeed, such patients are at a high risk of developing frank hypertension (>140/90 mm Hg) over a 4-year period (4), particularly black (Afro-Caribbean) subjects (5). Indeed, about 90% of those whose BP is normal at age 55 years ultimately develop hypertension over their lifetime (6).

2. Haemodynamic mechanism underlying essential/primary hypertension

Put at its simplest, essential, or primary, hypertension was considered to have no obvious cause. It comprises 90%–95% of all hypertension, with secondary hypertension (renal, endocrine, and vascular) comprising the remainder (**Figure 2-2**) (2).

Although the underlying cause of primary hypertension was unknown in the past, the actual hemodynamic mechanism of the high BP results from an increase of either cardiac output or peripheral resistance (or both) (**Figure 2-3**) (2). Some basic mechanisms responsible for a raised cardiac output or peripheral resistance (2) are shown in **Figures 2-4** and **2-5**.

3. Brachial and central blood pressure and age

A) Brachial clinic BP

The Framingham Heart Study provides insight into the effects of aging on systolic BP (SBP), DBP, and pulse pressure (P-P) (7). In a study of 2036 individuals followed up for 30 years (each individual had 15–16 BP measurements over that time), it was clear that SBP rose continu-

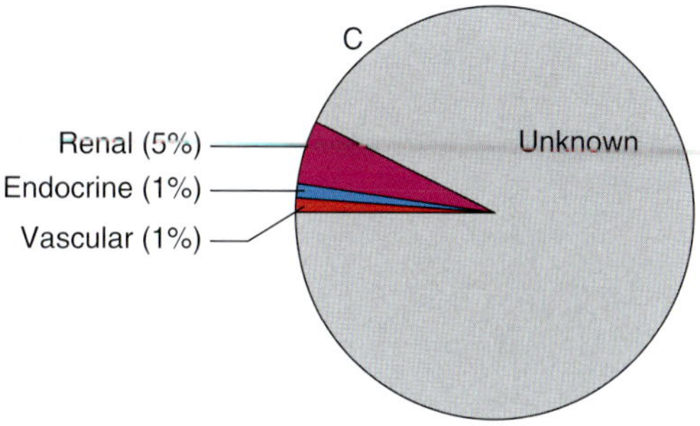

Fig. 2-2 In more than 90% of patients with hypertension, the cause is unknown; this is termed "primary" or "essential" hypertension. (From Fox KM, Shapiro LM. *Hypertension*. London: Wolfe Medical Publications Ltd.; 1986, p 13.)

1

Blood pressure = Cardiac output × peripheral vascular resistance

Fig. 2-3 BP is determined by a complex interplay of cardiac output and peripheral vascular resistance. (From Fox KM, Shapiro LM. *Hypertension*. London: Wolfe Medical Publications Ltd.; 1986, p 13.)

Increased Cardiac Output
1. Left ventricular factors
2. Fluid load { Mineralocorticoids, Sodium loading }

Fig. 2-4 In hypertension, a raised CO can be linked to increased heart rate and LV contractility (raised sympathetic nerve activity).

Increased Peripheral Vascular Resistance (PVR)
1. **Humoral, angiotensin and catecholamines**
2. **Sympathetic nervous system**

Fig. 2-5 An increased PVR occurs via the "aging" process, that is, stiff, poorly compliant blood vessels, and the factors shown in the figure.

ously over the whole time period (irrespective of initial BP), DBP rose up to the age 50–60 years and then declined, and P-P remained more or less constant up to the age 50–55 years and after that rose steeply up to the age of 80 years (**Figure 2-6**).

B) Central and peripheral BP (direct, intra-arterial)

In a group of patients (n = 175) undergoing coronary angiography, direct BP measurements were made in the radial artery, abdominal aorta, and aortic arch (8). Pressures in the radial artery, abdominal

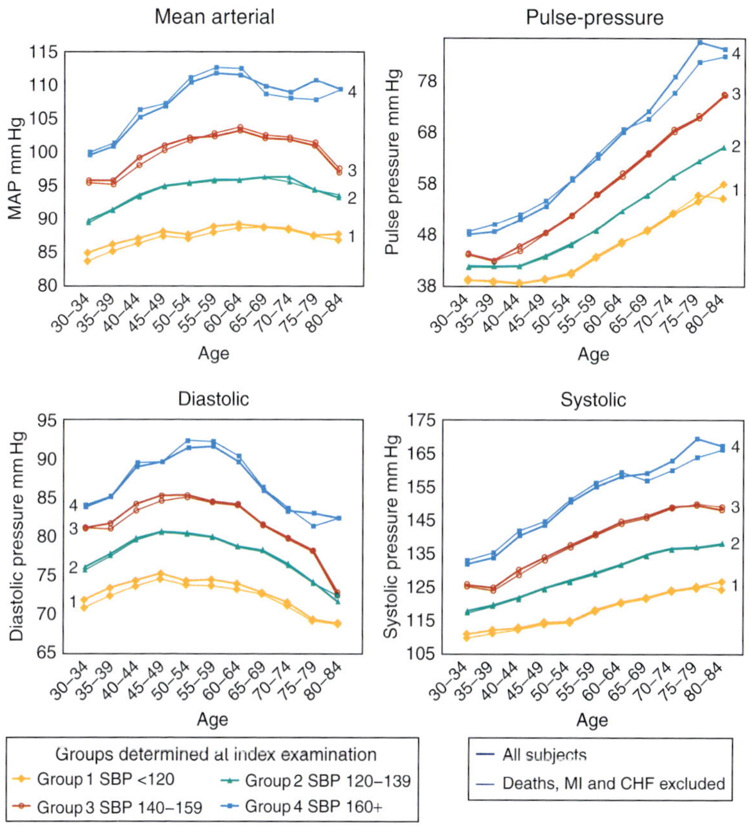

Fig. 2-6 Framingham Heart Study; effects of age upon BP and pulse pressure in 2036 subjects followed up for 30 years. (From Franklin SS, Gustin W, Wong N, et al. Haemodynamic patterns of age-related changes in blood pressure. The Framingham heart Study. *Circulation* 1997;96: 308–15.)

aorta, and aortic arch, in relation to age of the patient, are shown in **Figure 2-7**. It is apparent that aging has a greater effect on central rather than peripheral arterial hemodynamics, particularly in relation to P-P.

Thus, the difference between peripheral P-P and central P-P (P-P amplification) is greatest in the younger age groups (20–29 years) and least in the elderly (60–80 years+), for both men and women (**Figure 2-8**) (9). Hence, P-P amplification decreases with increasing age, because aging has a greater effect on central, rather than peripheral, haemodynamics.

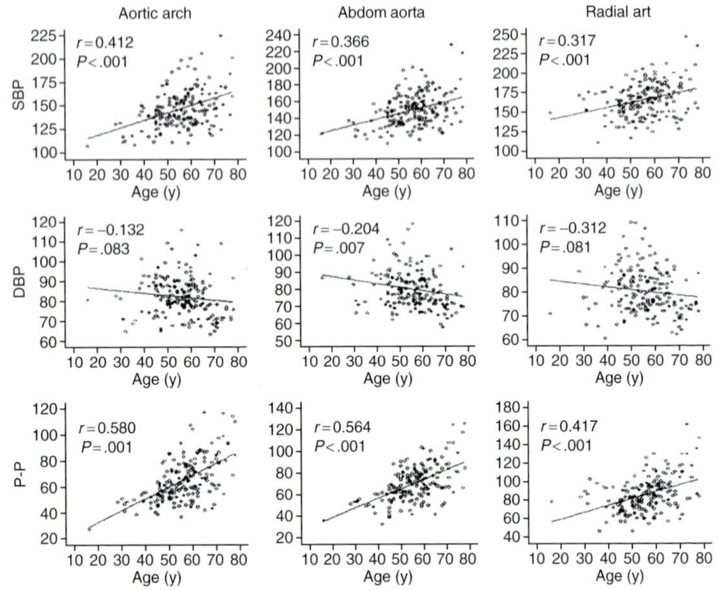

Fig. 2-7 Effects of age upon central and radial artery BP and pulse pressure (P-P) measured directly in 175 coronary angios. (From Choi CU, Kim EJ, Kim SH, et al. Differing effects of aging on central and peripheral blood pressures and pulse-wave velocity; a direct intraarterrial study. *J Hypertens* 2010;28:1252–60.)

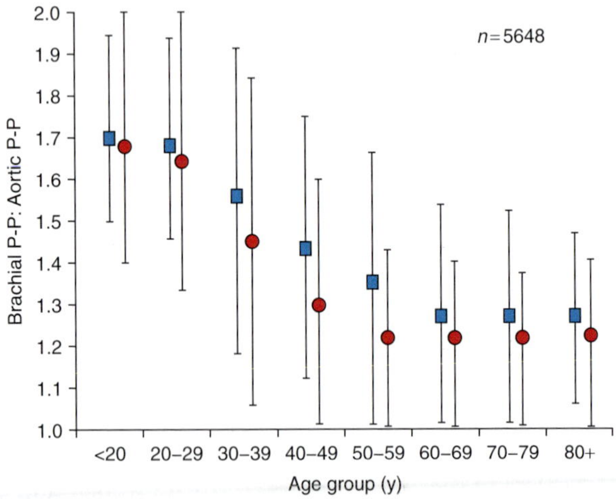

Fig. 2-8 Pulse pressure amplification (ratio of brachial P-P and aortic P-P) lessens with increasing age in both men (blue square) and women. (From Avolio AP, van Bortel LM, Boutouyrie JR, et al. Role of pulse-pressure amplification in arterial hypertension. Experts opinion on review of the data. *Hypertension* 2009;54:3375–83.)

METHODS OF MEASURING PERIPHERAL AND CENTRAL BLOOD PRESSURE

1. In the clinic—the mercury sphygmomanometer

For over a century, clinicians and research workers have used the mercury sphygmomanometer, a simple gravity-based instrument (10). Because of its accuracy and reliability, the mercury device has been generally regarded as the gold standard against which other devices should be compared (10).

However, there have been worries about the safety of the mercury sphygmomanometers (mercury is a toxic, poisonous substance), and these devices have been banned in several countries (11). The problem arises in replacing the mercury sphygmomanometer with other unreliable devices, for example, aneroid sphygmomanometers (using bellows and lever system, which become inaccurate on everyday use).

Automated devices relying on oscillometric techniques were initially unreliable, but recent models that have been rigorously validated are acceptable (see later) (11).

Assessing BP with a mercury sphygmomanometer is a skilled technique, and there are guidelines for obtaining the best, reproducible results (**Table 2-2**) (12). High BP levels (white coat hypertension) can arise inappropriately in the clinic (12) as illustrated in **Tables 2-3** and **2-4**. Of particular importance are cuff/bladder dimensions (**Table 2-5**) (13). Too small a cuff size results in inappropriate high BP readings. Ambient temperature is important, with higher BP readings in the cold (14, 15). BP is accordingly higher in the winter compared to the summer (**Figure 2-8a**) (16).

Nurse-led interventions in primary care are linked to lower BPs than usual care (doctor) (**Figure 2-9**) (17). The best results, in terms of BP control in primary care, arise when there is a telematic connection networking system between the general practice unit and the specialist unit (18).

The "white-coat" effect should not be underestimated. It is present in about 10% of Europeans (19) and may not be entirely benign (19). The white-coat effect can be of considerable magnitude, possibly as high as 27/14 mm Hg (20), as illustrated by clinic blood readings taken by either a physician or a technician (**Figure 2-10**) (19).

TABLE 2-2 Guidelines for measuring blood pressure in adults

- Seat the patient in a quiet, calm environment with a bared arm resting on a standard table or other support so the midpoint of the upper arm is at the level of the heart.
- Estimate the circumference of the bare upper arm at the midpoint between the shoulder and the elbow, by inspection or tape measure, and select an appropriate cuff. The bladder inside the cuff should encircle 80% of the arm.
- Place the cuff so that the midline of the bladder is over the arterial pulsation, then wrap and secure the cuff snugly around the subject's bare upper arm.
- The lower edge of the cuff should be 2.5 cm above the antecubital fossa where the head of the stethoscope is to be placed.
- Inflate the cuff rapidly to 70 mm Hg and then by 10 mm increments while palpating the radial pulse. Note the reading at which the pulse disappears and subsequently reappears during deflation.
- Place the low-frequency head (bell) of your stethoscope over the brachial artery pulsation.
- Inflate the bladder rapidly and steadily to a pressure 20–30 mm above the level previously determined by palpation, then allow the bladder to deflate at 2 mm/sec while listening for the appearance of the Korotkoff sounds.
- As the pressure in the bladder falls, note the manometer readings at the first appearance of repetitive sounds (phase I), at the muffling of these sounds (phase IV), and when they disappear (phase V). As long as the Korotkoff sounds are audible, the rate of deflation should be no more than 2 mm per pulse beat.
- After the last Korotkoff sound is heard, the cuff should be deflated slowly for at least another 10 mm to ensure that no further sounds are audible, and then rapidly and completely deflated; the subject should then be allowed to rest for 30 seconds.
- The systolic (phase I) and diastolic (phase V) pressures should be recorded immediately, to the nearest 2 mm Hg.
- The measurements should be repeated after at least 30 seconds have elapsed, and the 2 readings averaged. In clinical situations, additional measurements may be made in the same or opposite arm, in the same or an alternative position.
- Multiple visits are needed before the diagnosis of hypertension can be established; their exact number and frequency will depend on how much the blood pressure is raised and whether there are other cardiovascular risk factors.

From Mc Alister FA, Straus SE. Measurement of blood pressure on evidence based review. *BMJ* 2001;322:908–11.

TABLE 2-3 Effects of routine activities on clinic blood pressure

	Effect on blood pressure (mm Hg)	
Activity	Systolic blood pressure (mm Hg)	Diastolic blood pressure (mm Hg)
Attending a meeting	↑20	↑15
Commuting to work	↑16	↑13
Dressing	↑12	↑10
Walking	↑12	↑6
Talking on telephone	↑10	↑7
Eating	↑9	↑10
Doing desk work	↑6	↑5
Reading	↑2	↑2
Watching television	↑0.3	↑1

From Mc Alister FA, Straus SE. Measurement of blood pressure on evidence based review. *BMJ* 2001;322:908–11.

TABLE 2-4 Factors that can affect the accuracy of BP measurement

	Measured *V* actual blood pressure[a]		
Factor	Systolic blood pressure	Diastolic blood pressure	Highest quality of evidence[b]
Patient			
Talking	↑17 mm Hg	↑13 mm Hg	Level 1[3]
Acute exposure to cold	↑11 mm Hg	↑8 mm Hg	Level 2[4]
Acute ingestion of alcohol	↑8 mm Hg for ≤3 hr	↑7 mm Hg for ≤3 hr	Level 1[5]
Technique			
Patient supine rather than sitting	No effect; ↑3 mm Hg in supine position	↓2–5 mm Hg in supine position	Level 1[6]
Position of patient's arm	↓ (or ↑) 8 mm Hg for every 10 cm above (or below) heart level	↓ (or ↑) 8 mm Hg for every 10 cm above (or below) heart level	Level1[7]

TABLE 2-4 Factors that can affect the accuracy of BP measurement (*Continued*)

Factor	Measured *V* actual blood pressure[a] Systolic blood pressure	Diastolic blood pressure	Highest quality of evidence[b]
Failure to support arm	↑2 mm Hg	↑2 mm Hg	Level 1[7]
Cuff too small	↓8 mm Hg	↑2 mm Hg	Level 1[8]
Measurer			
Expectation bias (including end digit preference)	Rounding to nearest 5 or 10 mm Hg	Rounding to nearest 5 or 10 mm Hg	Level1[9]

[a] Mean values obtained from referenced studies.
[b] Using levels of evidence for diagnostic studies.
From Mc Alister FA, Straus SE. Measurement of blood pressure on evidence based review. *BMJ* 2001;322:908–11.

TABLE 2-5 Recommended sphygmomanometer cuff dimensions for adults

British Hypertension Society	
Standard cuff	Bladder 12 × 26 cm for the majority of adult arms
Large cuff	Bladder 12 × 40 cm for obese arms
Small cuff	Bladder 12 × 18 cm for lean adult arms and children
American Heart Association	
Small adult cuff	Bladder 10 × 24 cm for arm circumference 22–26 cm
Adult cuff	Bladder 13 × 30 cm for arm circumference 27–34 cm
Large adult cuff	Bladder 16 × 38 cm for arm circumference 35–44 cm
Adult thigh cuff	Bladder 20 × 42 cm for an circumference 45–52 cm

From O'brien E, Asmar R, Beilin L, et al. Practice guidelines of the European Society of Hypertension for clinic, ambulatory and self blood pressure measurement. *J Hypertens* 2005;23:697–701.

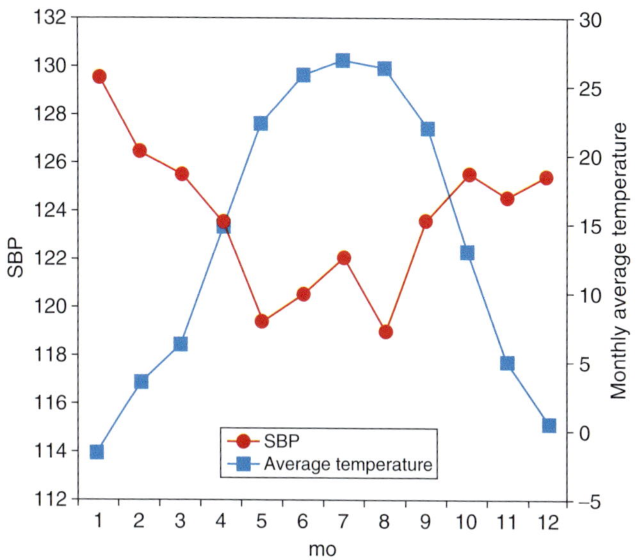

Fig. 2-8a Variation of SBP and monthly temperature. (From Handler J. Seasonal variability of blood pressure in California. *J Clin Hypertens* 2011;13:856–60.)

2. Home blood pressure recordings; avoiding the white-coat effect and unmasking "masked" hypertension

Automated home BP devices must be reliable and well validated (21). Techniques involving wrist or finger BP are not recommended (21). Automated devices for upper arm measurement, via oscillometric techniques, are now well accepted and cheap, and several devices have been well validated (mainly OMRON devices) (21). A typical automated home BP monitoring device is shown in **Figure 2-11**. A major advantage of home BP devices is that, unlike the mercury sphygmomanometer, no (or minimal) training is necessary. Indeed, a simple, low-cost, solar-powered, robust device (OMRON) is now available for low-income developing countries (22).

Home BPs avoid the white-coat response experienced in the clinic, particularly in the presence of a doctor. Thus, home BPs are lower than clinic BPs (**Figure 2-12**) (23), so that a normal home BP was considered to be less than 132/83 mm Hg (compared to less than

Study	Nurse led care			Usual care			Weight (%)	Mean difference (inverse variance, random, 95% CI)
	Mean	SD	Total	Mean	SD	Total		
Change in systolic blood pressure								
Hill 2003*	–7.5	22.2	125	3.4	25.0	106	11.7	–10.90 (–17.05 to –4.75)
Kastarinen 2002 (treatment)	–6.0	17.3	185	–4.7	14.0	189	26.5	–1.30 (–4.49 to 1.89)
Kastarinen 2002 (no treatment)	–2.0	11.5	175	0.4	10.8	166	33.6	–2.40 (–4.77 to –0.03)
O'Hare 2004	–6.7	21.2	41	–2.1	17.47	40	7.0	–4.60 (–13.05 to 3.85)
Woollard 1995	–8.0	31.1	46	–4.0	16.8	48	5.0	–4.00 (–14.17 to 6.17)
Woollard 2003	–3.1	10.0	54	0.2	15.9	57	16.2	–3.30 (–8.21 to 1.61)
Total (95% CI)			626			606	100.0	–3.48 (–5.88 to –1.08)

Mean difference (inverse variance, random, 95% CI)

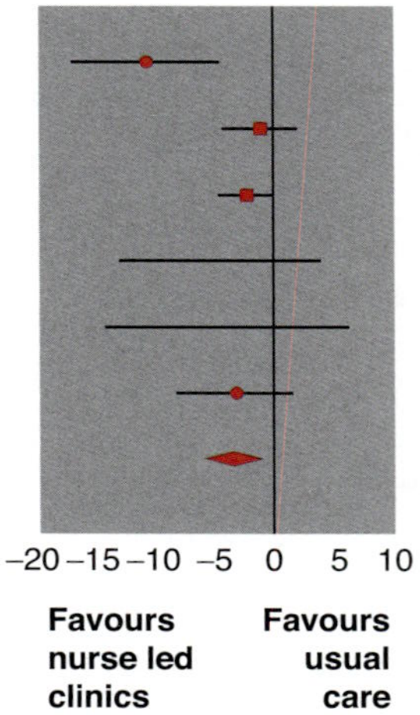

Test for heterogeneity: $\tau^2=3.00$, $\chi^2=7.86$, df=5, $P=.16$, $I^2=36\%$

Test for overall effect: z=2.84, $P=.005$

*Good quality study

Fig. 2-9 Changes in SBP for primary-care nurse led clinics compared with usual care (doctor). (From Clark CE, Smith LF, Taylor RS, et al. Nurse led interventions to improve control of blood pressure in people with hypertension: systematic review and meta-analysis. *BMJ* 2010;341:491.)

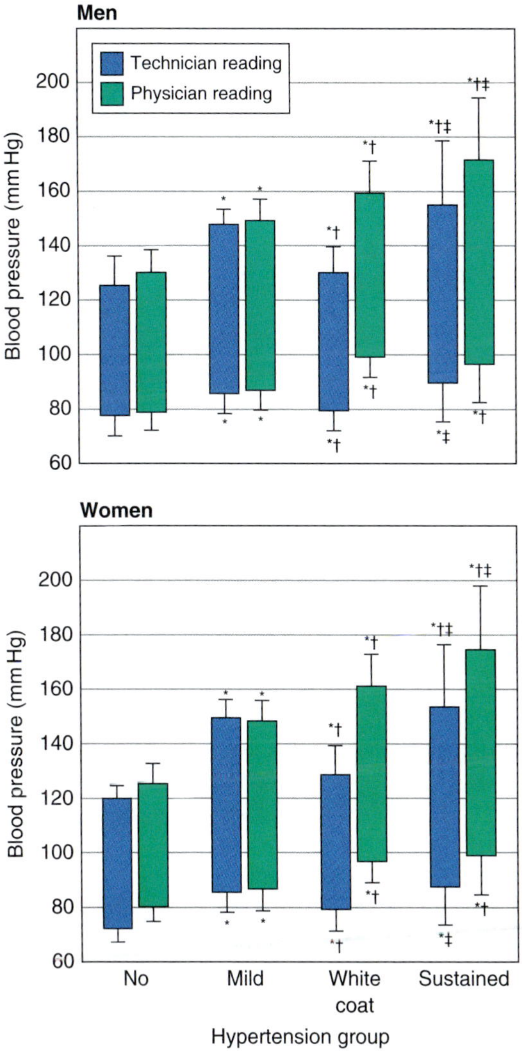

Fig. 2-10 BP values as measured in the clinic by a technician and a physician (MONICA). (From Muscholl MW, Hense H-W, Brockel U, et al. Changes in left ventricular structure and function in patients with white coat hypertension: cross sectional survey. *BMJ* 1998;317:565–70.)

140/90 mm Hg in the clinic). Controlled studies, comparing home BP with usual care BP, have shown a lower SBP of about 2.7 mm Hg in the former after 1 year (24). At 3 years, this difference in BP may be somewhat more, that is, at 4.4/2.4 mm Hg (25). Perhaps, the best results of all are when self-monitoring of BP is linked to

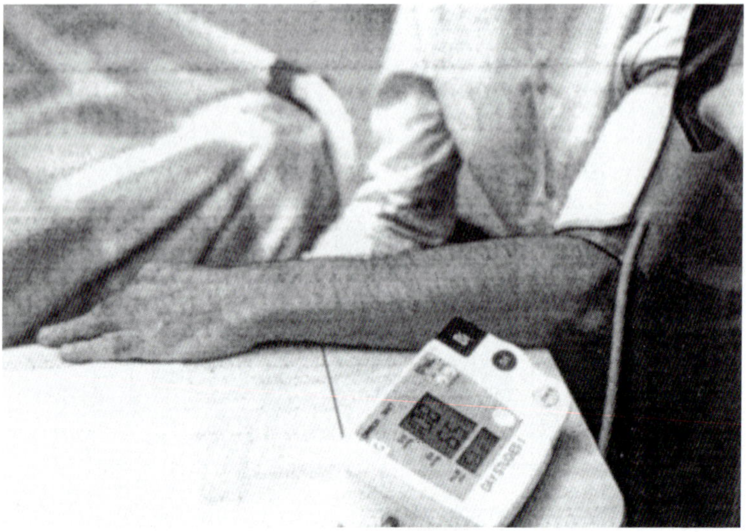

Fig. 2-11 Self-titration of BP using automated home BP monitoring device.

telemonitoring, where home readings are relayed by a health care professional (26). Even with automated BP, it is important that a doctor or nurse is not in the room when the patient takes his or her own BP; a quiet room is recommended, plus several readings (27).

Home BP monitoring is only for reliable, well-informed patients (28). For less reliable patients, self-monitoring in the clinic may be the answer (29), or 24-hour ambulatory monitoring (30). Elderly patients, undergoing home BP measurements, may require 3 days before a steady state is achieved (31). Perhaps, the best BP control, using home BP readings, is when a pharmacist is involved, and care can be delivered over a secure patient Web site (32).

There is US and European Guideline consensus on the advantages of home BP monitoring over conventional clinic BP measurement (33). These advantages are laid out in **Table 2-6**. Both guidelines suggest that normal home daytime BP is below 135/85 mm Hg. Such an approach is particularly suited to children and elderly. White-coat hypertension is avoided, as is "masked" hypertension (normal clinic pressure <140/90 mm Hg, but a high home BP, >135/85 mm Hg, possibly associated with high cardiovascular risk, is revealed. Masked hypertension is not uncommon, occurring in 8.1% of untreated population and being linked to prehypertension in the clinic, high body mass index, cigarette smoking, high alcohol intake, type 2 diabetes, and electrocardiogram left ventricular hypertrophy (34).

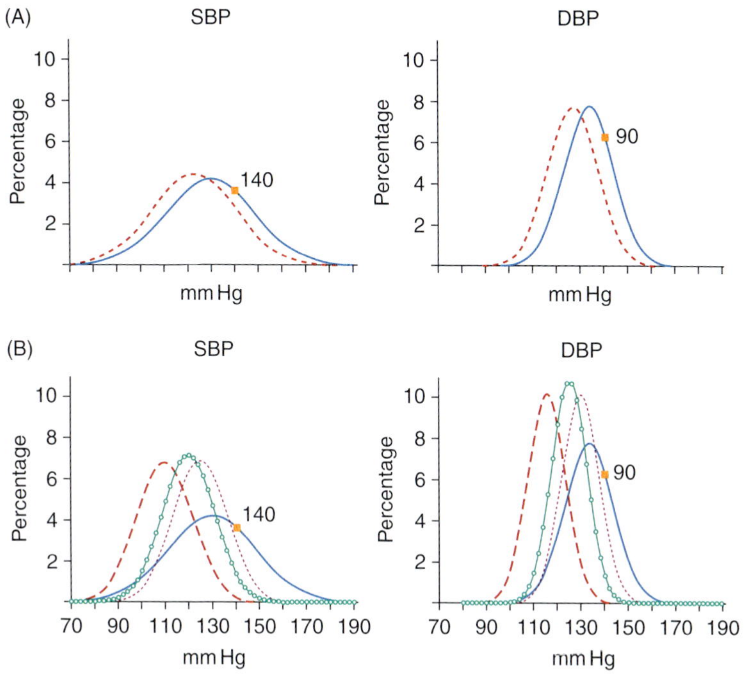

Fig. 2-12 (A) Frequency distribution of clinic (continuous line) and home (dashed line) BPs; (B) Clinic (continuous line) and mean 24 h (continuous line open circle), daytime mean (dotted line), and night (dashed line) mean BPs. (From Mancia G, Sega R, Grassi G, et al. Defining ambulatory and home blood pressure normality: further considerations based on data for the PAMELA study. *J Hypertens* 2001;19:995–9.)

TABLE 2-6 Advantage of home BP monitoring device over conventional clinic BP measurement

- More stable estimates of blood pressure (more readings)
- Better classification of hypertension (white coat and masked)
- Better prediction of cardiovascular risk
- Better estimates of blood pressure variability (daytime, wk, mo)
- Improved control of blood pressure during treatment
- Possible reduced costs of long-term care

Abbreviation: BP, blood pressure.
From Parati G, Pickering TG. Home blood pressure monitoring: US and European consensus. *Lancet* 2009;373:876–8.

3. Ambulatory blood pressure monitoring

Ambulatory monitoring has several advantages and disadvantages (**Table 2-7**) (35), and **Figure 2-13** illustrates a patient wearing such a device (35).

Indications for ambulatory BP monitoring are shown in Table 2-7 (13). A major advantage of 24-hour monitoring over clinic measurements of BP is low variability and high repeatability of the former (**Figure 2-14**) (36), and the fact that white-coat hypertension is avoided and masked hypertension is revealed (**Figure 2-15**) (36). White-coat hypertension is not rare, occurring in about 25% of the population (37). Masked hypertension can progress to frank hypertension and needs to be taken seriously (38), particularly as about 8%–10% in the general population have masked hypertension (34, 39). Patients with masked hypertension tend to be young and are probably at elevated risk of cardiovascular disease (39).

Similar to home BP readings, levels obtained by ambulatory monitoring can be substantially lower than clinic levels (**Figure 2-12**) (23).

Table 2-8 (40) illustrates the results of a prospective study in 8529 subjects (mean age 56 years). It is clear that for higher BPs assessed in the clinic, the equivalent values via 24-hour ambulatory BP are

TABLE 2-7 Clinical indications for ambulatory BP monitoring

Accepted indications	Suspected white-coat hypertension
	Suspected nocturnal hypertension
	Suspected masked hypertension
	To establish dipper status
	Resistant hypertension
	Hypertension of pregnancy
Potential indications	Elderly patient
	As a guide to antihypertensive drug treatment
	Type 1 diabetes
	Evaluation of symptoms suggesting orthostatic hypotension
	Autonomic failure

Abbreviation: BP, blood pressure.

From O'brien E, Asmar R, Beilin L, et al. Practice guidelines of the European Society of Hypertension for clinic, ambulatory and self blood pressure measurement. *J Hypertens* 2005;23:697–701.

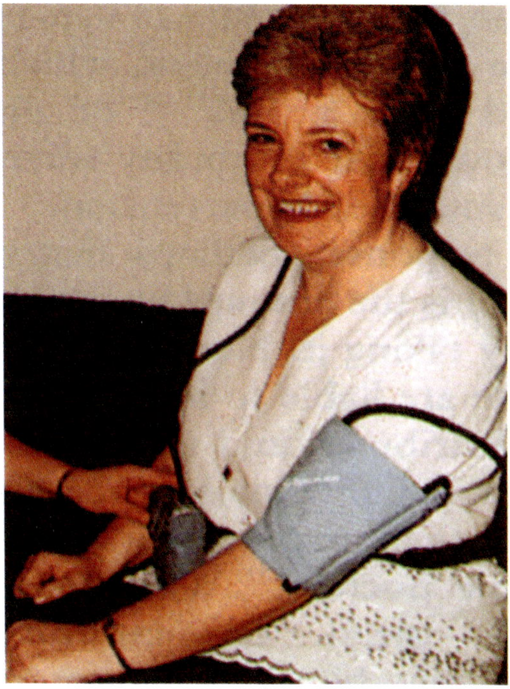

Fig. 2-13 Subject wearing an ambulatory blood pressure measuring device. (From Prasad N, Isles C. Ambulatory blood pressure monitoring: a guide for general practitioners. *BMJ* 1996;313:1535–41.)

markedly lower; for example, for daytime BP in severe hypertension, the difference is 12/5 mm Hg.

Weather conditions need to be taken into account, with higher daytime BPs being recorded in cold weather (**Figure 2-16**) (41). Daytime winter BP is 3/2 mm Hg greater than in summer and may be related to the higher incidence of myocardial infarction in winter (42).

Proposed normal and abnormal ambulatory BP measurements are shown in **Table 2-9** (43). Based on the 10-year cardiovascular risk in 5682 subjects, with a mean age of 59 years and followed up for 10 years, the threshold for normal daytime BP was 130/85 mm Hg, and nocturnal 110/70; optimal day BP 120/80 and nocturnal 100/65; and for hypertension, in daytime greater than 140/85 and nocturnal 120/70 mm Hg (44). Nocturnal BP normally decreases by 10%–30% (dipping), but this does not occur in about 30% of

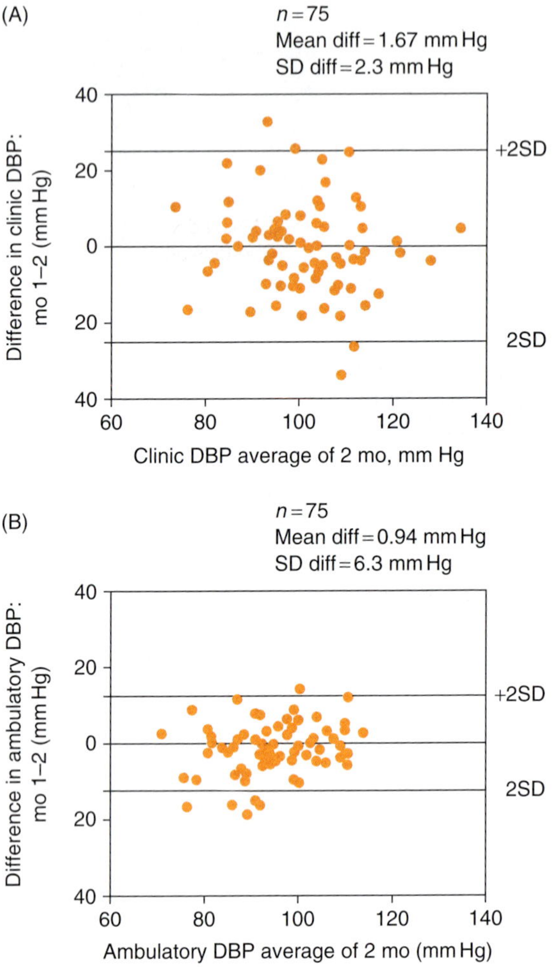

Fig. 2-14 Altman plots showing the 1-month repeatability (variability) of (A) clinic and (B) ambulatory recorded, DBP in 75 untreated hypertensives. (From Waeber B. What stands behind masked hypertension? *J Hypertens* 2008;26:1735–7.)

individuals (nondippers) (45), particularly in the elderly (46). In the early morning, on awakening, there is a surge in BP, coincident with an increase in sympathetic nerve activity and a peaking in cardiovascular risk (47). Various patterns of 24-hour ambulatory BP are shown in **Figure 2-17** (43).

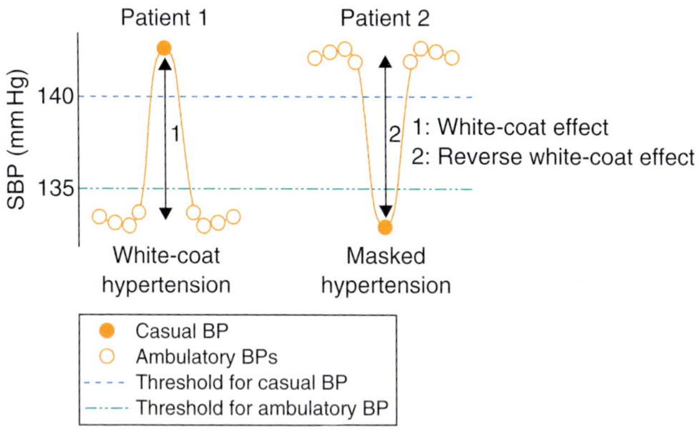

Fig. 2-15 Behaviour of casual (clinic) and ambulatory SBP in patient 1 with white-coat hypertension and patient 2 with masked hypertension. (From Waeber B. What stands behind masked hypertension? *J Hypertens* 2008;26:1735–7.)

TABLE 2-8 Ambulatory BP predicted from clinic BP measured by trained staff

	Seated clinic blood pressure threshold (mm Hg)	Predicted daytime ambulatory equivalent (mm Hg)	Predicted 24-h ambulatory equivalent (mm Hg)
Grade 3 (severe) hypertension	180/110	168/105	163/101
Grade 2 (moderate) hypertension	160/100	152/96	148/93
Grade 1 (mild) hypertension	140/90	136/87	133/84
Target blood pressure plus one condition	130/80	128/78	125/76
Target blood pressure with proteinuria	125/75	124/74	121/71
Normal blood pressure	120/80	120/78	117/76

Abbreviation: BP, blood pressure.

From Head GA, Mihaildon AS, Duggan KA, et al. Definition of ambulatory blood pressure targets for diagnosis and treatment of hypertension in relation to clinic blood pressure: a prospective study. *BMJ* 2010;340:849.

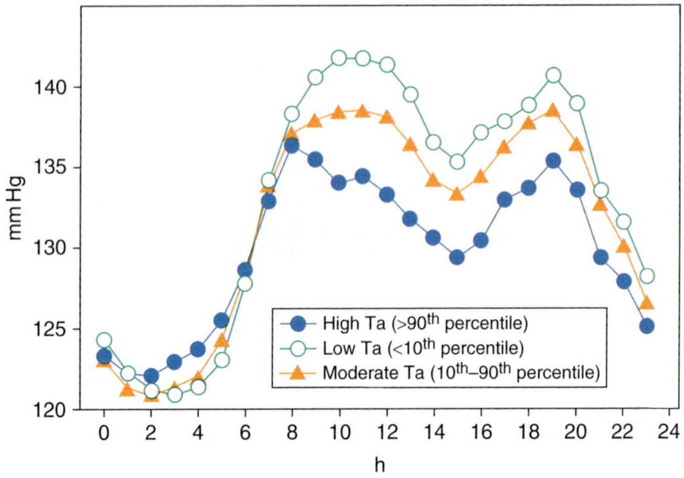

Fig. 2-16 Effect of temperature on 24 h BP; cold temperatures increase daytime BP. (From Modesti PA, Morabito M, Bertolozzi I, et al. Weather related changes in 24 hour blood pressure profile. *Hypertension* 2006;47:155–61.)

TABLE 2-9 Recommended standards for normal and abnormal BP during ambulatory measurement

	Normal BP (mm Hg)	Abnormal BP (mm Hg)
Day	≤135/85	>140/90
Night	≤120/70	>125/75
24 h	≤130/80	>135/85

Abbreviation: BP, blood pressure.
From O'brien EO, Coats A, Ownes P, et al. Use and interpretation of ambulatory blood pressure monitoring: recommendations of the British Hypertension Society. *BMJ* 2000;320:1128–34.

It has been proposed that ambulatory monitoring should be performed for most patients before starting antihypertensive drugs, because this approach reduces the chance of misdiagnosis and is cost effective due to better targeted treatment (48). Moreover, "out-of-office" approaches to high BP result in a reduction in morbid and fatal events attributable to cardiovascular disease (49).

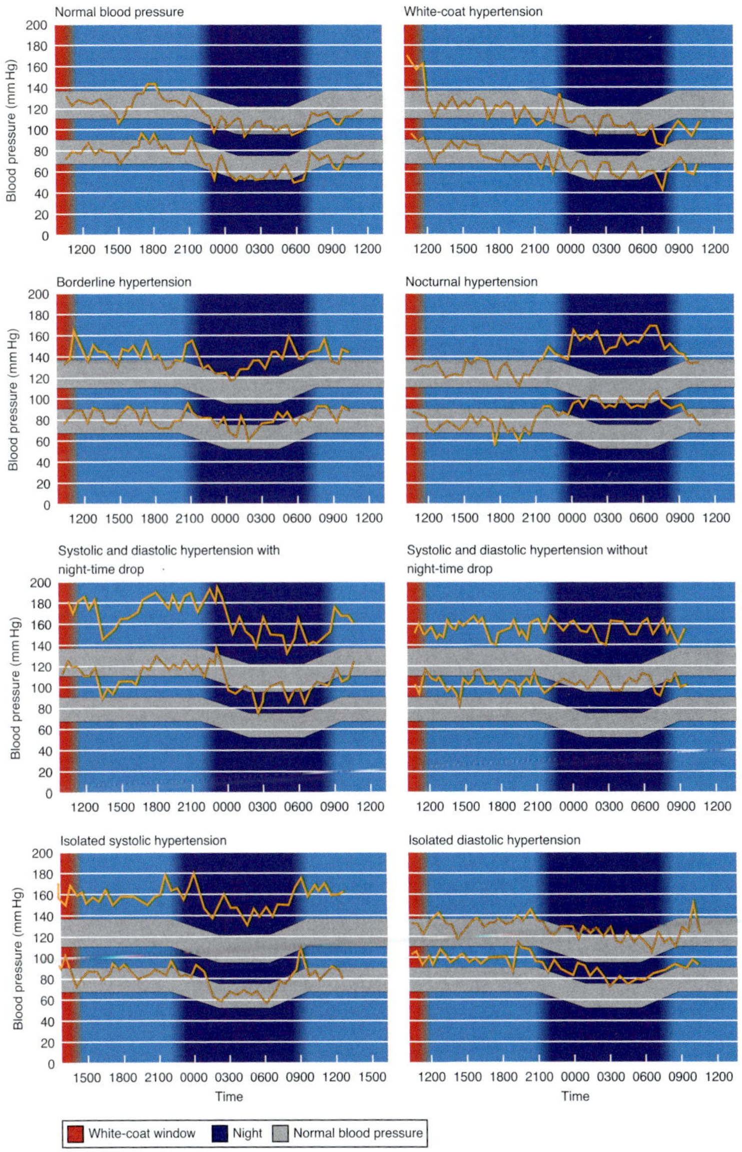

Fig. 2-17 Various patterns of 24 h ambulatory BP. (From O'brien EO, Coats A, Ownes P, et al. Use and interpretation of ambulatory blood pressure monitoring: recommendations of the British Hypertension Society. *BMJ* 2000;320:1128–34.)

4. Children and Adolescents (up to age 18 years)

Most information on children is based on clinic auscultatory data (50). Hypertension is defined as that pressure falling beyond the 95th percentile. Childhood BP tracts strongly into adulthood, so that high or high/normal BP need to be taken seriously, that is, avoid central obesity and do regular exercise (51). More recent data suggest that a more appropriate definition of hypertension is above the 98th percentile and that high-normal is between the 91st and 98th percentile (52). Now, there are preliminary data on ambulatory BP monitoring in children (53), and the fact that ambulatory BP values are similar to those derived from the home BP studies (54).

5. Central Blood Pressures

From a pathophysiological viewpoint, central BP, at least in the elderly, is likely to be more relevant than peripheral BP, regarding the risk left ventricular hypertrophy, heart failure, myocardial infarction, and stroke.

A) Vascular aging, increasing P-P, and P-P amplification

This is a complex area. Arterial distensibility decreases with age (**Figure 2-18**) (55), and the reduced distensibility is closely related to an increasing brachial P-P (**Figure 2-19**) (55). There is a complex relationship between brachial/central P-P and age. Myriads of pressure wave reflections are generated mainly at the aerial–arteriolar junctions, resulting in pressure amplification (56). This is well illustrated in **Figure 2-20** (57). In the young, this difference between central and peripheral P-P (and SBP) can be as high as 20–30 mm Hg (56), and the difference remains as high as 8–11 mm Hg in the very elderly (58). This phenomenon of P-P amplification is shown clearly in Figure 2-8 (59).

The stiffening of the arteries starts in adolescence, in males, and continues throughout the aging process (60), in contrast to females, where the process starts mainly post menopause (60), but earlier if oral contraceptives are being prescribed (61).

B) Augmentation of aortic pressures

In young subjects, with elastic, distensible vessels, a slow backward pressure wave (low pulse wave velocity [PWV]) returns from the distal

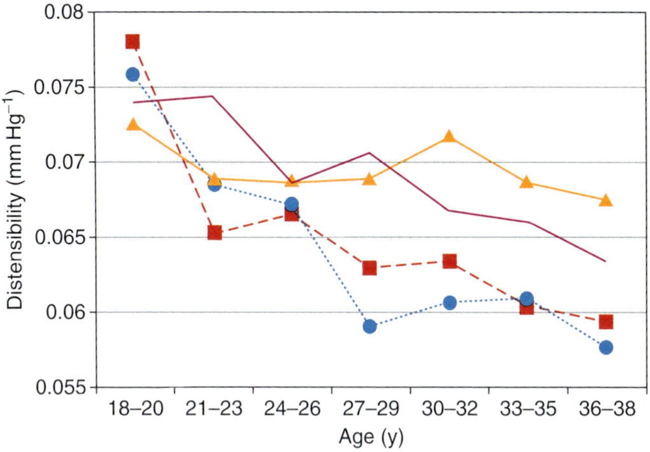

Fig. 2-18 Brachial artery distensiblity decreases with age—Bogalusa Heart Study; thick line, white men; triangles, black men; squares, white women; circles, black women. (From Urbina EM, Brinton T, Elkasabany A, et al. Brachial artery distensiblility and relation to cardiovascular risk factors in healthy young adults (The Bogalusa Heart Study). *Am J Cardiol* 2002;89:946–51.)

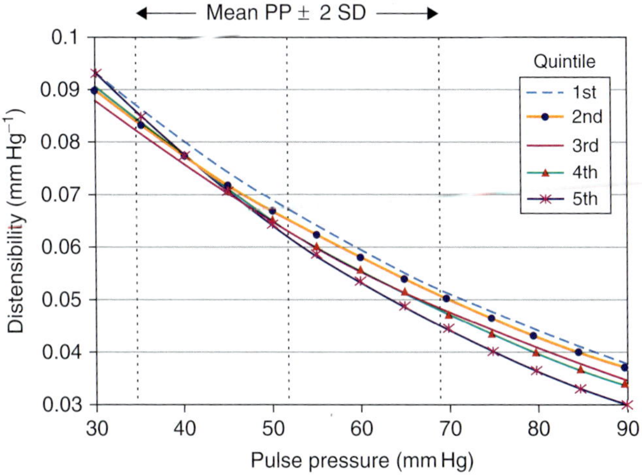

Fig. 2-19 As brachial artery distensibility increases pulse pressure increases—Bogalusa Heart Study. (From Urbina EM, Brinton T, Elkasabany A, et al. Brachial artery distensiblility and relation to cardiovascular risk factors in healthy young adults (The Bogalusa Heart Study). *Am J Cardiol* 2002;89:946–51.)

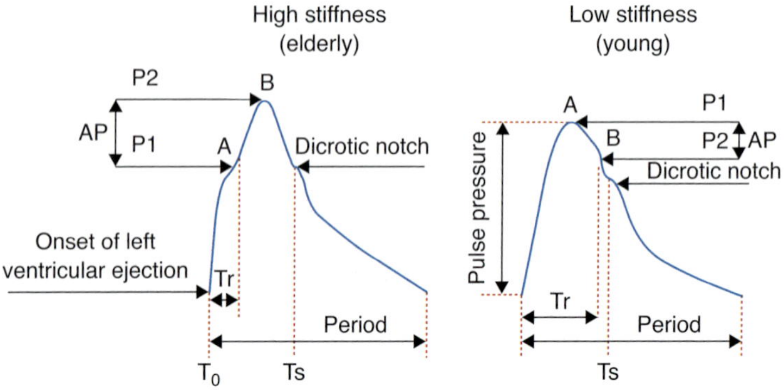

Fig. 2-20 Typical radial artery wave forms (reflecting central blood pressure) in the young and elderly; note in elderly an increased augmented SBP = AP × (P2 – P1). (From Protogerou AD, Pappaioannou TG, Blacher J, et al. Central blood pressures: do we need them in the management of cardiovascular disease? Is it a feasible target. *J Hypertens* 2007;25:265–72.)

arterial compartment and arrives centrally during diastole (thus aiding coronary filling) (**Figure 2-20a**) (59, 62). In older, stiffer arteries, the PWV is higher and the speeded reflected wave now arrives centrally during systole, resulting in an augmented systolic pressure (59). This phenomenon is shown in Figure 2-20 (57). Augmented systolic pressure, expressed as augmentation index (AIx), predictably increases with age (**Figure 2-20b**) (63), as does PWV (**Figure 2-20c**) (64).

C) "Spurious" systolic hypertension (wide P-P) in younger subjects

"Spurious,, or "pseudo," systolic hypertension was first described by O'Rourke et al. (65). In a study of 750 subjects aged 26–31 years (66), spurious systolic hypertension (SBP > 140 mm Hg and DBP < 90 mm Hg, and central SBP < 124 mm Hg for men and < 120 mm Hg for women) was found in 16% of men and 8% of women (66). Subjects with spurious hypertension were heavier than those without. The diagnosis need to be confirmed by ambulatory monitoring, to not confuse it with white-coat hypertension. In a study of 354 younger subjects (67), after 10 years of follow-up, individuals with a high brachial SBP, but low (less than median) central SBP (assessed by applanation tonometry), were at low risk of developing genuine hypertension requiring treatment, in contrast to those whose central pressures were above median values.

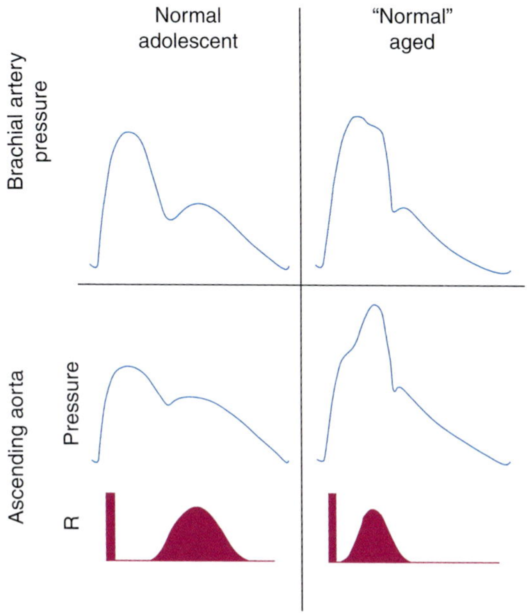

Fig. 2-20a In youth the reflected wave (R) arrives centrally in diastole; in aged, the reflected wave arrives in systole leading to augmented aortic SBP. (From O'Rourke M. From theory into practice: arterial haemodynamics in clinical hypertension. *J Hypertens* 2002;20:1901–15.)

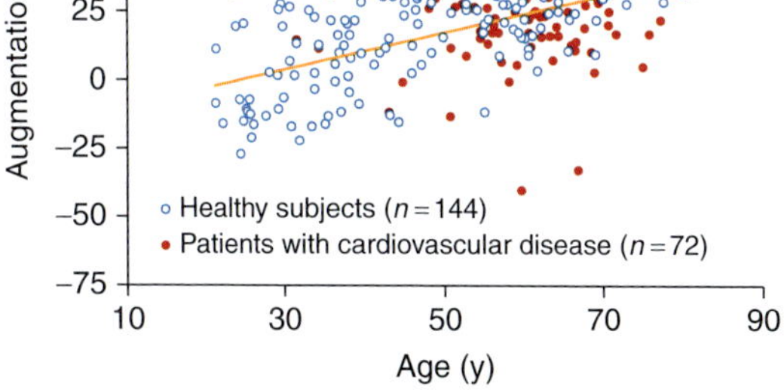

Fig. 2-20b Augmentation index (AIx) increases with age. (From Nurnberger J, Keflioglu-Schreiber A, Saez AM, et al. Augmentation index is associated with cardiovascular risk. *J Hypertens* 2002;20:2407–14.)

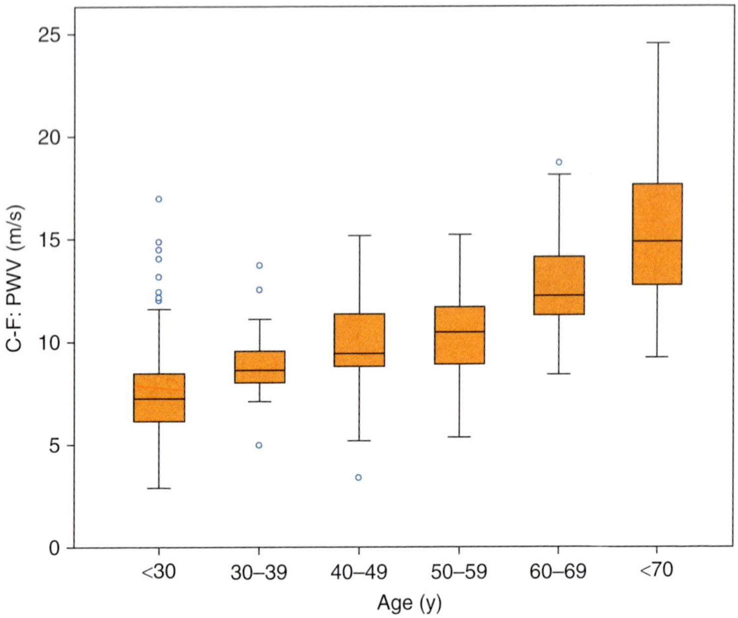

Fig. 2-20c Pulse wave velocity increases with age. (From Kostis V, Stabouli S, Karafillis I, et al. Early vascular aging and the role of central blood pressure. *J Hypertens* 2011;29:1847–53.)

D) Measurement of central blood pressures

It has been shown that central (aortic), assessed directly, and radial pressure wave forms measured simultaneously at cardiac surgery, can provide substantially equivalent values of BP (68). Two main methods have been developed for noninvasively measuring central BP using transcutaneous pressure transducers, involving either the carotid or the radial artery, the latter being more straight forward (69). Some favor a "finger cuff" methodology (70). The carotid is a surrogate for the aorta, but the radial artery is not and requires a "transfer function" to derive an aortic wave form (69). Differing results from different devices can be brought together by the use of the same transfer function algorithm (71, 72).

Figure 2-21 shows how radial artery applanation tonometry is performed (73), and a typical central P-P waveform is shown in **Figure 2-22**. The augmentation pressure is often expressed as an AIx, which in turn expressed as ±Ps – Pi/Ps – Pd (**Figure 2-23**) (74). This complex topic has been well reviewed (75).

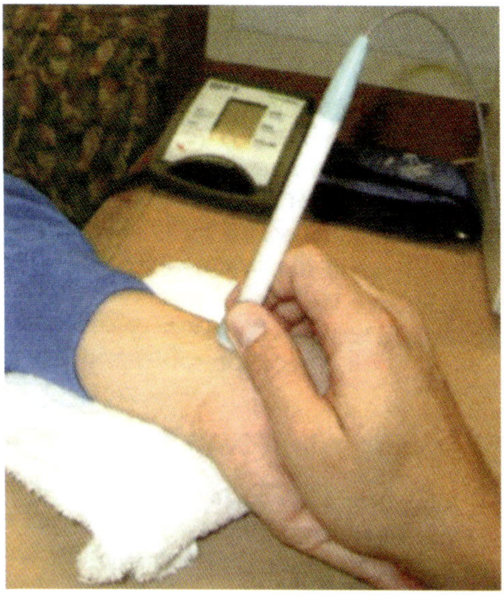

Fig. 2-21 Applanation tonometry is performed by placing a pressure sensor over the radial artery; pictured is the Sphygmocor device. (From Nelson MR, Stepanek J, Cevette M, et al. Non-invasive measurement of central vascular pressures with arterial tonometry: clinical review of the pulse pressure waveform. *Mayo Clin Proc* 2010;85:460–72.)

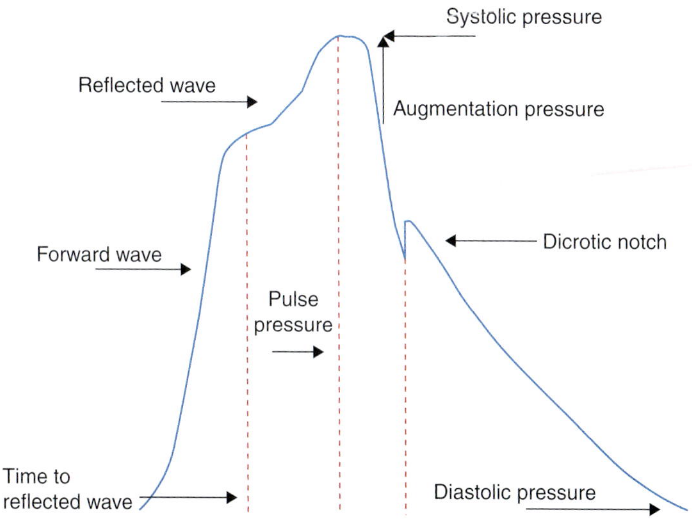

Fig. 2-22 Central pulse pressure waveform; SBP and DBP are the peak and trough of the waveform. (From Nelson MR et al. 2010.)

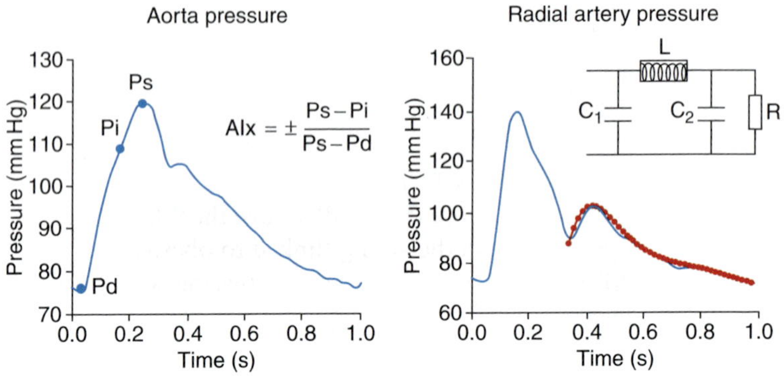

Fig. 2-23 Note radial artery peak SBP is about 20 mm Hg higher than aortic peak SBP; augmentation index (AIx) is derived from the ratio of augmented SBP (Ps – Pi) and pulse pressure (Ps – Pd). (From Segers P, Qasem A, De Backer T, et al. Peripheral "oscillatory" compliance is associated with aortic augmentation index. *Hypertension* 2001;37:1434–9.)

SUMMARY AND CONCLUSIONS

1. As indicated by George Pickering, the definition of hypertension, as measured in the clinic, is arbitrary; however, a rested, sitting BP in the clinic of 140/90 mm Hg or greater is widely regarded as "hypertension"; a BP of 130–9/80–89 mm Hg as "prehypertension"; and a SBP greater than 140 mm Hg plus a DBP less than 90 mm Hg as "isolated systolic hypertension."
2. High BP results from either an increased cardiac output, or an increased total peripheral resistance, or both.
3. SBP, whether measured via the sphygmomanometer in the clinic or centrally (aortic), increases continually with increasing age (due to stiffening of the arteries); by contrast, DBP increases up to age 50–60 years, then declines, resulting in a widened P-P.
4. Central (aortic) BP can be measured either directly or indirectly; in the young the peripheral SBP and P-P is substantially greater (10–30 mm Hg) than central values; this "P-P amplification" in the young, after the age of 40–50 years, diminishes markedly.
5. Clinic BP, as measured by the mercury sphygmomanometer, is variable, particularly when taken by a doctor ("white-coat" effect); the "white coat" effect can be minimized by good technique and by using the nurse/technician, or by utilizing home BP or ambulatory BP monitoring facilities.
6. Home BP and ambulatory BP measurements not only avoid "white-coat," but reveal "masked," hypertension, and are thus cost effective; normal home BP is less than 135/85 mm Hg.

7. Ambulatory BP over 24 hours markedly reduces "observer" variability and, like home BP, avoids the "white-coat" effect; information on nocturnal BP is useful e.g. dippers and non-dippers, as well as the "vulnerable" early morning surge in BP; normal daytime BP is 130–5/85 and nocturnal 110/70 mm Hg.
8. Childhood BP tracks into adulthood, thus the importance of recognizing hypertension, that is, BP above the 98th percentile, or pre-hypertension, in the young (linked to obesity).
9. Central BP increases markedly with increasing age, resulting in decreased P-P amplification; high central SBP and P-P in the elderly result from an "augmented" central SBP.
10. "Spurious" isolated hypertension of the young is usually associated with a low central SBP (unlike the elderly) and does not normally develop into hypertension.
11. Measuring central BP requires a specialist unit; it can be measured either directly (invasive) or indirectly by radial artery applanation tonometry plus a "transfer function."

REFERENCES

1. Pickering G. Hypertension: definitions, natural history and consequences. In: Laragh JH, Brenner BM, editors. *Hypertension*, vol. 1. New York: Raven Press; 1995, pp 3–16.
2. Fox KM, Shapiro LM. *Hypertension*. London: Wolfe Medical Publications Ltd; 1986, p 13.
3. Chobanian AV. Prehypertension revisited. *Hypertension* 2006;48:812–4.
4. Vasan RS, Larson MG, Leip EP, et al. Assessment of frequency of progression to hypertension in non-hypertensive participants in the Framingham Heart Study a cohort study. *Lancet* 2001;358:1682–6.
5. Selassie A, Wagner CS, Laken ML, et al. Progression is accelerated from prehypertension to hypertension in blacks. *Hypertension* 2011;56:579–87.
6. Vasan RS, Beiser A, Seshadri S, et al. Residual lifetime risk of developing hypertension in middle-aged women and men; the Framingham heart Study. *JAMA* 2002;287:1003–10.
7. Franklin SS, Gustin W, Wong N, et al. Haemodynamic patterns of age-related changes in blood pressure. The Framingham Heart Study. *Circulation* 1997;96:308–15.
8. Choi CU, Kim EJ, Kim SH, et al. Differing effects of aging on central and peripheral blood pressures and pulse-wave velocity; a direct intraarterrial study. *J Hypertens* 2010;28:1252–60.
9. Avolio AP, van Bortel LM, Boutouyrie JR, et al. Role of pulse-pressure amplification in arterial hypertension. Experts opinion on review of the data. *Hypertension* 2009;54:3375–83.
10. Jones DW, Appel LJ, Sheps SG, et al. Measuring blood pressure accurately. New and persistent challenges. *JAMA* 2003;289:1027–30.

11. O'Brien E. Replacing the mercury sphygmomanometer. *BMJ* 2000;320: 815–6.
12. Mc Alister FA, Straus SE. Measurement of blood pressure on evidence based review. *BMJ* 2001;322:908–11.
13. O'Brien E, Asmar R, Beilin L, et al. Practice guidelines of the European Society of Hypertension for clinic, ambulatory and self blood pressure measurement. *J Hypertens* 2005;23:697–701.
14. Barnett AG, Sans S, Salomaa V, et al. The effect of temperature on systolic blood pressure. *Blood Press Monit* 2007;12:196–203.
15. Halonen JI, Zanobetti A, Sparrow D, et al. Relationship between outdoor temperature and blood pressure. *Occup Environ Med* 2011;68:296–301.
16. Handler J. Seasonal variability of blood pressure in California. *J Clin Hypertens* 2011;13:856–60.
17. Clark CE, Smith LF, Taylor RS, et al. Nurse led interventions to improve control of blood pressure in people with hypertension: systematic review and meta-analysis. *BMJ* 2010;341:491.
18. De Luca N, Izzo R, Iaccarino G, et al. The use of telematic connection for the follow-up of hypertensive patients improves the cardiovascular prognosis. *J Hypertens* 2005;23:1414–23.
19. Muscholl MW, Hense H-W, Brockel U, et al. Changes in left ventricular structure and function in patients with white coat hypertension: cross sectional survey. *BMJ* 1998;317:565–70.
20. Parati G, Mancia G. White coat effect: semantics, assessment and pathophysiological implications. *J Hypertesn* 2003;21:481–6.
21. O'Brien E, Waeber B, Parati G, et al. Blood pressure measuring devices; recommendations of the European Society of Hypertension. *BMJ* 2001;322:531–6.
22. Sliwa K, Stewart S. A low cost solar-powered blood pressure device. *Lancet* 2011;378:647–8.
23. Mancia G, Sega R, Grassi G, et al. Defining ambulatory and home blood pressure normality: further considerations based on data for the PAMELA study. *J Hypertens* 2001;19:995–9.
24. McMannus RJ, Mant J, Roalfe A, et al. Targets and self-monitoring in hypertension randomised controlled trial and cost-effective analysis. *BMJ* 2005;331:493–6.
25. Cappuccio FP, Kerry SM, Forbes L, et al. Blood pressure control by home monitoring a meta-analysis of randomised trials. *BMJ* 2004;329:145–8.
26. McMannus RJ, Mant J, Braq EP, et al. Telemonitoring and self management in the control of hypertension (TASMINH2): a randomised trial. *Lancet* 2010;376:163–72.
27. Myers MG, Godwin M, Dawes M, et al. Conventional versus automated measurements of blood pressure in primary care patients with systolic hypertension: a randomised parallel design controlled trial. *BMJ* 2011;342:d286.
28. Ogedegbe G. Self-titration for treatment of uncomplicated hypertension. *Lancet* 2010;376:144–6.

29. Bakx JE, van der Wel MC. Self monitoring of high blood pressure. *BMJ* 2005;331:466–7.
30. Nordmann A, Frach B, Walker T, et al. Reliability of patients measuring blood pressure at home. *BMJ* 1999;319:1172.
31. Celis H, De Cort P, Fagard R, et al. For how many days should blood pressure be measured at home in older patients before steady state levels are obtained. *J Hum Hypert* 1997;11:673–7.
32. Green BB, Cook AJ, Ralston J, et al. Effectiveness of home blood pressure monitoring, web communication and pharmacist care on hypertension control. *JAMA* 2008;299:1857–67.
33. Parati G, Pickering TG. Home blood pressure monitoring: US and European consensus. *Lancet* 2009;373:876–8.
34. Hanninen M-R, Niirinen TJ, Puukka PJ, et al. Determinants of masked hypertension in the general population: the Finn-Home study. *J Hypertens* 2011;29:1880–8.
35. Prasad N, Isles C. Ambulatory blood pressure monitoring: a guide for general practitioners. *BMJ* 1996;313:1535–41.
36. Waeber B. What stands behind masked hypertension? *J Hypertens* 2008;26:1735–7.
37. Hoegholm A, Kristensen KS, Madsen H, et al. White coat hypertension diagnosed by 24-hour ambulatory monitoring. *Am J Hypertens* 1992;5:64–70.
38. Messerli FH, Mackini H. Relentless progression towards hypertension. *Hypertension* 2009;54:217–8.
39. Pickering TG, Gerin W, Schwartz JE, et al. Franz Volkard lecture: should doctors still measure blood pressure? The missing patients with masked hypertension. *J Hypertens* 2008;26:2259–67.
40. Head GA, Mihaildon AS, Duggan KA, et al. Definition of ambulatory blood pressure targets for diagnosis and treatment of hypertension in relation to clinic blood pressure: a prospective study. *BMJ* 2010;340:849.
41. Modesti PA, Morabito M, Bertolozzi I, et al. Weather related changes in 24 hour blood pressure profile. *Hypertension* 2006;47:155–61.
42. Gatzka CD. Activity, environment and blood pressure. *J Hypertens* 2006;24:1239–41.
43. O'brien EO, Coats A, Ownes P, et al. Use and interpretation of ambulatory blood pressure monitoring: recommendations of the British Hypertension Society. *BMJ* 2000;320:1128–34.
44. Kikuya M, Hansen TW, Thijs L, et al. Diagnostic threshold for ambulatory blood pressure monitoring based on 10-year cardiovascular risk. *Circulation* 2007;115:2145–52.
45. White WB, Larocca GM. Improving the utility of the nocturnal hypertension definition by using absolute sleep blood pressure rather than the "dipping" proportion. *Am. J Cardiol* 2003;92:1439–41.
46. O'Sulllivan C, Duggan J, Atkins N, et al. Twenty four hour ambulatory blood pressure in community-dwelling elderly men and women, aged 60–102 years. *J Hypertens* 2003;21:1641–7.

47. Kaplan NM. Morning surge in blood pressure. *Circulation* 2003;107:1347.
48. Lovibond K, Jowett S, Barton P, et al. Cost-effectiveness of options for the diagnosis of high blood pressure in primary care: a modelling study. *Lancet* 2011;378:1219–30.
49. Gaziano TA. Accurate hypertension diagnosis is key in efficient control. *Lancet* 2011;378:1199–200.
50. National High Blood Pressure Education Program Working Group on High Blood Pressure in Children and Adolescents. The fourth report on the diagnosis, evaluation and treatment of high blood pressure in children and adolescents. *Paediatrics* 2004;114:555–74.
51. Gidding SG. Measuring children's blood pressure matters. *Circulation* 2008;117:3163–4.
52. Bird C, Michie C. Measuring blood pressure in children. *BMJ* 2008;336:1321.
53. Urbina E, Alpert B, Flynn J, et al. Ambulatory blood pressure monitoring in children and adolescents: recommendations for standard assessment. *Hypertension* 2008;52:433–51.
54. Stergiou GS, Nasothimiou E, Giovas P, et al. Diagnosis of hypertension in children and adolescents based on home versus ambulatory blood pressure monitoring. *J Hypertens* 2008;26:1556–62.
55. Urbina EM, Brinton T, Elkasabany A, et al. Brachial artery distensiblility and relation to cardiovascular risk factors in healthy young adults (The Bogalusa Heart Study). *Am J Cardiol* 2002;89:946–51.
56. Protogerou AD, Papaioannou TG, Lekakis JP, et al. The effect of antihypertensive drugs on central blood pressure beyond peripheral blood pressure. Part I—Pathophysiology, rationale and perspective on pulse-pressure amplification. *Curr Pharm Des* 2009;15:267–71.
57. Protogerou AD, Pappaioannou TG, Blacher J, et al. Central blood pressures: do we need them in the management of cardiovascular disease? Is it a feasible target. *J Hypertens* 2007;25:265–72.
58. Mc Eniery CM, McDonnell B, Yasmin, et al. Central pressure: variability and impact of cardiovascular risk factor. The Anglo-Cardiff Collaborative Trial II. *Hypertension* 2008;51:1476–82.
59. Safar ME, Levy B, Struijker-Boudier H. Current perspectives on arterial stiffness and pulse pressure in hypertension and cardiovascular disease. *Circulation* 2003;107:2864–9.
60. Rossi P, Frances Y, Kingwell BA, et al. Gender differences in artery wall biomechanical properties throughout life. *J Hypertens* 2011;29:1023–33.
61. Hickson SS, Miles KC, McDonnell BJ, et al. Use of the oral contraceptive pill is associated with increased large artery stiffness in young women: the ENIGMA Study. *J Hypertens* 2011;29:1155–9
62. O'Rourke M. From theory into practice: arterial haemodynamics in clinical hypertension. *J Hypertens* 2002;20:1901–15.
63. Nurnberger J, Keflioglu-Schreiber A, Saez AM, et al. Augmentation index is associated with cardiovascular risk. *J Hypertens* 2002;20:2407–14.

64. Kostis V, Stabouli S, Karafillis I, et al. Early vascular aging and the role of central blood pressure. *J Hypertens* 2011;29:1847–53.
65. O'Rourke M, Vlachopoulos C, Graham R. Spurious systolic hypertension in youth. *Vasc Med* 2000;5:141–5.
66. Hulsen HT, Nijdam M-E, Bos W-J, et al. Spurious systolic hypertension in young adults; prevalence of high brachial systolic blood pressure and low central pressure and its determinants. *J Hypertens* 2006;24:1027–32.
67. Saladini F, Santonastaso M, Mos L, et al. Isolated systolic hypertension of young-to-middle-age individuals implies a relatively low risk of developing hypertension needing treatment when central blood pressure is low. *J Hypertens* 2011;29:1311–9.
68. Pauca AL, O'Rourke MF, Kon ND. Prospective evaluation of a method for estimating ascending aortic pressure from the radial artery pressure waveform. *Hypertension* 2001;38:932–7.
69. Payne RA, Webb DJ. Peripheral augmentation index. *Hypertension* 2008;51:37–8.
70. Guilcher A, Brett S, Munir S, et al. Estimating central SBP from the peripheral pulse: influence of waveform analysis and calibration error. *J Hypertens* 2011;29:1357–66.
71. Kips JG, Schutte AE, Vermeerch J, et al. Comparison of central pressure estimates obtained from SphygmoCor, Omron HEM-9000AI and carotid applanation tonometry. *J Hypertens* 2011;29:1115–20.
72. Boutouyrie P, Alivon M, Herbert A. Precision, accuracy and added value of central pressure measurement. *J Hypertens* 2011;29:1059–60.
73. Nelson MR, Stepanek J, Cevette M, et al. Non-invasive measurement of central vascular pressures with arterial tonometry: clinical review of the pulse pressure waveform. *Mayo Clin Proc* 2010;85:460–72.
74. Segers P, Qasem A, De Backer T, et al. Peripheral "oscillatory" compliance is associated with aortic augmentation index. *Hypertension* 2001;37:1434–9.
75. Laurant S, Cockcroft J, Van Bortel L, et al. Expert consensus document on arterial stiffness: methodological issues and clinical applications. *Europ Heart J* 2006;27:2588–605.

Epidemiology of Hypertension

CHAPTER 3

INTRODUCTION

The Framingham Heart Study Group (1) has shown that, till 1998, the life-time risk of developing hypertension (>140/90 mm Hg) was about 90% (**Figure 3-1**), and of developing stage-2 hypertension (>169/100 mm Hg) was about 35%–44% for both men and women aged 65 years. This high risk of developing hypertension was linked to lifestyle factors, particularly obesity. The increased risk for men up to 1988 (vs. 1975) seems at odds with the WHO MONICA data (2), which reported on a fall in the prevalence of hypertension at that time (possibly due to an increased likelihood of effective treatment).

The increased risk of hypertension for women occurs mainly at the postmenopausal period (estrogen is a vasodilator), where, in the United States, 75% of older women are hypertensive (3).

1. Global perspective

The global burden of hypertension (>140/90 mm Hg) in 2000 was about 26%, which is predicted to increase to about 29% in 2025 (**Figure 3-2**) (4). Interestingly, in developed countries (such

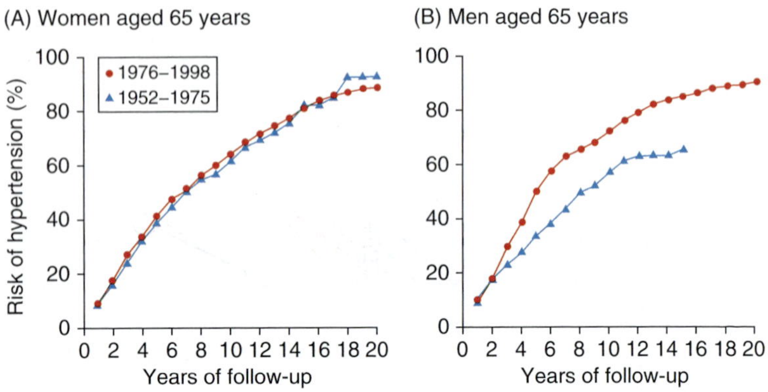

Fig. 3-1 Framingham; residual lifetime risk of hypertension in women and men aged 65 years. (From Vasan RS, Beiser A, Seshadri S, et al. Residual lifetime risk for developing hypertension in middle-aged men and women. The Framingham Heart Study. *JAMA* 2002;287:1003–10.)

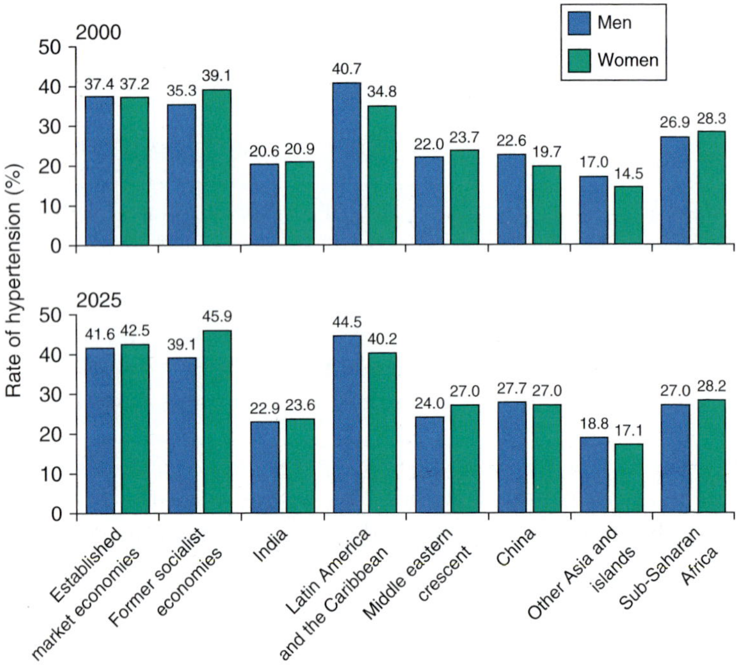

Fig. 3-2 Frequency of hypertension in people aged greater than 19 years by world region and sex in year 2000 (upper) and 2025 (lower). (From Kearney PM, Whelton M, Reynolds K, et al. Global burden of hypertension: analysis of worldwide data. *Lancet* 2005;365:217–25.)

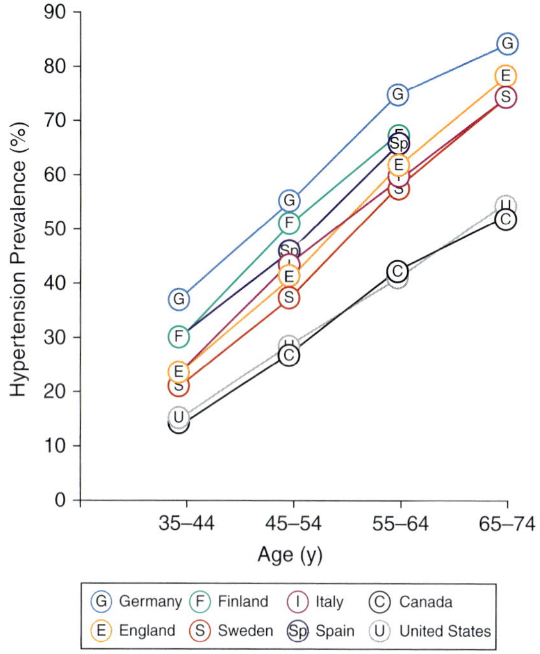

Fig. 3-3 Hypertension prevalence in six European and two North American countries, men and women combined, by age group. (From Wolf-Maier K, Cooper RS, Banegas JR, et al. Hypertension prevalence and blood pressure level in 6 European countries, Canada and the United States. *JAMA* 2003;289:2363–9.)

as United States of America, Canada, and Europe), the prevalence of hypertension was higher in Europe than in the United States/Canada (44% vs. 28%), possibly due to a lower treatment threshold in the United States/Canada (**Figure 3-3**) (5). This lower prevalence of hypertension in the United States/Canada is reflected in fewer strokes (**Figure 3-4**) (5). The prevalence of hypertension in Australia, at 34%, falls between that in Europe and Canada/United States (6).

When the focus is on isolated systolic hypertension (ISH) (SBP > 140 and DBP < 90 mm Hg), its prevalence increases with age, with about 50% having hypertension aged greater than 60 years (7) and about 75% aged greater than 75 years (8). The distribution of the different types of essential hypertension according to age is shown in **Figure 3-4a** (9).

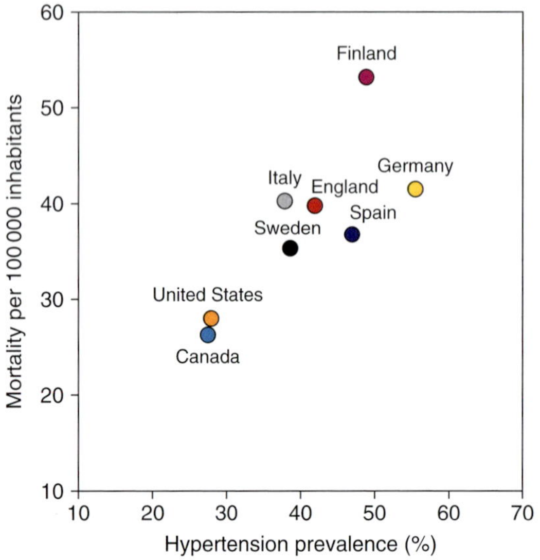

Fig. 3-4 Hypertension prevalence versus stroke-mortality in six European and two North American countries (men and women combined, age is adjusted). (From Wolf-Maier K, Cooper RS, Banegas JR, et al. Hypertension prevalence and blood pressure level in 6 European countries, Canada and the United States. *JAMA* 2003;289:2363–9.)

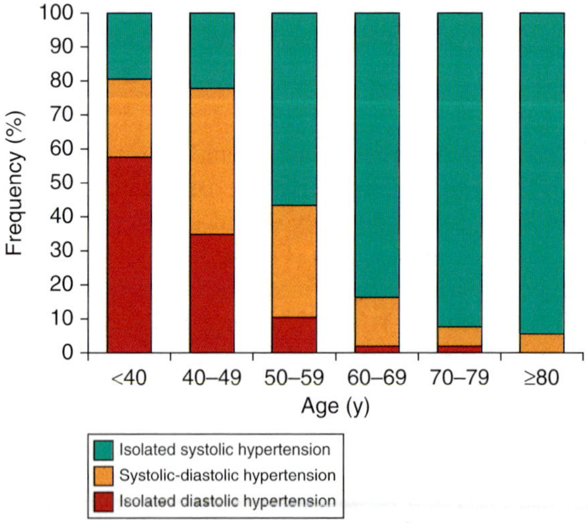

Fig. 3-4a Types of hypertension in untreated cases according to age. (From Franklin SS, Jacobs MJ, Wong ND, et al. Predominance of isolated systolic hypertension among middle-aged and elderly US hypertensives: analysis based on Nation Health and Nutrition Examination Survey [NHANES III]. *Hypertension* 2001;37:869–74.)

2. Low-income countries

Although 90% of expenditure on antihypertensive drugs occurs in the high-income developed world (10), about 75% of hypertensives live in low-income developing countries (11). It is level of income, and not educational status, that is related to incidence of hypertension (12).

In sub-Saharan Africa, there is a high prevalence of hypertension in middle age (**Figure 3-5**) (13). This prevalence is increasing in low-income countries compared with richer developed countries (**Figure 3-6**) (14).

3. Racial aspects in the United States of America and other countries

In 2000, the prevalence of hypertension in the United States of America was 31%, 3% (15) being considerably higher (40% in females and 37% in males) in non-Hispanic black subjects (**Figure 3-7**). This racial disparity continues into old age (**Figure 3-8**) (16), and is thought to be due to environmental and behavioral (particularly obesity) characteristics rather than genetic (17).

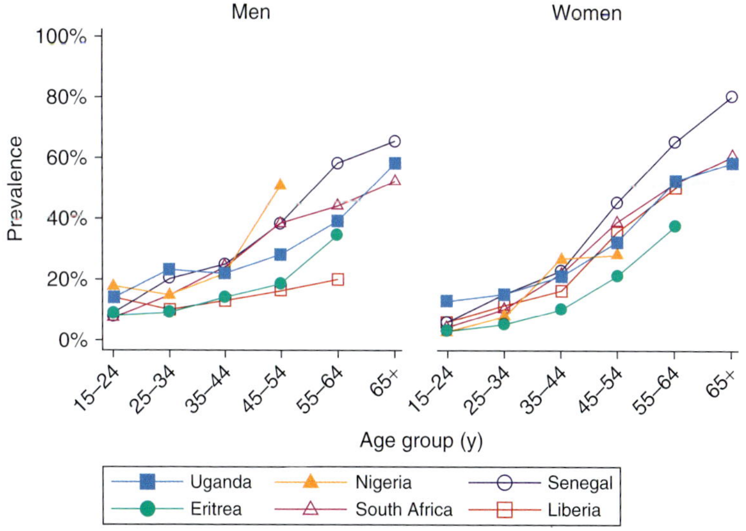

Fig. 3-5 Age-specific prevalence of hypertension by sex, in countries in sub-Saharan Africa. (From Maher D, Waswa L, Baisley K, et al. Epidemiology of hypertension in low-income countries: a cross-sectional population based survey in rural Uganda. *J Hypertens* 2011;29:1061–8.)

(A) Men

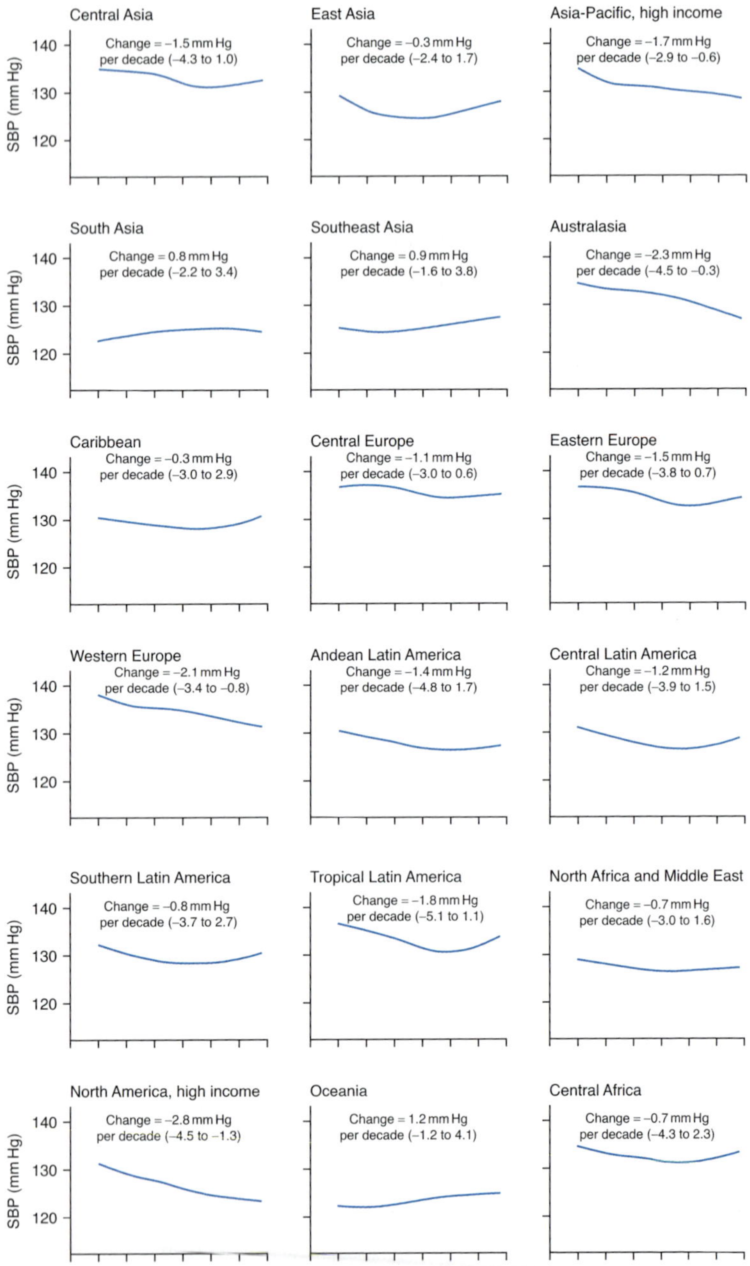

Fig. 3-6 Trends in age-standardized mean SBP by subregion between 1980 and 2008 for men (A) and women (B). (From Danaei G, Finucane MM, Lin JK, et al. National, regional and global trends in SBP since 1980: systematic analysis of health examination surveys s and epidemiological studies with 786 country-years and 5.4 million participants. *Lancet* 2011;377:568–77.)

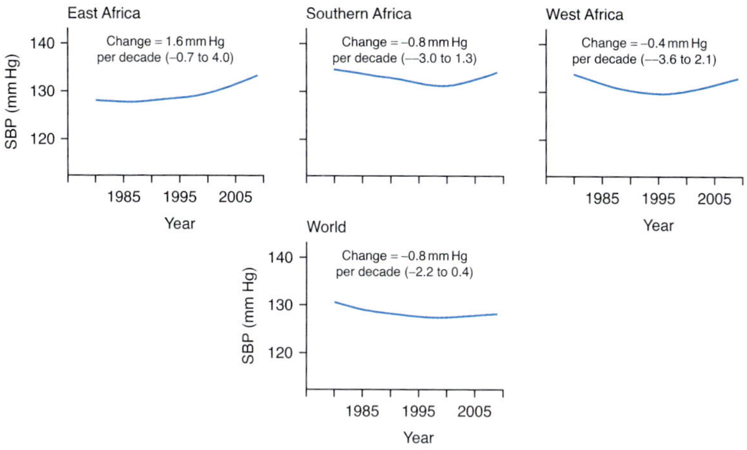

(B) Women

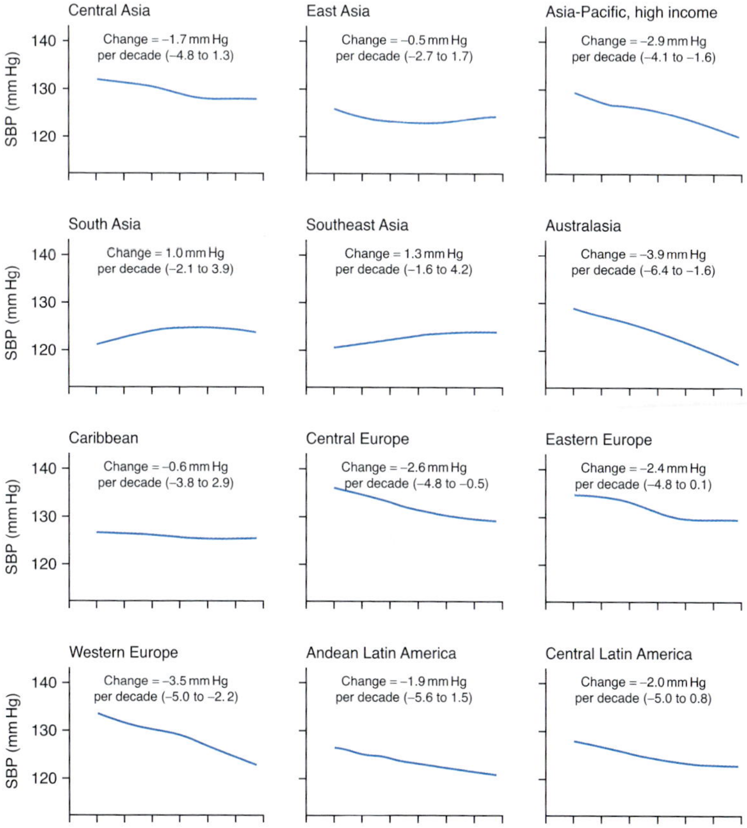

Fig. 3-6 *continued*

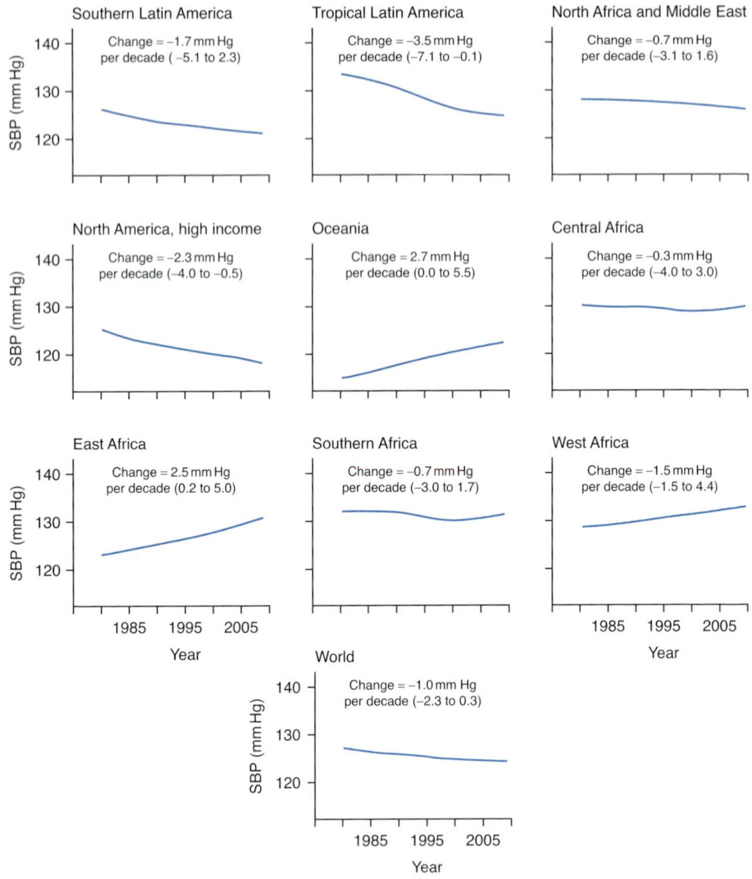

Fig. 3-6 *continued*

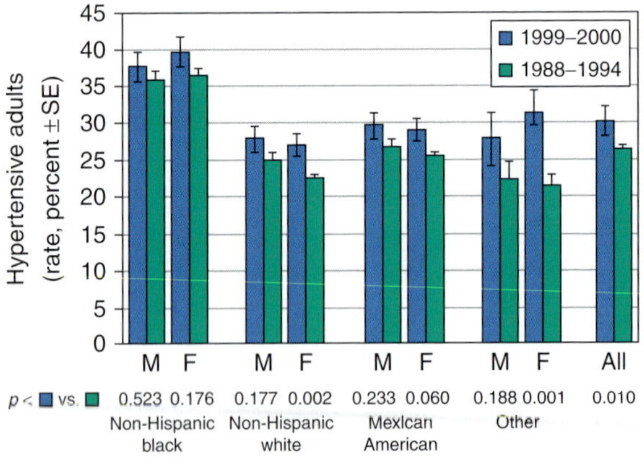

Fig. 3-7 Estimated percent of US adults with hypertension by sex, race, and ethnicity from 1999 to 2000. (From Fields LE, Burt VL, Cutler JA, et al. The burden of adult hypertension in the United States 1999–2000: a rising tide. *Hypertension* 2004;44:398–404.)

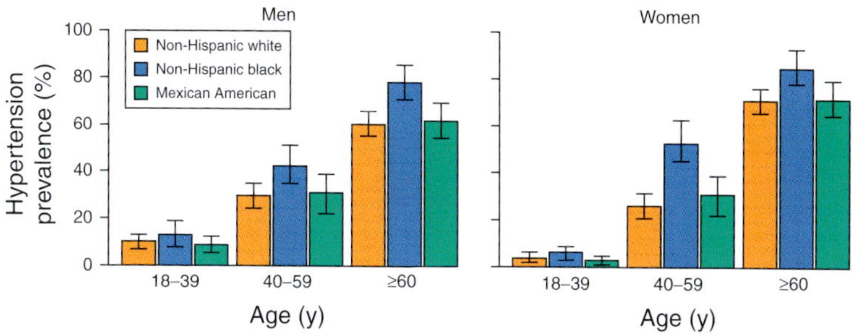

Fig. 3-8 Hypertension prevalence in the United States by age and race/ethnicity in men and women. (From Hajjar I, Kotchen TA. Trends in prevalence, awareness, treatment and control of hypertension in the United States, 1988–2000. *JAMA* 2003;290:199–206.)

In young adults (mean age 29 years) in the United States, a high systolic blood pressure (SBP) (plus high heart rates) was closely linked to low-income/low-education groups, who were more likely to be overweight, centrally obese, and smokers with high intake of alcohol (18).

4. Children and young adults

In children, hypertension is diagnosed when the levels are above the 95th centile, and prehypertension reflects the levels between the 90 and 95th centiles (some favor 98th and 95–98th centiles, respectively). There are data from the United Kingdom that suggest that in young adults, declines in blood pressure over time were taking place up to 50 years ago (19). Likewise, in adolescents, substantial decreases in systolic and diastolic blood pressure (about 2/2 mm Hg) occurred over the decade 1990–2000 (20).

In children and adolescents (age 3–18 years), hypertension is frequently underdiagnosed (21), with just under 4% being hypertensive. In overweight/obese children, the frequency of hypertension can be as high as 30% (21). In 13-year-olds, prehypertension occurs in 20% of boys and 13% of girls, which after 2 years develops into frank hypertension in 12%–14% (22).

Central augmentation index (AIx) in both men and women increases with age in various racial groups (**Figure 3-8a**) (23), and this increase is most marked in African and Hispanic subjects (**Figure 3-8b**).

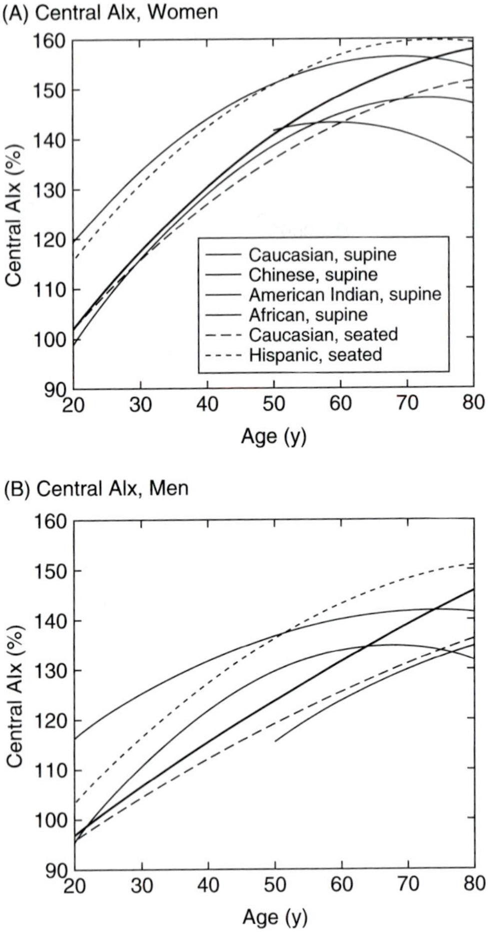

Fig. 3-8a Central augmentation index (AIx) increases with age in women (A) and men (B), in all ethnic groups. (From Chirinos JA, Kips JG, Roman MJ, et al. Ethnic differences in arterial wave reflections and normative equations for augmentation index. *Hypertension* 2011;57:1108–16.)

In younger adults (18–39 years), a surprising fact shown in Nation Health and Nutrition Examination Survey (NHANES) is that ISH is more common than diastolic/systolic hypertension (24). The prevalence of ISH is increasing, particularly in patients of low education, smokers, and the obese (**Figure 3-9**).

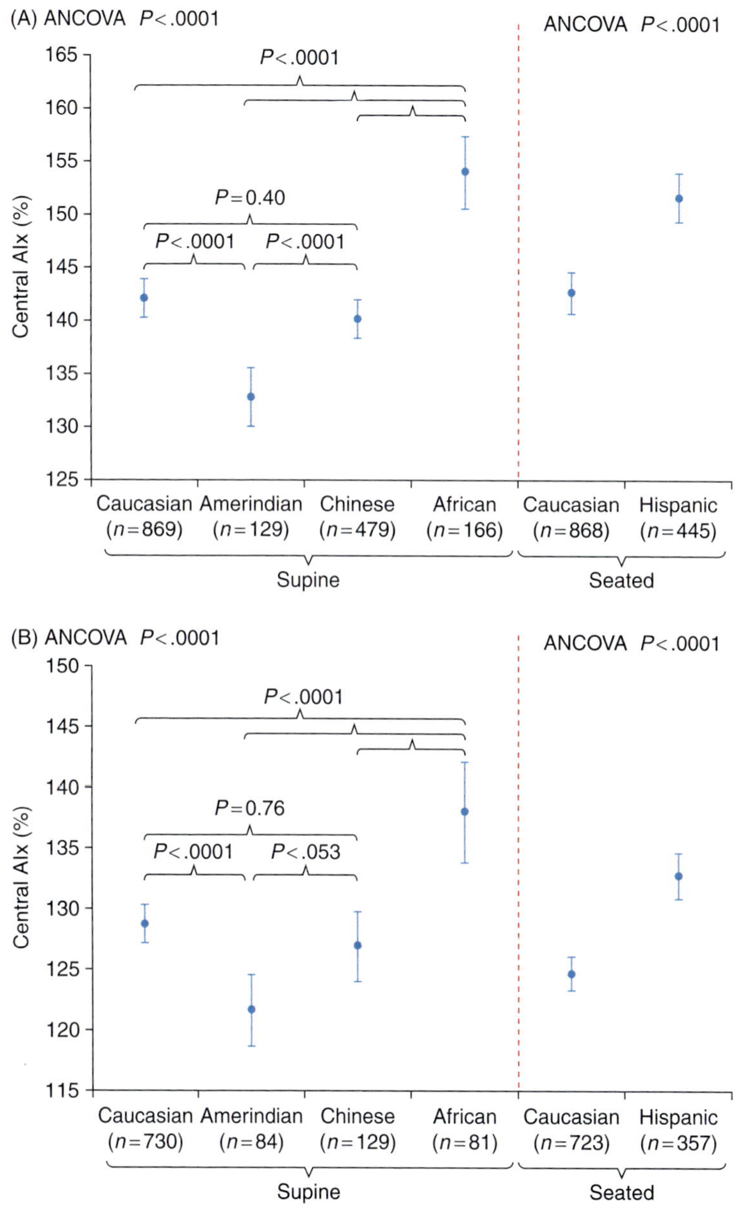

Fig. 3-8b Ethnic comparisons of central augmentation index (AIx) in women (A) and men (B). (From Chirinos JA, Kips JG, roman MJ, et al. Ethnic differences in arterial wave reflections and normative equations for augmentation index. *Hypertension* 2011;57:1108–16.)

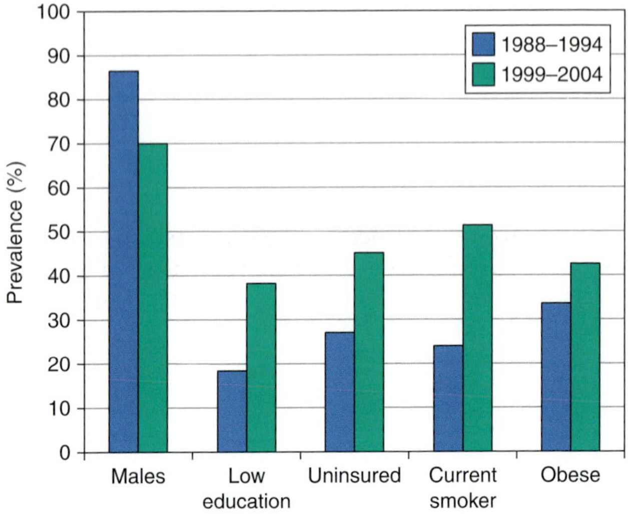

Fig. 3-9 Isolated systolic hypertension prevalence among adults aged 18–39 years in NHANES 111 and 1999–2004. (From Grebla RC, Rodriguez CJ, Borrell LN, et al. Prevalence and determinants of isolated systolic hypertension among young adults: the 1999–2004 US National Health and Nutrition Examination Survey. *J Hypertens* 2010;28:15–23.)

SUMMARY AND CONCLUSIONS

1. The lifetime risk of developing hypertension (>140/90 mm Hg) in subjects aged 65 years is about 90%.
2. In women, the risk of hypertension occurs mainly in the post-menopausal period, where about 75% of women are hypertensive in the United States.
3. Globally, in 2000, about 20% of the adults had hypertension.
4. The prevalence of hypertension is higher in Europe (44%) than in Canada/United States (28%).
5. Most of the world's hypertension occurs in low-income developing countries, where the prevalence is increasing faster than that in high-income developed countries.
6. The prevalence of hypertension (in the United States of America) is particularly high in non-Hispanic black subjects, due to environmental/behavioral factors.
7. ISH increases with age, the prevalence being about 50% at age greater than 50 years and 75% at age greater than 75 years.

8. In children/adolescents, hypertension (>95th centile) occurs in only less than 4% of the subjects, although prehypertension (between 90 and 95th centile) occurs in 20% boys and 13% girls.
9. In younger adults (aged 18–39 years), surprisingly, ISH is more common than diastolic/systolic hypertension (SDH) with a rising prevalence, particularly in low-education, smoking, and obese groups.
10. All the above "prevalence" figures are based on clinical blood pressures; these figures would be lower based on home or daytime 24-hour ambulatory monitoring that would avoid the "white-coat" effect.

REFERENCES

1. Vasan RS, Beiser A, Seshadri S, et al. Residual lifetime risk for developing hypertension in middle-aged men and women. The Framingham Heart Study. *JAMA* 2002;287:1003–10.
2. Tunstall-Pedoe H, Connaghan J, Woodward M, et al. Pattern of declining blood pressure across replicate population surveys of the WHO MONICA project, mid 1980's to mid-1990s, and the role of medication. *BMJ* 2006;332:629–32.
3. Barton M, Meyer MR. Postmenopausal hypertension. *Hypertension* 2009;54:11–18.
4. Kearney PM, Whelton M, Reynolds K, et al. Global burden of hypertension: analysis of worldwide data. *Lancet* 2005;365:217–25.
5. Wolf-Maier K, Cooper RS, Banegas JR, et al. Hypertension prevalence and blood pressure level in 6 European countries, Canada and the United States. *JAMA* 2003;289:2363–9.
6. Carrington MJ, Jennings GL, Stewart S. Pattern of blood pressure in Australian adults: results from a National Blood Pressure Screening Day of 13,825 adults. *Intern J Cardiol* 2010;145:461–7.
7. Wilkinson IB, Christison DJ, Cockcroft JR. Isolated systolic hypertension: a radical rethink. *BMJ* 2000;320:1685.
8. Basile JN. Systolic blood pressure. *BMJ* 2002;325:917–18.
9. Franklin SS, Jacobs MJ, Wong ND, et al. Predominance of isolated systolic hypertension among middle-aged and elderly US hypertensives: analysis based on Nation Health and Nutrition Examination Survey (NHANES III). *Hypertension* 2001;37:869–74.
10. MacMahon S, Alderman MH, Lindholm LH, et al. Blood-pressure-related diseases is a global health priority. *Lancet* 2008;371:1480–1.
11. Kaplan NM, Opie LH. Controversies in hypertension. *Lancet* 2006;367:168–76.
12. Vathesatogkit P, Woodward M, Tanomsup S, et al. Long-term effects of socioeconomic status on incident hypertension and progression of blood pressure. *J Hypertens* 2012;30:1347–53.

13. Maher D, Waswa L, Baisley K, et al. Epidemiology of hypertension in low-income countries: a cross-sectional population based survey in rural Uganda. *J Hypertens* 2011;29:1061–8.
14. Danaei G, Finucane MM, Lin JK, et al. National, regional and global trends in SBP since 1980: systematic analysis of health examination surveys s and epidemiological studies with 786 country-years and 5.4 million participants. *Lancet* 2011;377:568–77.
15. Fields LE, Burt VL, Cutler JA, et al. The burden of adult hypertension in the United States 1999–2000: a rising tide. *Hypertension* 2004;44:398–404.
16. Hajjar I, Kotchen TA. Trends in prevalence, awareness, treatment and control of hypertension in the United States, 1988–2000. *JAMA* 2003;290:199–206.
17. Fuchs FD. Why do black Americans have higher prevalence of hypertension? *Hypertension* 2011;57:379–80.
18. Brummett BH, Babyak MA, Siegler IC, et al. Systolic blood pressure, socio economic status and behavioural risk factors in a nationally representative US young adult sample. *Hypertension* 2011;58:161–6.
19. McCarron P, Okasha M, McEwen J, et al. Changes in blood pressure among students attending Glasgow University between 1948 and 1960: analyses of cross sectional surveys. *BMJ* 2001;322:885–9.
20. Watkins D, McCarron P, Murray L, et al. Trends in blood pressure over 10 years in adolescents: analysis of cross sectional surveys in Northern Island Young Hearts project. *BMJ* 2004;329:139–41.
21. Hansen ML, Guna PW, Kaelber DC. Underdiagnosis of hypertension in children and adolescents. *JAMA* 2007;298:874–9.
22. Falkner B, Gidding SS, Portman R, et al. Blood pressure variability and classification of prehypertension and hypertension and adolescence. *Pediatrics* 2008;122:238–42.
23. Chirinos JA, Kips JG, Roman MJ, et al. Ethnic differences in arterial wave reflections and normative equations for augmentation index. *Hypertension* 2011;57:1108–16.
24. Grebla RC, Rodriguez CJ, Borrell LN, et al. Prevalence and determinants of isolated systolic hypertension among young adults: the 1999–2004 US National Health and Nutrition Examination Survey. *J Hypertens* 2010;28:15–23.

CHAPTER 4

Pathophysiology of Essential Hypertension

GENETIC COMPONENTS

The development of hypertension is linked to various combinations of genetic and environmental factors (1). From the studies on monozygotic and dizygotic twin children, as well as their other children and adopted children, genetic factors accounted for about 30% of the pathophysiology of essential hypertension (2, 3). Normotensive children of hypertensive parents have peripheral and central blood pressures which are higher than normal (4). Hypertension is associated with 7 genetic loci in the Japanese population (5). Certain genes are related to obesity-associated hypertension (6), and such hypertension possibly has a genetic basis different from lean-associated hypertension (7).

1. Telomere dysfunction, aging, and pulse pressure

It has been noted that there are marked similarities between aging and hypertension (8). Both conditions share alterations in telomerase activity and shortening of the DNA component of telomeres, and these events are influenced by genetic factors (8). There are genetic links to pulse wave velocity (PWV) (9), arterial stiffness (9–11), and pulse pressure (P-P) (12).

2. Sodium reabsorption in loop of Henle

One aspect of the origin of hypertension is a pressure–natriuresis relationship that achieves a balance between sodium intake and output.

There are associations of rare mutations and common variants in genes, which encode for determinants of sodium reabsorption in the thick ascending limb (TAL) of the loop of Henle, and are associated with the risk of hypertension (13). Certainly, salt sensitivity in hypertension appears to be under genetic control (14).

3. β-2 Receptor and ACE genotypes

Blunted β-2 adrenoceptor-mediated vasodilatation has been implicated in the pathogenesis of hypertension. Interestingly, a certain haplotype 1 of the β-2 receptor is linked to low blood pressure (BP) in young subjects, but not in the elderly where β-2 receptor desensitization occurs (15). There are also β-2 receptor locus variants (with attenuated vasodilatory properties) that are associated with hypertension in the Chinese population (16).

Most, although not all, studies have shown no association between angiotensin-converting enzyme (ACE) genotype and hypertension (17). However, many hypertensive patients have a decreased fibrinolytic capacity (leading to an increased risk of myocardial infarction), and this is linked to the ACE/DD genotype (18).

4. Sympathetic nerve activity and angiotensin I and II

Adrenergic regulation of BP may be altered not only in the hypertensives themselves but also in their (normotensive) first-degree relatives (siblings and offspring), and family history of hypertension is a powerful risk factor for the development of the disease (19). Multiple genetic loci are likely to contribute to common variations in autonomic function (19).

In young/middle-aged, non-overweight hypertensives, muscle sympathetic nerve activity (MSNA) is expressed more than twice that in aged-matched normotensives (**Figure 4-1**) (20); and the increased sympathetic activity (noradrenaline spillover) is expressed in heart and kidney (**Figure 4-2**) (20) and lumbar region (21). Interestingly, there is no relationship between sympathetic activity and the renin–angiotensin system; indeed, angiotensin I and II

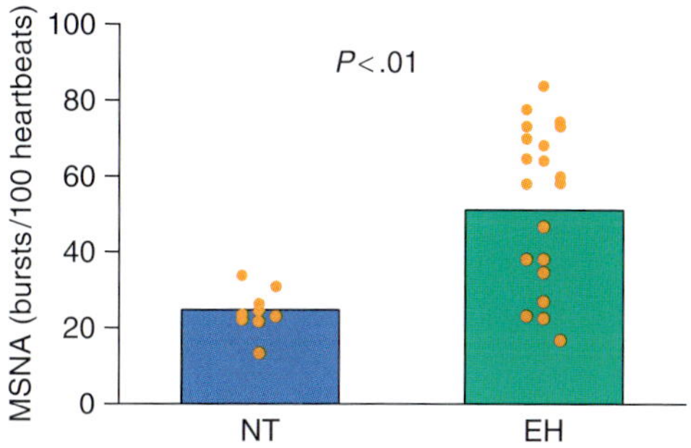

Fig. 4-1 Muscle sympathetic nerve activity (MSNA) in young/middle-aged, normal-weight hypertensives (EH) and normotensives (NT). (From Schlaich MP, Lambert E, Kaye DM, et al. Sympathetic augmentation in hypertension. *Hypertension* 2004;43:169–75.)

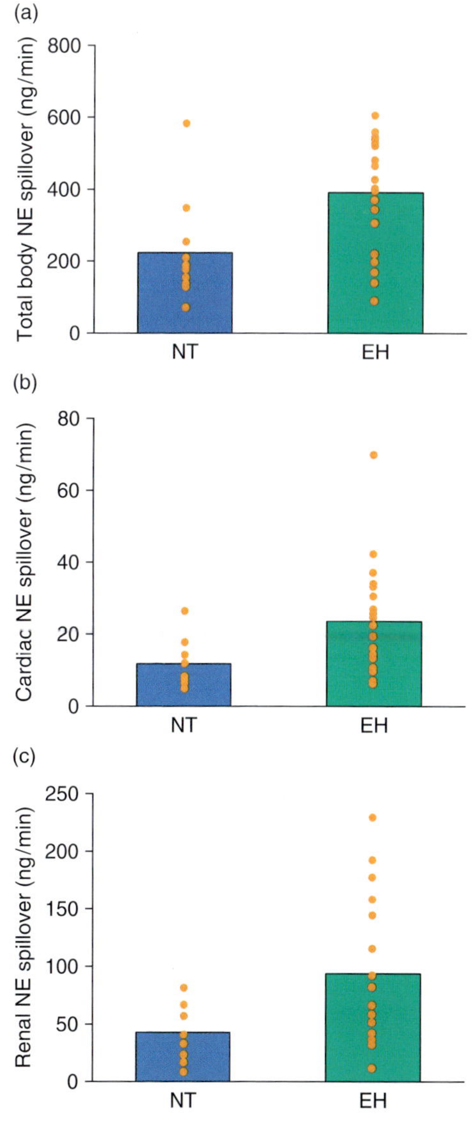

Fig. 4-2 Whole body (A), cardiac (B), and renal (C) noradrenaline spillover in young/middle-aged, normal-weight normotensive (NT) and hypertensive (EH) subjects. (From Schlaich MP, Lambert E, Kaye DM, et al. Sympathetic augmentation in hypertension. *Hypertension* 2004;43:169–75.)

are not increased (**Figure 4-3**). The increased levels of MSNA in normal-weight hypertensives are not as high as in age-matched, middle-aged obese hypertensives (**Figure 4-4**) (22), but, unlike

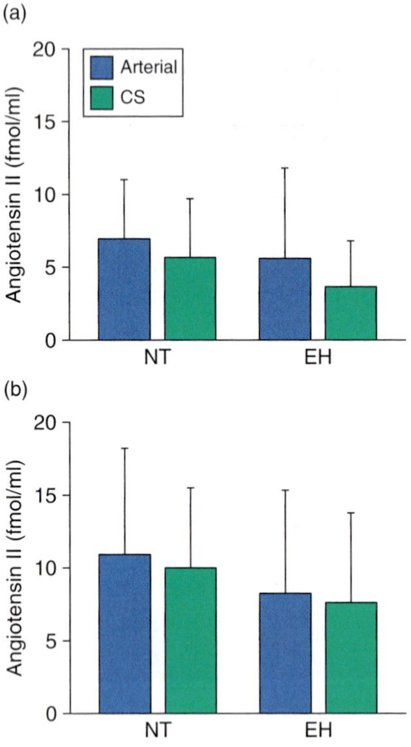

Fig. 4-3 Angiotensin 11 (A) and 1 (B) arterial and coronary sinus (CS) levels in young/middle-aged, normal-weight normotensive (NT) and hypertensive (EH) subjects. (From Schlaich MP, Lambert E, Kaye DM, et al. Sympathetic augmentation in hypertension. *Hypertension* 2004;43:169–75.)

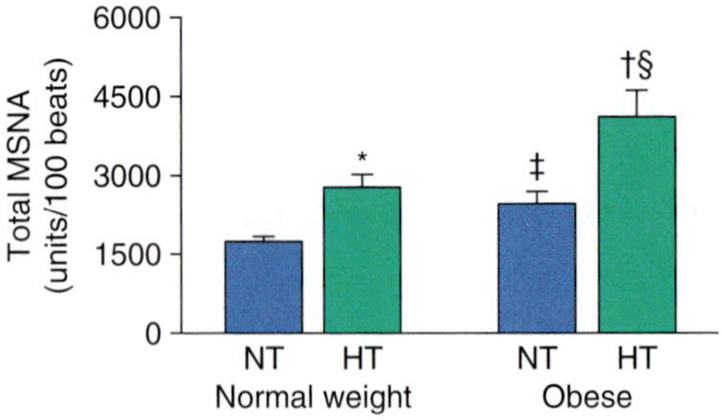

Fig. 4-4 Muscle sympathetic nerve activity (MSNA) in normal-weight and obese, young/middle-aged normotensives (NT) and hypertensives (EH). (From Lambert E, Straznicky N, Schlaich M, et al. Differing pattern of sympathoexcitation in normal-weight and obesity-related hypertension. *Hypertension* 2007;50:862–8.)

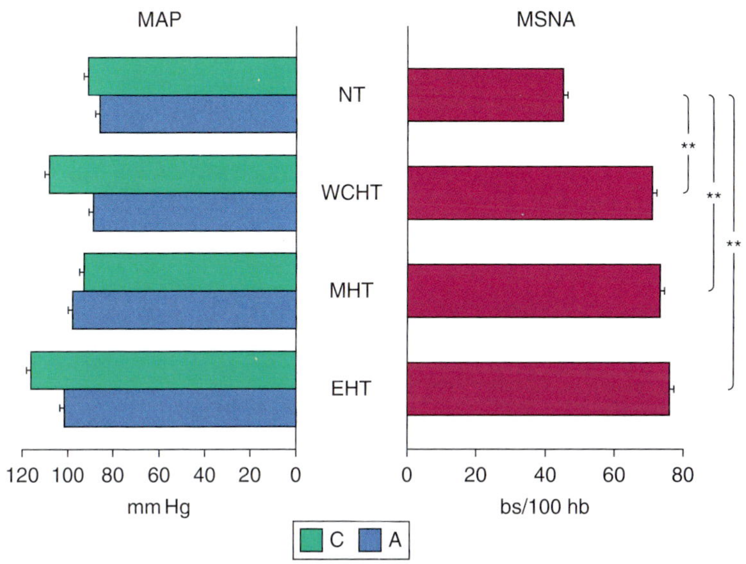

Fig. 4-4a Muscle sympathetic nerve activity (MSNA) is raised in white-coat hypertension (WCHT) and masked hypertension (MHT), as well as sustained hypertension (EHT) versus normotension (NT); BP assessed in clinic (C) and by ambulatory monitoring (A). (From Grassi G. Sympathetic neural activity in hypertension and related diseases. *Am J Hypertens* 2010;23:1052–60.)

obesity-related hypertension, cardiac sympathetic nerve activity is increased. It is worth noting that sympathetic nerve activity is raised not only in sustained hypertension but also in "white-coat" and "masked" hypertension (**Figure 4-4a**) (23). Tyrosine hydroxylase (TH) plays a rate-limiting key role in the formation of catecholamines, and a variant *TH* gene is present in some cases of younger/middle-aged, nonobese hypertensives (25).

5. Hypertension drug-target genes

Achieving BP control in patients often requires multiple medications and trial and error switching of drugs. This suggests that interindividual differences in BP and response to treatment may be influenced by genetic variations. Thirty drug-target genes have been identified, including targets of α-blockers, ACE inhibitors, angiotensin receptor blockers, β-blockers, calcium channel blockers, diuretics, and vasodilators (26). This discovery provides the potential for more intelligent use of drugs in controlling BP.

ENVIRONMENTAL COMPONENTS

Lifestyle factors are thought to be responsible for about 70%–80% of cases of hypertension (27), where 10–20 mm Hg of average systolic BP (SBP) of a typical western population can be attributed to various combinations of overweight, physical inactivity, high salt intake, high alcohol consumption, and typical Western diet, that is, low consumption of fruit, vegetables, and fish but high intake of saturated fat and sugar.

1. Overweight/obesity in young/middle-aged subjects

A) Obesity epidemic—link to hypertension

Overweight/obesity is undoubtedly the most important environmental risk factor for hypertension, being responsible for 60%–70% of hypertension in adults (28). In the United States in 2000, in those aged 60 years, 65% were overweight, 31% were obese, and 4%–5% were morbidly obese (29). In black women older than 40 years, 80% were overweight (29). By 2030, in the United States, it has been estimated that 42% of adults will be obese (body mass index [BMI] > 40 kg/m^2) and 11% will be morbidly obese (BMI > 40 kg/m^2) (30). Obesity is set to overtake smoking as the primary preventable cause of death (31). Central obesity, as expressed by either waist circumference or waist-to-hip ratio, is linked to total mortality, cardiovascular mortality, and cancer mortality in women, as evidenced in the Nurses' Health study involving 44 636 middle-aged women followed up for 16 years (**Figure 4-4b**) (32).

As BMI increases, so does the frequency of hypertension in middle-aged subjects (**Figure 4-5**) (33). The higher BP is particularly evident at night (**Figure 4-6**) (34), as is a higher heart rate. The relationship between BMI, or central obesity, and hypertension seems greater in Aboriginal, East Asian, and Southern Asian populations than in White counterparts (35).

As shown in the Framingham Heart Study, the marked relation between obesity and diastolic/systolic hypertension is evident only in the young/middle-aged subjects; in elderly, isolated systolic hypertension is a function of aging and stiffening of the arteries (**Table 4-1**) (36).

B) Obesity and sympathetic nerve activity

As already noted, sympathetic nerve activity is markedly increased in young/middle-aged obese hypertensives (Figure 4-4) (22), and the degree of hypertension is matched by the degree of increased

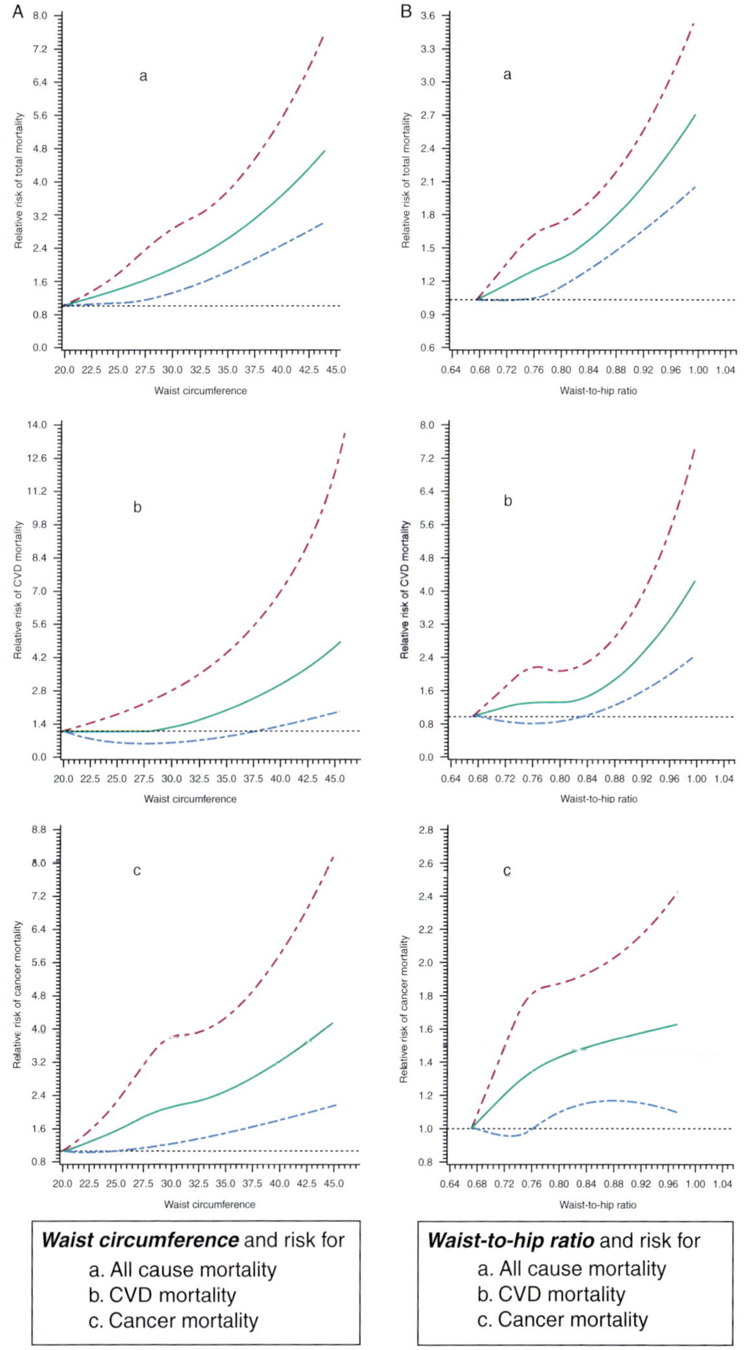

Fig. 4-4b Nurses Health Study; effect of central obesity [waist circumference (A) and waist-to-hip ratio (B)] on total, cardiovascular, and cancer mortality over 16 years. (From Zhang C, Rexrode KM, van Dam RM, et al. Abdominal obesity and the risk of all-cause, cardiovascular and cancer mortality. *Circulation* 2008;117:1658–67.)

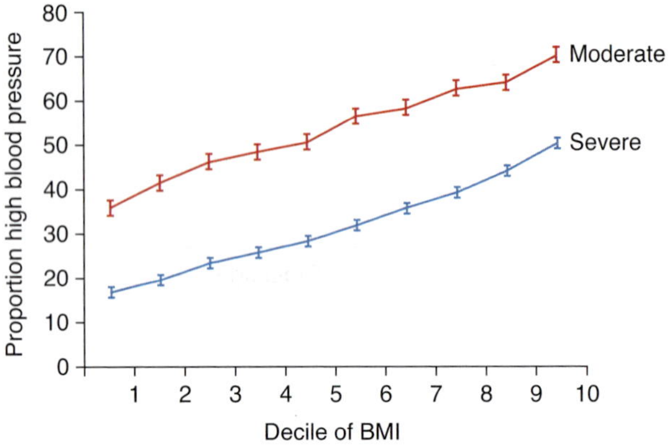

Fig. 4-5 Adiposity and blood pressure in middle-aged (mean 58 y) subjects (n = 37 027). (From Timpson NJ, Harbord R, Davey-Smith G, et al. Does greater adiposity increase blood pressure and hypertension risk? *Hypertension* 2009;54:84–90.)

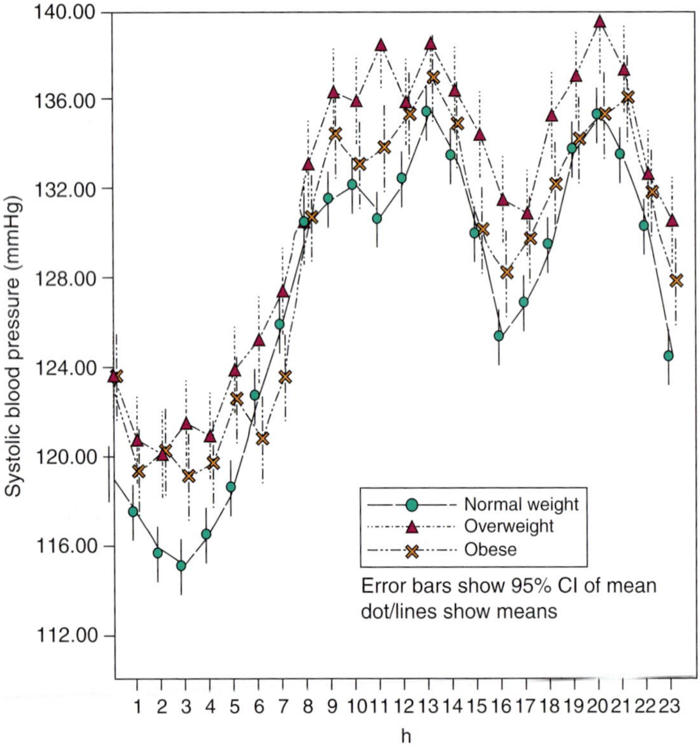

Fig. 4-6 Twenty-four hour SBP in normal-weight, overweight, and obese subjects. (From Kotsis V, Stabouli S, Bouldin M, et al. Impact of obesity on 24-hour ambulatory blood pressure and hypertension. *Hypertension* 2005;45:602–7.)

TABLE 4-1 Different predictors of DH (±raised SDH) and ISH—Framingham study

Predictors of diastolic hypertension (±systolic hypertension) = DBP ≥ 90 mm Hg (±SBP ≥ 140 mm Hg)	Predictors of isolated systolic hypertension = SBP ≥ 140 mm Hg + DBP < 90 mm Hg (wide P-P)
Young age	Older age
Male sex	Female sex
High BMI at baseline	Increased BMI during follow-up (weak)
Increased BMI during follow-up	ISH arises more commonly from normal and high normal BP, than "burned out" diastolic hypertension
Main mechanism of DH and SDH is raised peripheral resistance	Only 18% with new-onset ISH had a previous DBP ≥ 95 mm Hg
	Main mechanism of ISH is increased arterial stiffness = aging of arteries

Abbreviations: DBP, diastolic blood pressure; SBP, systolic blood pressure; P-P, pulse pressure; BMI, body mass index; BP, blood pressure; ISH, isolated systolic hypertension; DH, diastolic hypertension; SDH, systolic–diastolic hypertension.
From Franklin SS, Pio JR, Wong ND, et al. Predictors of new-onset diastolic and systolic hypertension. The Framingham Heart Study. *Circulation* 2005;111:1121–7.

sympathetic nerve activity, especially in nondippers (23). This increased sympathetic activity occurs mainly in muscle and kidney, with little or no increase in the heart [unlike nonobese hypertensives (20)], gut, and liver; but adrenaline level is not raised (**Figure 4-7**) (37). The process is very rapid, where in rats fed a high-fat diet renal sympathetic nerve activity is increased within 1 week (38). The increased sympathetic stimulation is of a greater magnitude with central obesity when compared with peripheral obesity (**Figure 4-8**) (39). Therefore, it is not surprising that in patients with the metabolic syndrome (40, 41) or type 2 diabetes (42), where central obesity is the norm, there is a marked increase in sympathetic nerve activity (**Figures 4-9** and **4-10**). The increased plasma noradrenaline levels are particularly notable at night (43), especially in "nondippers" (23). The diurnal increase in noradrenaline is markedly reduced by loss of weight (43). In men, there is a powerful linear relationship between waist circumference and sympathetic nerve activity (**Figure 4-11**) (44). In younger subjects, the degree of increased BP is matched by an increased level of sympathetic nerve activity(23, 24).

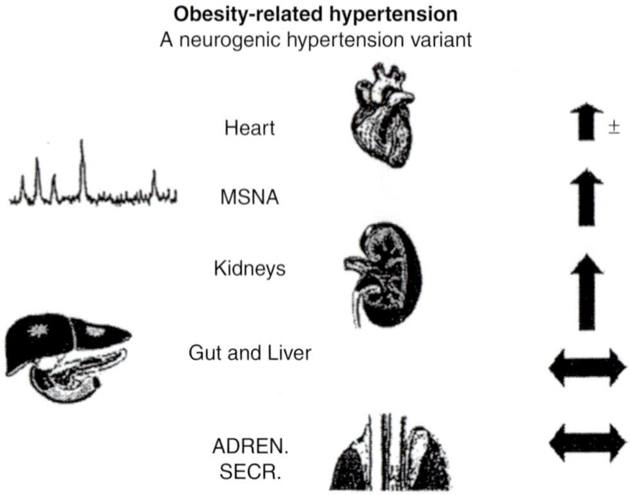

Fig. 4-7 In obesity-related hypertension, increased sympathetic nerve activity occurs mainly in muscle (MSNA) and kidney. (From Esler M, Straznicky N, Eikelis N, et al. Mechanisms of sympathetic activation in obesity-related hypertension. *Hypertension* 2006;48:787–96.)

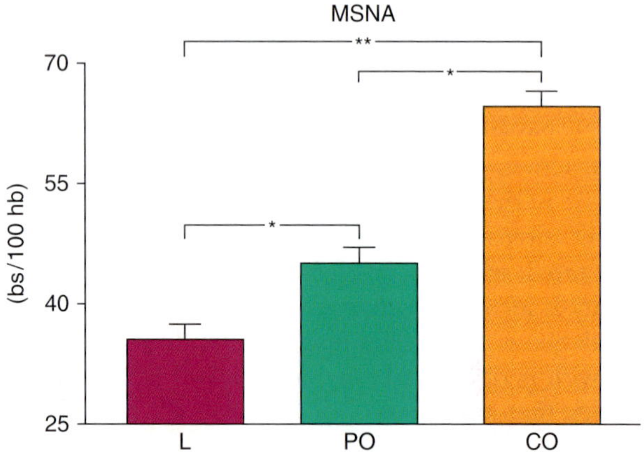

Fig. 4-8 In 30 lean (L), 20 peripherally obese (PO), and 26 centrally obese (CO) subjects (mean age 36 years), muscle sympathetic nerve activity (MSNA) was significantly higher in CO than PO and L subjects. (From Grassi G, Dell'Oro R, Facchini A, et al. Effect of central and peripheral body fat distribution on sympathetic and baroreflex function in obese normotensives. *J Hypertens* 2004;22:236–9.) *Statistically significant.

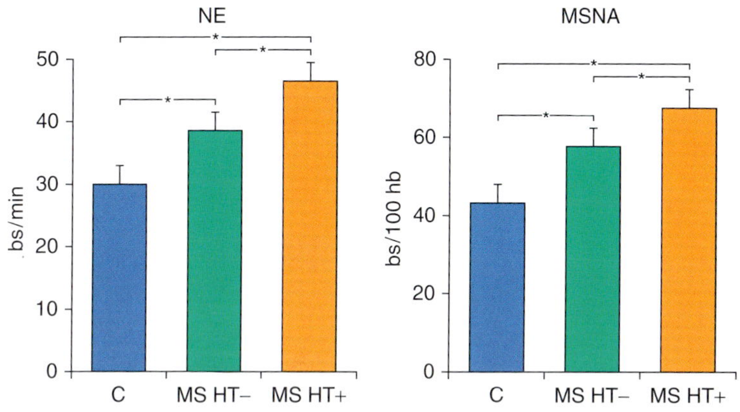

Fig. 4-9 Plasma noradrenaline levels (NE) and muscle sympathetic nerve activity (MSNA) in control, metabolic syndrome without hypertension (MSHT–) and with hypertension (MSHT+). (From Mancia G, Bousquet P, Elghozi JL, et al. The sympathetic nervous system and the metabolic syndrome. *J Hypertens* 2007;25:909–20.)

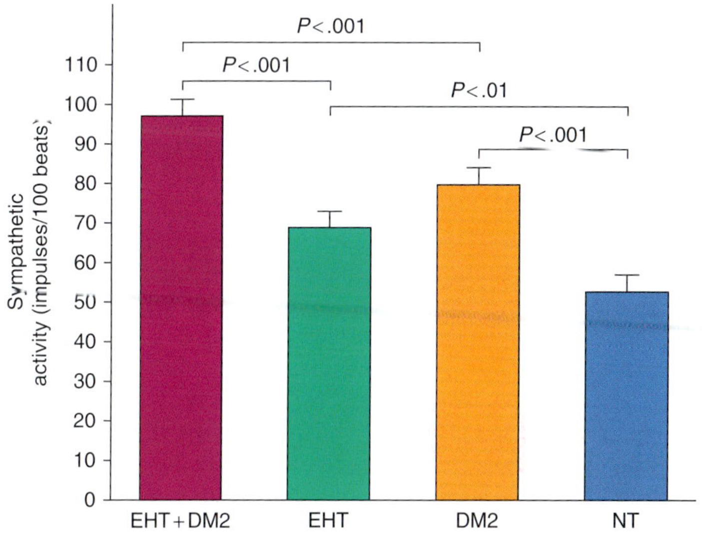

Fig. 4-10 In 68 matched subjects (17 NT, 17 DM2, 17 HT, and 17 DM2 + HT), sympathetic activity markedly raised in DM2 + HT and correlated with high insulin levels. (From Huggett RJ, Scott EM, Gilbey SG, et al. Impact of type 2 diabetes on sympathetic neural mechanisms in hypertension. *Circulation* 2003;108:3097–101.)

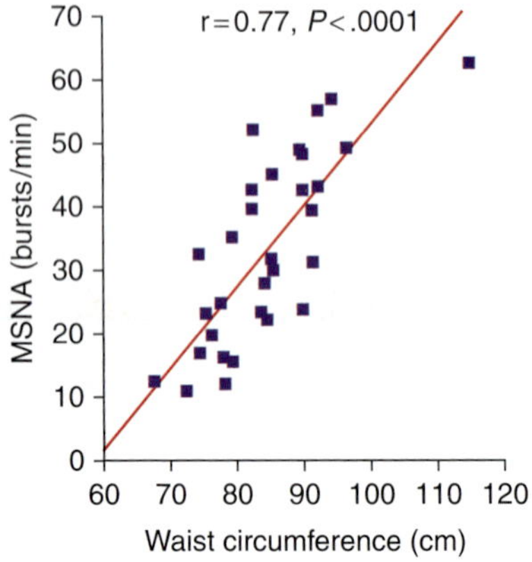

Fig. 4-11 Relationship between waist circumference and muscle sympathetic nerve activity (MSNA) in men. (From Joyner MJ, Charkoudian N, Wallin G. Sympathetic nervous system and blood pressure in humans. *Hypertension* 2010;56:10–16.)

C) How does high sympathetic activity increase blood pressure—hemodynamic and kidney

Young/middle-aged hypertension is closely linked to central obesity, a high cardiac output, a high heart rate, and an increased peripheral resistance (**Figure 4-12**) (45). Thus, high sympathetic nerve activity acts via increasing both cardiac output and total peripheral resistance.

The kidney is closely involved in the development of hypertension (46). Mechanisms involve a reduction in glomerular filtration rate, resulting in reduced sodium excretion, and tubular mechanisms (47), again involving sodium retention and angiotensin I receptors (46). Increased renal sympathetic nerve activity is also associated with sodium retention (48, 49), reversed by renal denervation (50).

The active β-receptor appears to be of the β-1 variety (51), residing in the TAL of Henle. Stimulation of this receptor by noradrenaline results in sodium retention (leading to blood volume expansion), whereas β-1 blockade promotes diuresis and natriuresis (51, 52).

Weight gain in young/middle-aged subjects is associated with a decrease in arterial compliance (53) and a widening of P-P (54). An increased sympathetic nerve activity is related to increased wave reflection amplitude in young men, but not in women, resulting in an increased central augmentation index (AIx) (**Figure 4-13**) (55). Women may be "protected" by oestrogens.

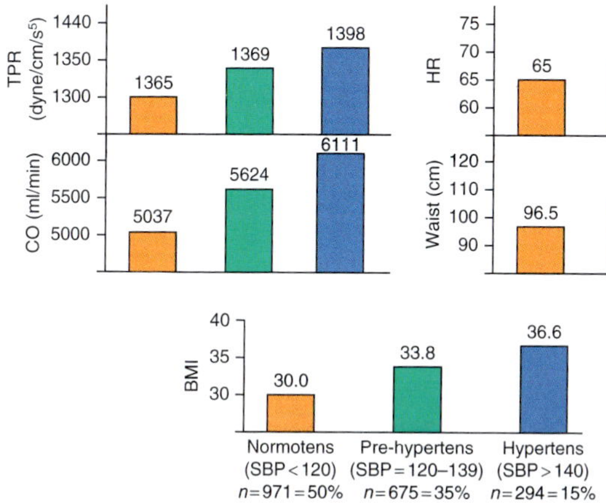

Fig. 4-12 STRONG Heart study—1940 US adolescent/young subjects (age 14–39 years)—50% were normotensive, 35% prehypertensive, and 15% hypertensive. (From Druktenis JS, Roman MJ, Fabsitz RR, et al. Cardiac and systemic hemodynamic characteristics of hypertension and prehypertension in adolescents and young adults. The Strong Heart Study. *Circulation* 2007;115:221–7.)

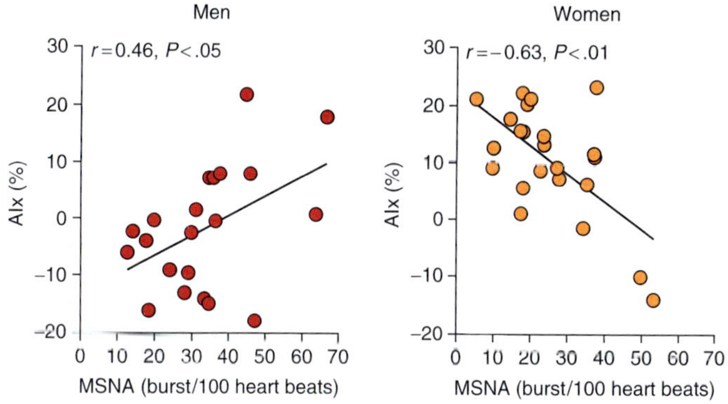

Fig. 4-13 Relationship between muscle sympathetic nerve activity (MSNA) and central augmentation index (AIx) in men and women. (From Casey DP, Curry TB, Joyner MJ, et al. Relationship between muscle sympathetic nerve activity and aortic wave reflection characteristics in young men and women. *Hypertension* 2011;57:421–7.)

D) What is the likely mechanism for the association between obesity and high sympathetic nerve activity?

There is a "chicken-egg" debate (56, 57), which suggests that rather than obesity preceding increased sympathetic nerve activity, the reverse is true. Thus, initial high sympathetic activity results in downregulation of β-receptors, thereby resulting in a decreased thermogenic response and a propensity to gain weight. Most would accept the reverse argument, that is, that obesity precedes the increased sympathetic nerve activity. What is the possible mechanism for this relationship?

The likely series of events linking central obesity with high sympathetic activity and hypertension were set out by Cruickshank (58) and later refined (59). Briefly, centrally located adipocytes produce several vasculotoxic adipokinins [e.g., tumor necrosis factor (TNF)-α and interleukin (IL)-6 (60, 61)], which act on the liver that, in turn, releases C-reactive protein (CRP), an indicator of acute inflammation. In middle-aged hypertensives, CRP levels relate to the level of BP (**Figure 4-13a**) (62). The adipokinins also set in motion an endothelial inflammatory response, resulting in insulin resistance (**Figure 4-14**). Insulin resistance is accompanied by a compensatory increase in insulin secretion that acts centrally, resulting in an increased sympathetic outflow (63) and renin release (via β-1 stimulation of the renal juxtaglomerular apparatus) (64). Central adipocytes also produce the "thin hormone" leptin that, like insulin, also acts centrally, resulting in an increased sympathetic outflow (65). The high renin levels result in increased angiotensin II production, which (like leptin and insulin) also act centrally (hypothalamic region), resulting in an increased sympathetic outflow (66, 67, 68), in addition to effecting marked renal vasoconstriction and sodium retention. Thus, there is a vicious cycle that results in high noradrenaline activity, leading to chronic β-1 stimulation and its concomitant injurious effects on the periphery [e.g., cardiac necrosis and apoptosis (69)], increased risk of ventricular fibrillation and sudden death (70), increased atheroma formation (71), and left ventricular hypertrophy (**Figure 4-15**) (72). All these problems are, at least theoretically, solved by chronic β-1 blockade.

More recent information has linked sympathetic nerve overactivity in obese subjects to selective leptin resistance (Figure 4-16) (73), and in particular, the high sympathetic activity is evident in the kidneys (**Figure 4-17**) (73, 74). The high leptin levels, associated with hypertension/obesity, are especially evident in women (75), particularly in older black and white women (76). Leptin, as well as insulin and angiotensin II, acts centrally by activating a specific melanocortin-dependent pathway that alters hypothalamic paraventricular nucleus activity, thereby increasing glutaminergic drive to the rostral ventrolateral medulla and increasing BP via increased sympathetic outflow (77).

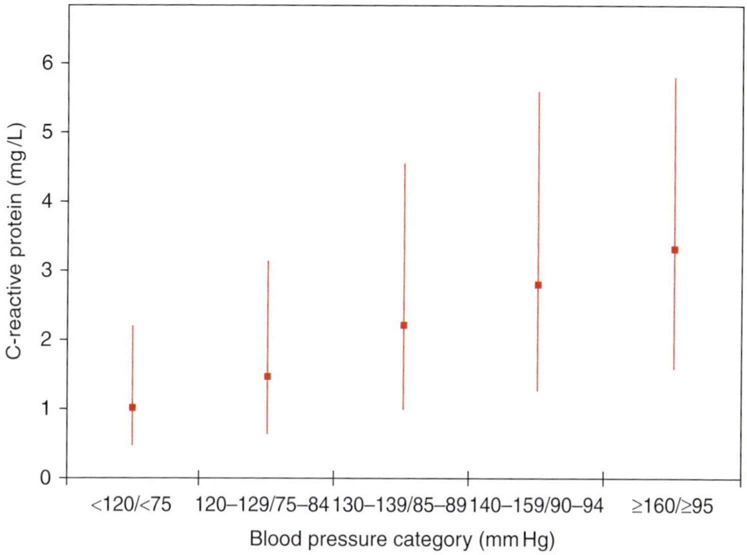

Fig. 4-13a In middle-aged hypertensives, CRP levels rise in accordance with increasing BP. (From Blake GJ, Rifai N, Buring JE, et al. Blood pressure, C-reactive protein and risk of future cardiovascular events. *Circulation* 2003;108:2993–9.)

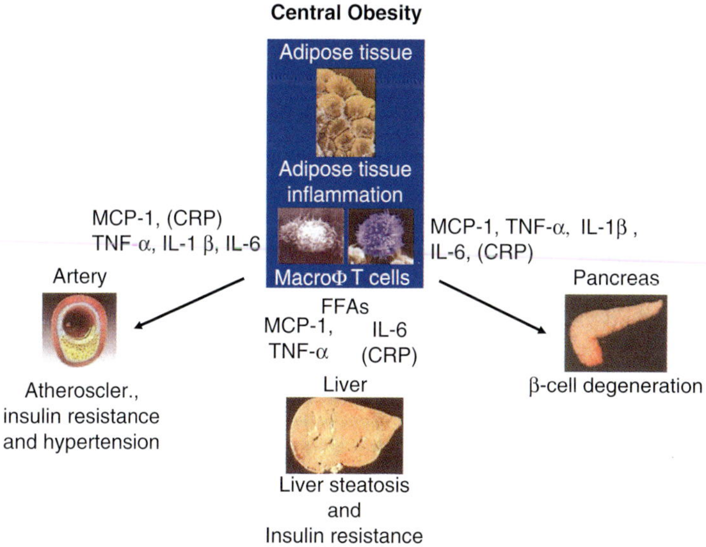

Fig. 4-14 Central obesity, inflammation, adipokinins and the immune response, and the possible effects on the blood vessels, liver, and pancreas. (From Cruickshank JM. *The Modern Role of Beta-Blockers in Cardiovascular Medicine*. Shelton, Connecticut: People's Medical Publishing House; 2011; pp 84–9.)

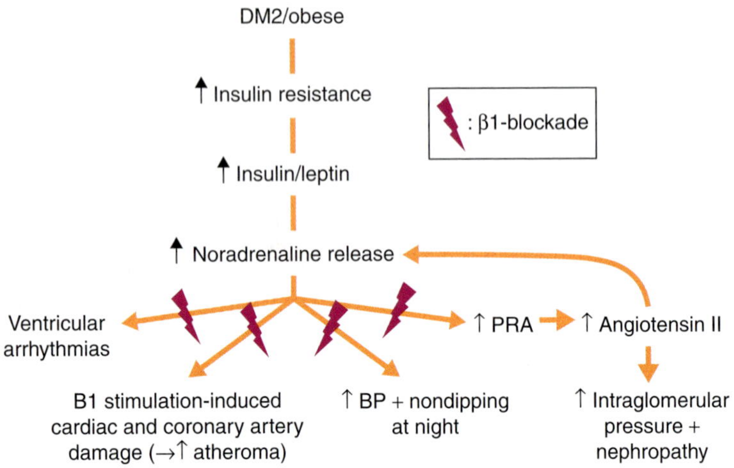

Fig. 4-15 β1-Blockade benefits in central obesity/insulin resistance/DM2 with hypertension. (From Cruickshank JM, 2011.)

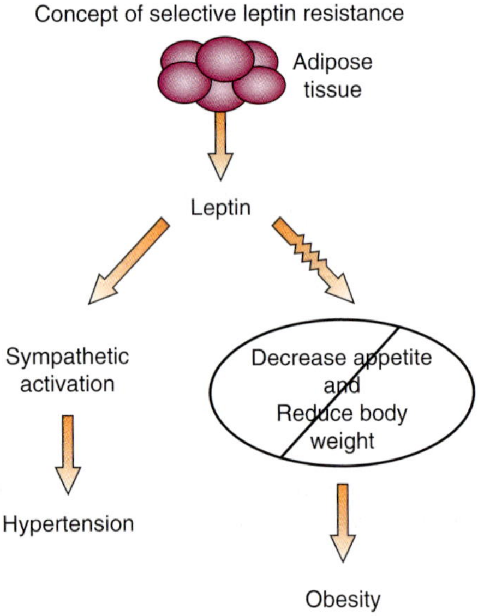

Fig. 4-16 Leptin resistance may be confined to the satiety and weight-reducing action of leptin and not to its ability to induce sympathetic nerve overactivity and hypertension. (From Mark AL, Correia ML, Rahmouni K, et al. Selective leptin resistance: a new concept in leptin physiology with cardiovascular implications. *J Hypertens* 2002;20:1245–50.)

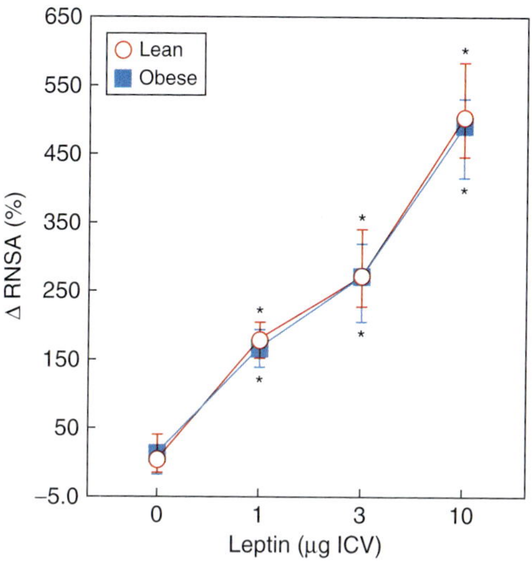

Fig. 4-17 Positive relationship between intracerebroventricular administration of leptin and renal sympathetic nerve activity (RNSA) in lean and obese mice. (From Mark AL, Correia ML, Rahmouni K, et al. Selective leptin resistance: a new concept in leptin physiology with cardiovascular implications. *J Hypertens* 2002;20:1245–50.)

Adiponectin is secreted predominantly by adipocytes (78), and its expression is reduced in obesity and insulin resistance. Treatment with adiponectin improves insulin sensitivity (79) and lowers BP (probably via lowering insulin concentration and thus sympathetic nerve activity). High adiponectin levels are linked to low inflammatory markers such as TNF-α, IL-6, and CRP (78). However, the role of adiponectin in the development of hypertension remains unclear (80).

Clearly, hypertension involved with obesity is closely linked to an inflammatory response and an increased sympathetic activity (Figures 4-14 and 4-15). Not only are central adipocytes implicated but also T cells are involved in the immune response (81, 82). Certainly, T cells can be powerful producers of cytokines (83). The ability of noradrenaline to induce inflammation may be via stimulation of receptive T cells (83).

Perivascular adipose tissue may be involved in the pathophysiology of primary hypertension (84). Under normal circumstances, methyl palmitate is released spontaneously from perivascular adipose tissue, causing vasorelaxation, but when hypertension is present, release of the vasorelaxant is diminished at the same time as angiotensin II release from the perivascular adipose tissue is increased.

2. Systolic hypertension in the elderly

In contrast to diastolic hypertension in younger subjects (and its link with obesity), the Framingham Study showed that elderly systolic hypertension was a quite separate condition arising from aging, stiffening of the vasculature (Table 4-1) (36). The development of elderly systolic hypertension did not, in particular, arise from "burned out" diastolic hypertension, but it was a quite separate entity (36). This observation is at odds with the opinion that there was an evolutionary phase from younger diastolic hypertension to elderly systolic hypertension (85). Others have shown that systolic hypertension in younger and older subjects is a quite different condition, with normal vascular compliance in the young, and decreased vascular compliance in the older individuals (86).

A) Elderly systolic hypertension and the sympathetic nervous system, renin/angiotensin, and salt retention

In younger subjects, sympathetic nerve activity is greater in men compared with women (87, 88). However, with increasing age, MSNA increases in normotensive and hypertensive subjects (89); the increase being greater in women than in men (90). Interestingly, in premenopausal women, sympathetic nerve activity is significantly higher in those with hypertension, a difference that disappears in the postmenopausal period (91) (**Figure 4-17a**). Unlike MSNA, renal sympathetic outflow (noradrenaline) decreases with age (**Figure 4-17b**) (92).

With increasing age, β-receptor affinity/sensitivity declines (93, 94, 95, 96), resulting in a decrease in the cardiac output (85, 97). This loss of β-receptor affinity/sensitivity is less in women than men (87). The loss of β-receptor affinity/sensitivity in the kidney results in a decrease in plasma renin-angiotensin activity (stimulation of β-1 receptors in the juxtaglomerular apparatus results in release of renin). The combination of reduced renin-angiotensin activity and reduced β-1 receptor sensitivity would account for the salt retention (46, 51, 52), as noted in elderly systolic hypertension. Salt retention leads to sympathetic nerve activation mediated by the effects of sodium on α-2 adrenergic receptors in the brainstem, leading to increased peripheral resistance and BP (quite independent of volume overload) (98).

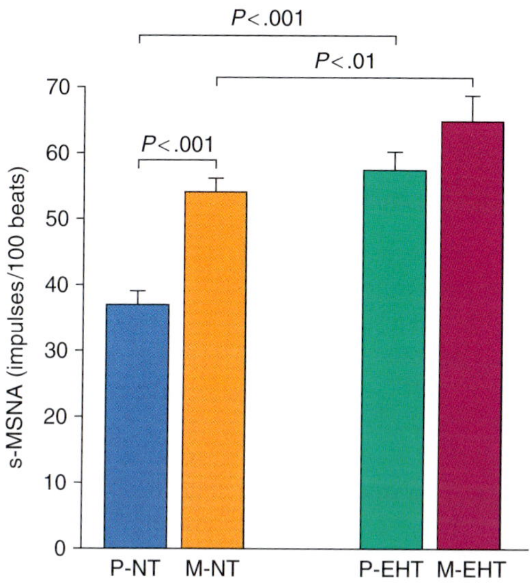

Fig. 4-17a Muscle sympathetic nerve activity (MSNA) in premenopausal (P) and menopausal (M) women, with (EHT) and without (NT) hypertension. (From Hogarth AJ, Graham LN, Corrigan JH, et al. Sympathetic nerve activity and its effect in postmenopausal women. *J Hypertens* 2011;29:167–75.)

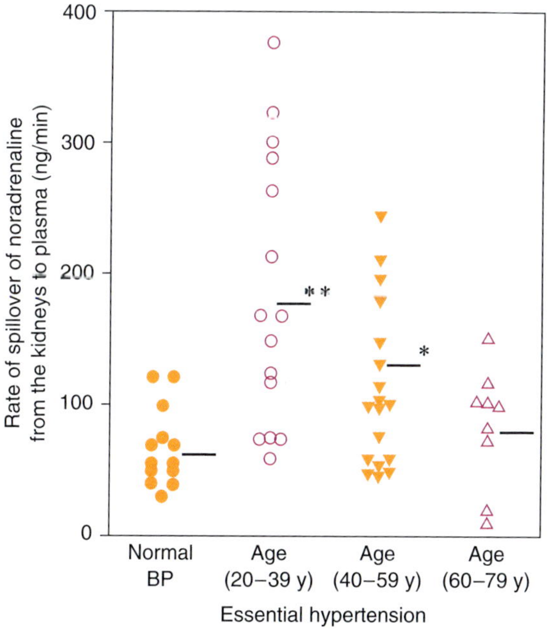

Fig. 4-17b Renal sympathetic nerve activity is raised in hypertension up to the age of 60 years. (From Esler M, Jennings G, Korner P, et al. Measurement of total and organ-specific norepinephrine kinetics in humans. *Am J Physiol* 1984;247:E21–E28.)

B) Elderly systolic hypertension and vascular stiffness (compliance)—P-P and amplification and augmentation index

This is a complex area as indicated in **Figure 4-18** (99). The upper panel shows that the pulse wave generated in the heart travels down the arterial tree with a certain velocity (PWV), which in turn depends on the distensibility of the arterial wall (increased PWV with stiff arteries). Eventually, the pulse wave is reflected at branch points and travels backward toward the heart. Peripheral P-P is the summation of the forward and reflected waves. The middle panel (Figure 4-18) shows that the amplitude of P-P increases toward the periphery, especially in younger subjects, because these points are closer to reflection sites, and the reflected wave has to travel back a lesser distance. The lower panel (**Figure 4-18**) shows that in subjects with a stiff aorta, the reflected wave returns earlier (arriving in systole) and superimposes on the forward wave at the inflection point, which results in an augmentation of the aortic SBP and P-P.

These points were alluded to Chapter 2 where it was shown that (a) arterial distensibility decreases with age (Figure 2-18), (b) the reduced distensibility was closely related to an increasing P-P (Figure 2-19), (c) pressure amplification decreases with increasing age (Figure 2-8), and (d) the concept of the AIx is shown in Figure 2-23.

The AIx increases with age (**Figure 4-19**) (100).

C) Elderly and pulse wave velocity

The Framingham group showed that in middle-aged subjects, increasing PWV leads to premature return of the reflected wave to the central aorta during systole, which augments central SBP and P-P, and reduces peripheral amplification; PWV increases with age (**Figure 4-20**) (101), particularly in the obese (102). However, in young/middle-aged subjects, PWV is strongly related to the degree of sympathetic nerve activity (Figure 4-20a) (103).

D) Arterial stiffness and inflammation

Inflammation is related not only to the development of hypertension in young/middle-aged subjects but also to the systolic hypertension and wide P-P in the elderly. It has been shown that infection (*Salmonella*) increases arterial stiffness and PWV, and

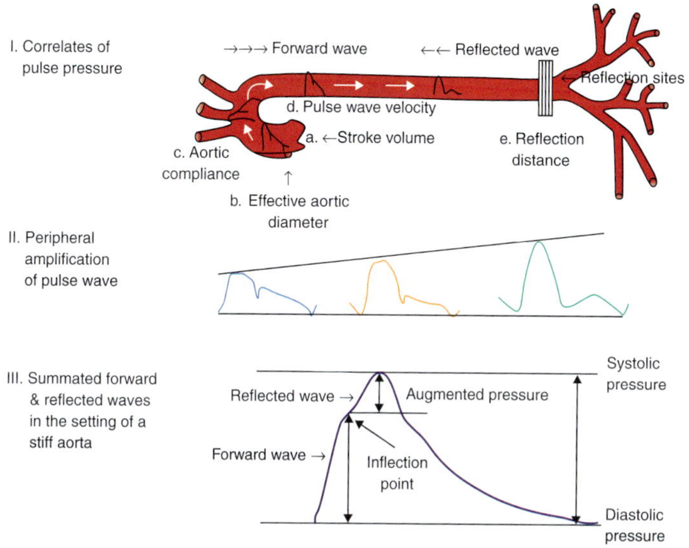

Fig. 4-18 Concept of forward and reflected pulse waves, peripheral amplification of pulse wave, and central augmented SBP. (From Vasan RS. Pathogenesis of elevated peripheral pulse pressure. *Hypertension* 2008;51:33–6.)

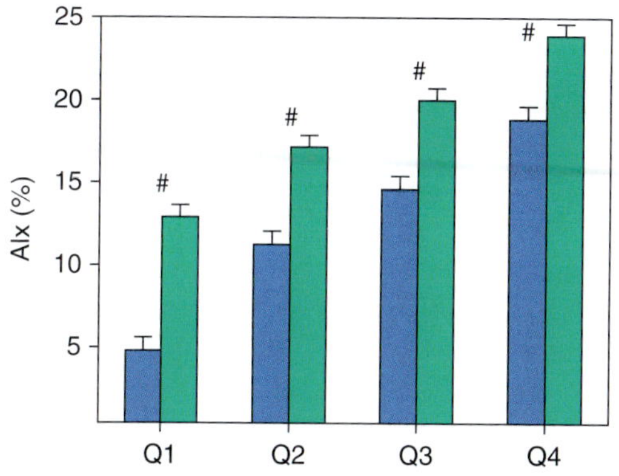

Fig. 4-19 Central augmentation index (AIx) increases with age (Q), particularly in women (light bars). (From Segers P, Rietzschel ER, De Buyzere ML, et al. Non-invasive input impedance, pulse wave velocity, and wave reflection in healthy middle-aged men and women. *Hypertension* 2007;49:1248–55.) # = Statistically Significant.

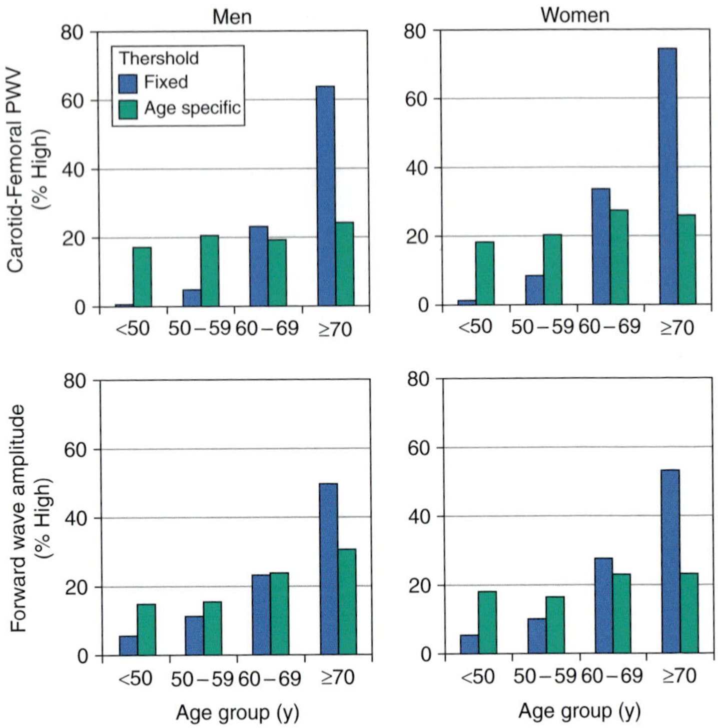

Fig. 4-20 Pulse wave velocity (PWV) and forward wave amplitude increase with increasing age. (From Mitchell G, Praise H, Benjamin EJ, et al. Changes in arterial stiffness and wave reflection with advancing age in healthy men and women. *Hypertension* 2004;43:1239–45.)

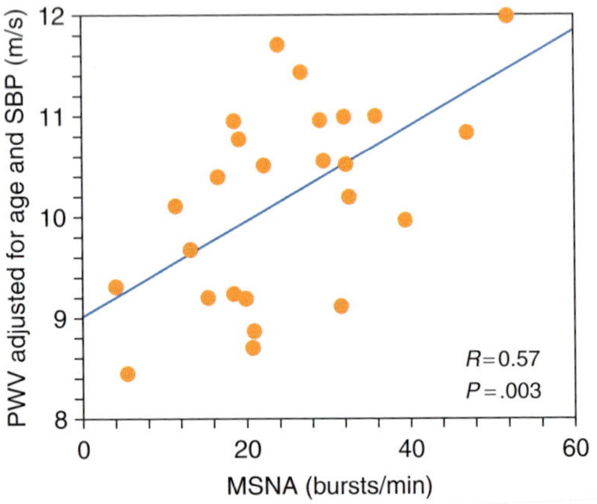

Fig. 4-20a Relationship between muscle sympathetic nerve activity (MSNA) and PWV in young/middle-aged subjects. (From Swierblewska E, Hering D, Kara T, et al. An independent relationship between muscle sympathetic nerve activity and pulse wave velocity in normal humans. *J Hypertens* 2010;28:979–84.)

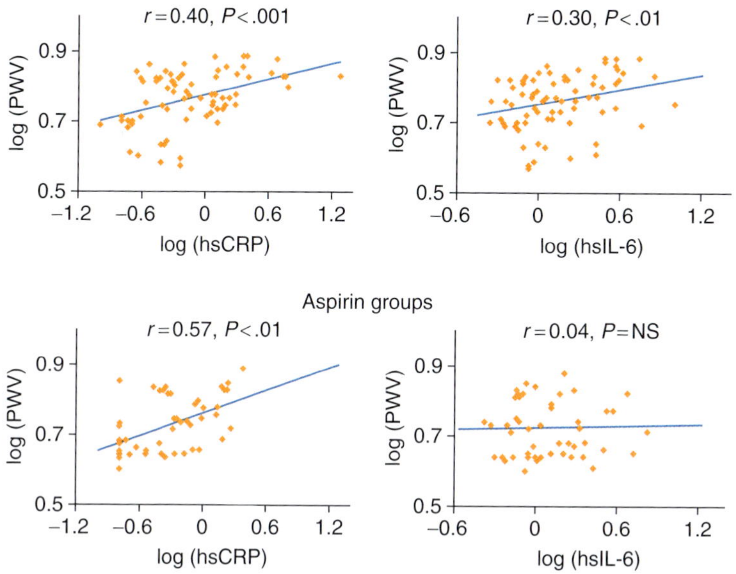

Fig. 4-21 *Salmonella* vaccination-induced inflammation (CRP and IL-6) was associated with an increase in pulse wave velocity (PWV). (From Vlachopoulos C, Dima I, Aznaouridis K, et al. Acute systemic inflammation increases arterial stiffness and decreases wave reflection in healthy individuals. *Circulation* 2005;112:2193–200.)

the increase in PWV is associated with increased levels of CRP (**Figure 4-21**) (104). Similarly, in essential hypertension, a high CRP level correlates with an increased PWV (**Figure 4-22**), central AIx, and the adipokinins IL-6 and TNF-α (105). Interestingly, patients with rheumatoid arthritis (who have a high cardiovascular risk) have a high PWV, which is reduced by anti-TNF-α therapy (106).

E) Salt and arterial stiffness

There is strong evidence that high dietary salt intake increases arterial stiffness, independent of BP (107). Sodium intake may be a predictor of systolic, but not diastolic, hypertension (108). Thus, sodium consumption and P-P are positively associated, particularly in men. Certainly, sodium restriction lowers SBP. High-salt diets induce phenotypic changes in vascular smooth muscle cells, which develop secretory properties resulting in collagen accumulation within the large artery wall (108).

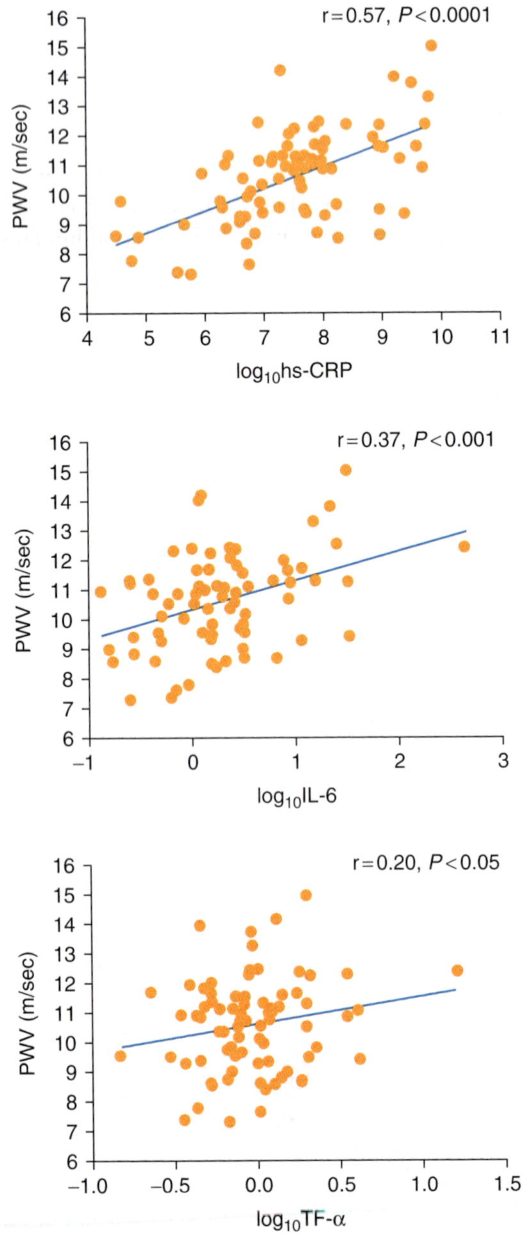

Fig. 4-22 In middle-aged hypertensives, arterial stiffness (PWV) is linked to inflammation (CRP, IL-6, and TNF-α). (From Mahmud A, Feely J. Arterial stiffness is related to systemic inflammation in essential hypertension. *Hypertension* 2005;46:1118–22.)

3. Children

A) Obesity and hypertension

In the United States, overweight and obesity in children and adolescents are a major public health concern (109); nearly, one-third of children and adolescents aged 2–19 years are overweight or obese (30). Not surprisingly, obese children tend to become obese adults (110). Twenty percent of obese children have blood lipid disturbances and hypertension (110). This trend is increasing (111). In 8-year-old children, the link between obesity and hypertension is clear (**Figure 4-23**) (112), but appears to affect only the SBP (**Figure 4-24**) (113). Children with high adiposity scores from birth to adolescence have more than a 6-fold increase in risk of developing hypertension by the age of 14 years, so that about 60% of boys in this group have either prehypertension or frank hypertension (114). This is particularly evident in non-Hispanic black subjects and Mexican Americans (115).

The high BP in childhood tracks into young adulthood (**Figure 4-25**) (116, 117), particularly for boys (118). High-risk children, including high BP, develop stiff arteries as adults, manifest as a high PWV (119). However, obese children who become normal-weight adults assume a low-risk status (120).

The high BP in 10-year-old obese children is closely related to high heart rates and leptin levels, probably linked to high sympathetic nerve activity (121).

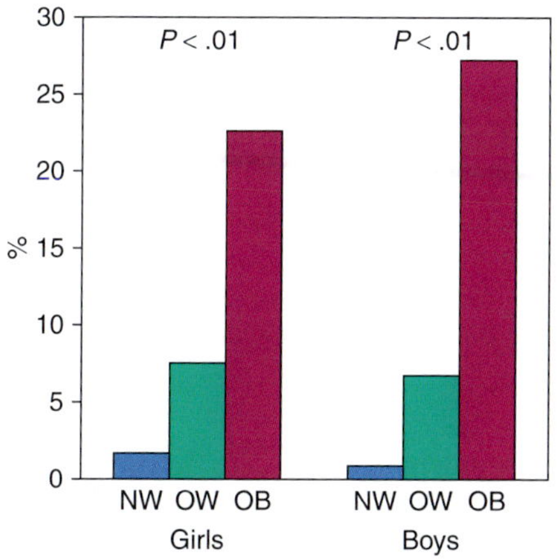

Fig. 4-23 Prevalence of hypertension in 5- to 11-year-old children (Italy). NW, normal weight; OW, overweight; OB, obese. (From Genovesi S, Antolini L, Giussani M, et al. Usefulness of waist circumference for the identification of childhood hypertension. *J Hypertens* 2008;26:1563–70.)

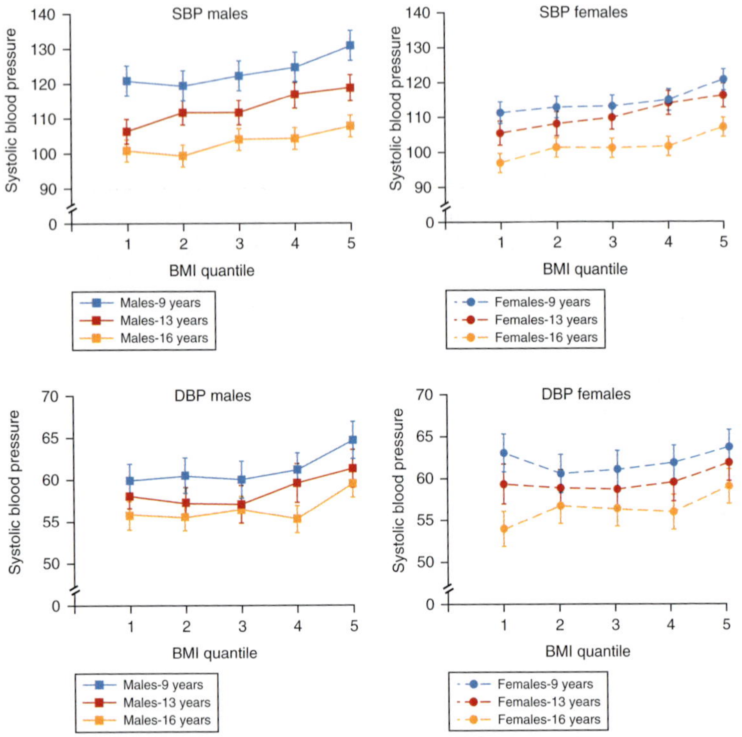

Fig. 4-24 Relationship between BMI and BP in 9 to 16 year olds. (From Parades G, Lambert M, O'Louglin J, et al. Blood pressure and adiposity in children and adolescents. *Circulation* 2004;110:1832–8.)

B) Physical activity and hypertension in children

Hypertension was inversely associated with physical activity in adolescents (122). Girls are generally less active than boys, but high cardiorespiratory fitness in girls, unlike boys, is linked to low BP (**Figure 4-26**) (123). High cardiorespiratory fitness is also linked to low stiffness of the arteries, that is, lower PWV (**Figure 4-27**) (124).

C) Hypertension and sympathetic nerve activity in children

Overweight or obese children (mean age 11 years) were noted to have high nocturnal BP, closely linked to high heart rates and insulin levels (**Figure 4-28**) (125). High insulin levels act centrally to increase sympathetic nerve outflow (63), and the high nocturnal

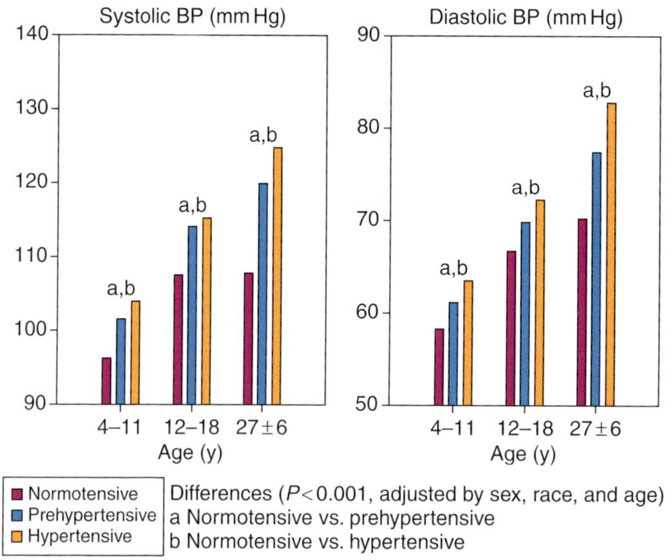

Fig. 4-25 Bogalusa Heart study; BP levels from childhood to young adulthood by adult hypertension status. (From Srinivason S, Myers L, Berenson GS. Changes in metabolic syndrome variables since childhood in prehypertensive and hypertensive subjects. The Bogalusa Heart Study. *Hypertension* 2006;48:33–9.)

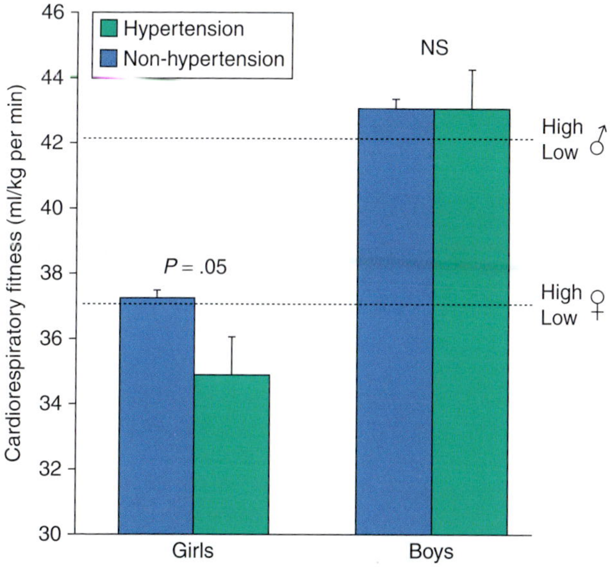

Fig. 4-26 Cardiorespiratory fitness levels by BP in 9- to 10-year-old boys and girls. (From Ruiz JR, Ortega FB, Loit HM, et al. Body fat is associated with blood pressure in school-aged girls with low cardiorespiratory fitness: the European Youth Heart Study. *J Hypertens* 2007;25:2027–34.)

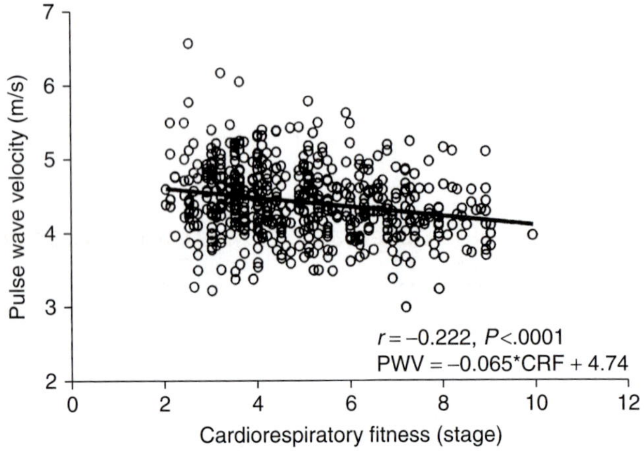

Fig. 4-27 Relationship between cardiorespiratory fitness and pulse wave velocity in 10- to 11-year-old children. (From Sakuragi S, Abhayaratna K, Gravemaker KH, et al. Influence of adiposity and physical activity on arterial stiffness in healthy children. *Hypertension* 2009;52:611–6.)

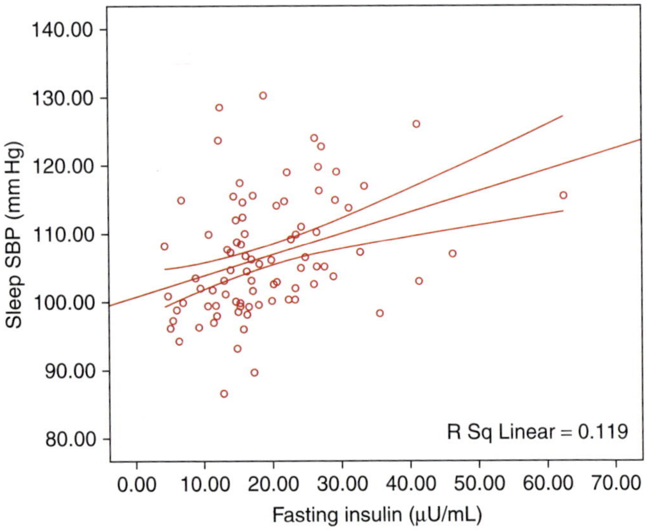

Fig. 4-28 Relationship between fasting blood insulin levels and nocturnal SBP in overweight/obese 11-year-old children. (From Lurbe E, Torro I, Aguilar F, et al. Added impact of obesity and insulin resistance in nocturnal blood pressure elevation in children and adolescents. *Hypertension* 2008;51:635–41.)

BP is a powerful predictor of cardiovascular events (126). Older children, aged up to 16 years, have also shown a strong relationship between BMI, insulin levels, and BP (127). In 19-year olds, there was a clear positive relationship between arterial noradrenaline levels and BP (128). Sympathoadrenal stress reactivity is a powerful predictor of future hypertension in 19-year olds (129).

D) Birth weight and other factors and future hypertension

A low birth weight was associated with a high SBP [not diastolic BP (DBP)] at the age of 8–11 years in girls but not boys (**Figure 4-29**) (130). This phenomenon is particularly evident in those of low socioeconomic status, for both boys and girls (131). Immaturity at birth, connected with prematurity, is important in

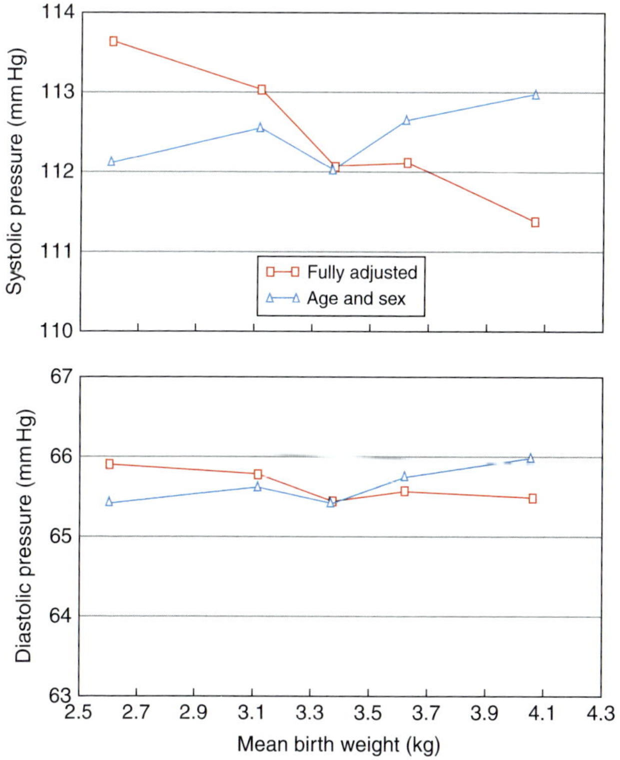

Fig. 4-29 Low birth-weight relates to high BP only in girls aged 8 to 11years- (squares). (From Taylor SJ, Whincup PH, Cook DG, et al. Size at birth and blood pressure: a cross sectional study in 8–11 year old children. *BMJ* 1997;314:475–80.)

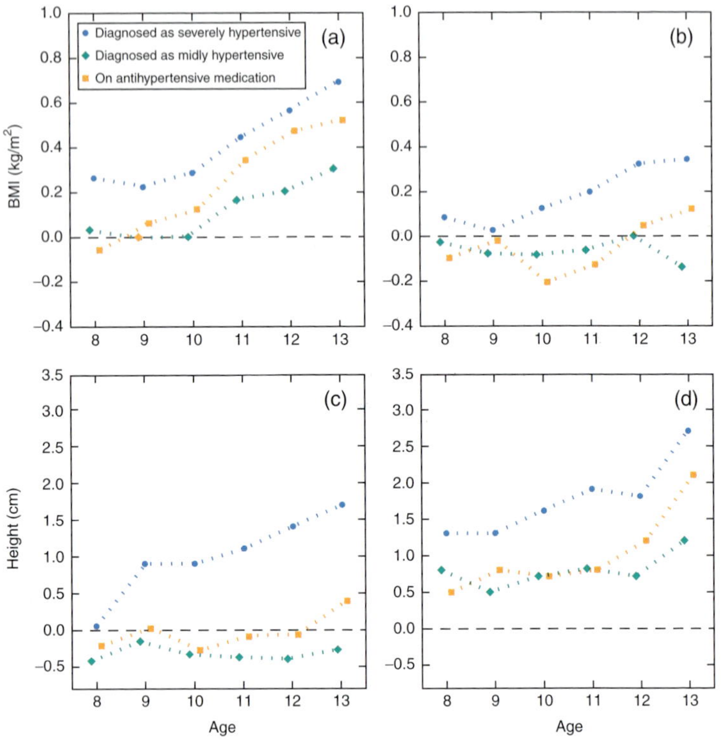

Fig. 4-30 Rapid growth from 8- to 13-year old is linked to severe hypertension in girls only (d). The graphs (a) and (c) relate to males, whereas (b) and (d) relate to females. (From Halldorsson TI, Gunnarsdottir, I, Birgisdottir BE, et al. Childhood growth and adult hypertension in a population of high birth weight. *Hypertension* 2011;58:8–15.)

predicting high BP in young men (132). Low placental weight, particularly in those of low socioeconomic status, is associated with high BP in 11-year olds (133). Smoking during pregnancy results in the development of high BP in the 5-year-old child (134), and smoking during breast feeding was associated with lower BP (134, 135).

Rapid growth of an infant is associated to hypertension 31 years later (136), similar to the rapid growth of child between the 8 and 13 years, despite high birth weight (**Figure 4-30**) (137).

The mechanism regarding the relation between low birth weight and later high BP is open to speculation, but programming within the foetus could be linked to both high sympathetic nerve activity (138) and arterial stiffness (139).

4. Miscellaneous

A) Salt sensitivity and hypertension in black subjects

Hypertension in black Afro-Caribbean subjects, as with whites, is associated with obesity (140) and increased sympathetic nerve activity (141). However, in black hypertensives, there is a high degree of β-receptor desensitization (142). Thus, β-1 stimulation induced increases in plasma renin will be blunted, accounting for the fact that, compared with young/middle-aged white hypertensives, plasma renin activity is reduced (**Figure 4-31**) (2).

So what is the mechanism of hypertension in black subjects? High salt (low potassium) is known to increase BP (**Figure 4-32**) (143). However, not all patients react to high salt intake with a rise in BP (salt resistant), but those who do are termed salt sensitive (144). Interestingly, salt-sensitive normotensive subjects have a high cumulative mortality (144). Many, but not all, black subjects are salt sensitive. Salt-sensitive, unlike nonsensitive, black subjects experience an increase in BP, systemic vascular resistance, and cardiac output in response to a high salt diet (**Figure 4-33**) (145). Thus, salt-sensitive individuals have an impaired vasodilatory capacity.

B) Mental stress/depression

Epidemiologic studies support the idea that behavioral and psychological factors can be important in the development of essential hypertension. There are data linking chronic mental stress in the workplace (146, 147) and in community life (148) with the development of hypertension. Depression appears to be an independent risk factor for hypertension (149).

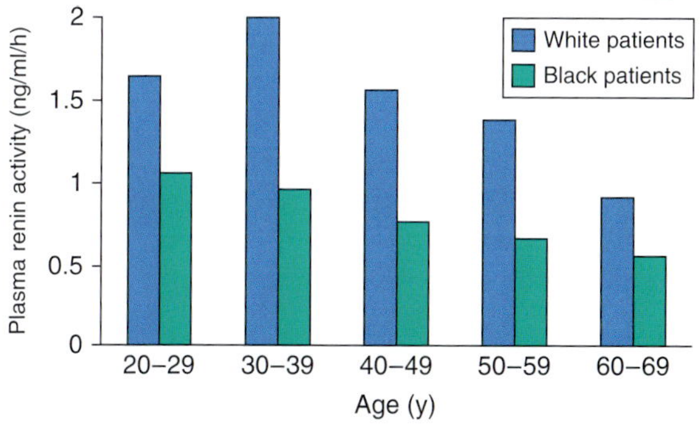

Fig. 4-31 Plasma renin levels in black and white hypertensive patients. (From Beevers G, Lip GY, O'brien E. The pathophysiology of hypertension. *BMJ* 2001;322:912–6.)

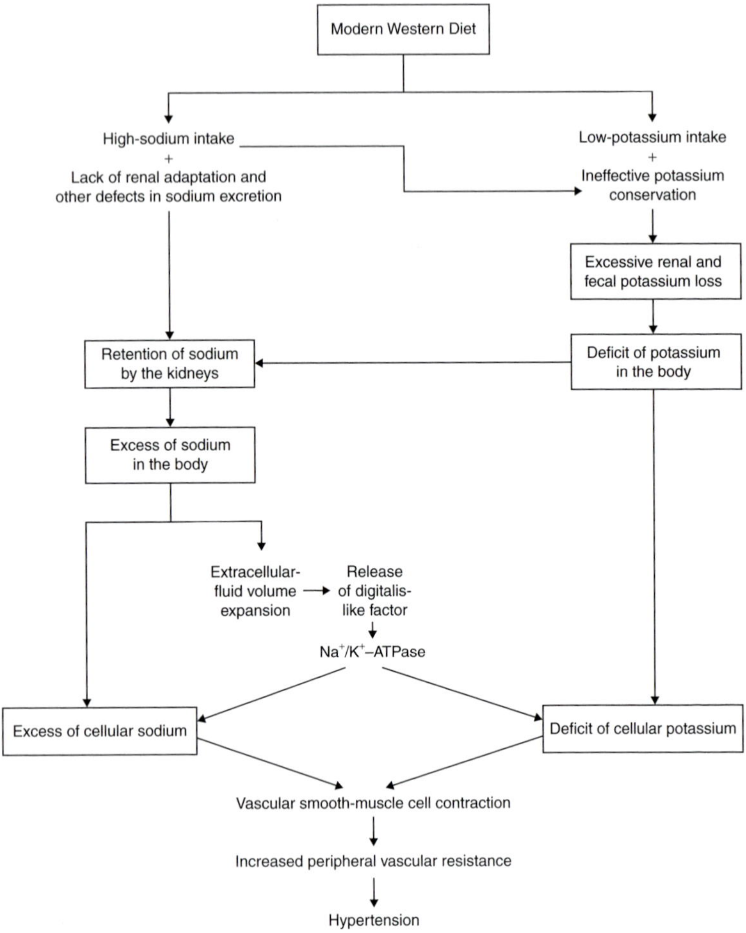

Fig. 4-32 Interaction of the modern Western diet and the kidneys with accent on sodium and potassium in the development of high BP. (From Adrogue HK, Madias NE. Sodium and potassium in the pathogenesis of hypertension. *NEJM* 2007;356:1966–78.)

Interestingly there is a lay perspective that hypertension is linked to stress, such that when the symptoms of stress subside the patient stops taking the antihypertensive therapy (150).

C) Alcohol intake and hypertension

Regular small amounts of alcohol are known to increase longevity (151). However, higher intake of alcohol is known to increase BP in both westernized (152) and Asian (153) subjects. The

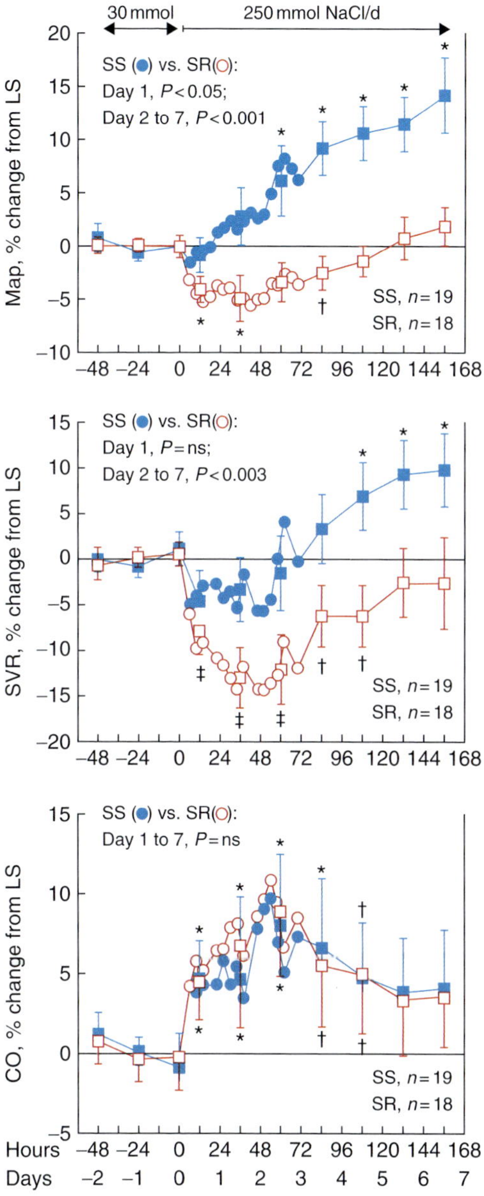

Fig. 4-33 Effect of high-salt diet on mean BP, vascular resistance (SVR), and cardiac output (CO) in salt-sensitive (black circles) and salt-insensitive (white circles) black subjects. (From Schmidlin O, Forman A, Leone A, et al. Salt sensitivity in blacks. *Hypertension* 2011;58:380–5.)

alcohol-induced hypertension is particularly evident in the early morning, which is the so-called vulnerable period to stroke and myocardial infarction (154). The type of alcohol, that is, beer, wine, or spirits, is unimportant; all are linked to an increase in BP (155).

Alcohol drinking outside meal times appears to markedly increase the risk of an increase in BP (156). The mechanism of alcohol-induced hypertension is speculative (157), but increases in endothelin concentration may be relevant (151).

D) Cigarette smoking and caffeine intake

Smoking is associated with the development of hypertension, independent of inflammation, and other confounders (158). Certainly, smoking increases vascular stiffness, increasing PWV and central AIx (159).

Although caffeine intake was not associated with hypertension in women (160), it has been shown to decrease aortic compliance and increase PWV (161).

E) Dietary factors

There is good evidence that vegetarians have lower BP than meat eaters (27). High fibre/soy protein diet is linked to low BP (27). Certainly, a high intake of fruit and vegetables is linked to improved endothelial function in hypertensives (162). Fish meals in daily diet are linked to lower BPs (27).

Diets high in sugar and sugar-sweetened beverages are linked to hypertension (161, 163), a phenomenon independent of obesity, but correlated with urinary sodium excretion (164). Certainly, in 12 year-old girls, high glycemic index and glycemic load diets are linked to increases in blood pressure (165). However, the most recent data, based on systematic review/meta-analysis, indicate that fructose intake has no significant effect on BP (166).

F) Physical activity and blood pressure

Physical activity is associated with lower BPs (27), and low aerobic fitness is associated with hypertension (167, 168) and high levels of visceral adiposity (168). The correlation of hypertension and low physical activity/high levels of TV watching is independent of BMI (169). Low aerobic fitness, as well as obesity, stress, and smoking, contributes to the higher BPs observed those with lower education (170).

G) Hormones

High androgen levels are linked to hypertension in men and also in women with polycystic ovaries (171). BP increases in many women after the menopause and is accompanied by an increase in plasma

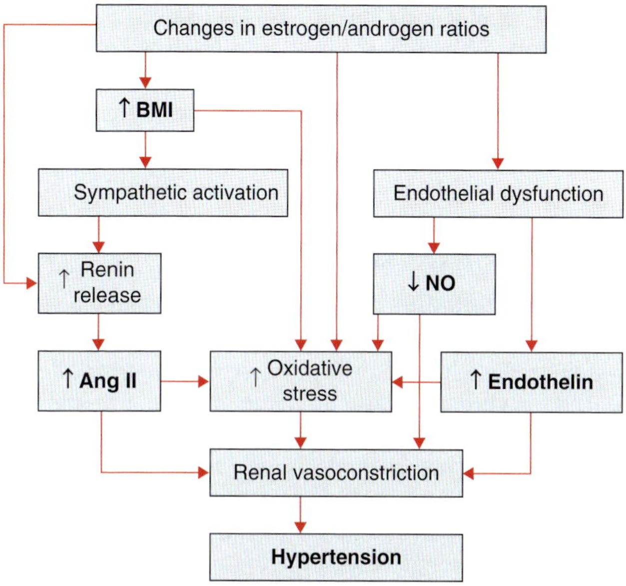

Fig. 4-34 Possible contribution of sex hormones to postmenopausal hypertension. (From Coylewright M, Reckelhoff JF, Ouyang P. Menopause and hypertension. *Hypertension* 2008;51:952–9.)

renin activity, as well as increased sympathetic tone associated with obesity (172). In the postmenopausal period, there is impairment of endothelial function, with diminished nitric oxide (NO) production (173). Acute oestrogen deprivation after oopherectomy results in impaired endothelium-dependent vasodilatation due to reduced NO availability, and this deficit is corrected by oestrogen therapy (173).

H) Other possible links

Short sleep duration (regularly less than 5 hours per night) is associated with an increased risk of hypertension (174). Obstructive sleep apnoea is linked to increased sympathetic nerve activity, independent of obesity (175). In subjects younger than 60 years, sleep-disordered breathing is associated with diastolic hypertension (176). The hypertension associated with obstructive sleep apnea is relieved by continuous positive airway pressure (177), though not all agree (178).

There is a weak relationship between uric acid levels and hypertension (179), particularly in adolescents (180). Air pollution possibly has a weak association with the incidence of hypertension (181), although a 2-hour exposure to diesel fumes (vs. filtered air) increased SBP significantly (**Figure 4-34**) (182). In perimenopausal and postmenopausal women, blood lead levels are associated with DBP and SBP (183). High serum selenium concentrations have been linked to hypertension (184). Essential hypertension has been linked to human cytomegalovirus infection (185).

SUMMARY AND CONCLUSIONS

1. The pathophysiology of essential hypertension in adults involves about 30% genetic factors, which control telomere dysfunction, sodium reabsorption in the loop of Henle, β-2 and ACE genotypes, sympathetic nerve activity, and angiotensin I and II.
2. Environmental factors comprise the remaining 70% of essential hypertension, which lead to obesity and sympathetic nerve and renin/angiotensin activity in the young/middle-aged subjects, and involve the vascular aging process in the elderly.
3. Obesity, particularly central, is a major problem in westernized cultures; central adipocytes produce adipokinins (e.g., IL-6 and TNF-α), which induce an inflammatory process and insulin resistance, which results in increased insulin and leptin levels that stimulate the hypothalamic region of the brain, resulting in high sympathetic nerve activity (noradrenaline), high BP, and high heart rate.
4. High BP results not only from the direct effects of obesity-related increases in sympathetic nerve activity on cardiac output and peripheral resistance but also from chronic stimulation of the β-1 receptors in the TAL of Henle, resulting in sodium reabsorption (β-1 blockade promotes diuresis and naturesis); resultant high sodium levels stimulate α-2 receptors in the mid-brain, leading to a further increased sympathetic outflow and raised peripheral resistance (quite unrelated to plasma volume overload).
5. β-1 stimulation also acts on the juxtaglomerular apparatus in the kidney, resulting in renin release and angiotensin II formation, which, in addition to effecting vasoconstriction directly, acts centrally, resulting in a further activation of the sympathetic nervous system.
6. Systolic hypertension in the elderly is a function of aging/stiffening of the vasculature, resulting in low compliance of the vascular wall, a low DBP, and a widened P-P.
7. Poor arterial compliance results in a speeding of the reflected wave and a high PWV, leading to augmentation of central SBP and P-P.

8. Muscle, but not renal, sympathetic nerve activity is high in the elderly; but due to β-receptor desensitization, unlike in the young/middle-aged, BP is no longer directly dependent on β-1 stimulation and increased cardiac output but is a function of arterial stiffness and increased peripheral resistance.
9. Childhood hypertension, like that in young/middle-aged adults, is closely linked to obesity and low birth weights, and tracts into adulthood; high sympathetic nerve activity appears to be the underlying cause.
10. Hypertension in black subjects, like whites, is often linked to obesity and high sympathetic nerve activity, but β-receptor desensitization and low renin levels are common, similar to salt sensitivity.
11. Other factors that can be associated with the development of hypertension are mental stress/depression, high alcohol intake, cigarette smoking, high caffeine intake, high sugar intake, physical inactivity, hormonal factors, diesel fumes, high blood lead or selenium levels, and obstructive sleep apnoea.

REFERENCES

1. Staessen JA, Wang J, Bianchi G, et al. Essential hypertension. *Lancet* 2003;361:1629–41.
2. Beevers G, Lip GY, O'Brien E. The pathophysiology of hypertension. *BMJ* 2001;322:912–6.
3. Cowley AE, Nadau JH, Baccarelli A, et al. Report of the National Heart, Lung, and Blood Institute Working Group on epigenetics and hypertension. *Hypertension* 2012;59:899–905.
4. Othman AS, Othman NI, Rosman A, et al. Central and peripheral blood pressure profile of young offspring with hypertensive and normotensive parents. *J Hypertens* 2012;30:1552–5.
5. Takeuchi F, Isono M, Katsuya T, et al. Blood pressure and hypertension are associated with 7 loci in the Japanese population. *Circulation* 2010;121:2302–9.
6. Pausova Z, Gaudet D, Gossard F, et al. Genome-wide scan for linkage to obesity—associated hypertension in French Canadians. *Hypertension* 2005;46:1280–5.
7. Morris BJ. Dissecting hypertension by obesity identifies a locus at 1p36. *Hypertension* 2005;46:1256–8.
8. Fuster JJ, Diez J, Andres V. Telomere dysfunction in hypertension. *J Hypertens* 2007;25:2185–92.
9. Mitchell GF, De Stefano AL, Larson MG, et al. Heritability and genome-wide linkage scan for arterial stiffness, wave reflection and mean arterial pressure. The Framingham Heart Study. *Circulation* 2005;112:194–9.

10. Laurent S, Boutougrie P, Lacolley P. Structural and genetic basis of arterial stiffness. *Hypertension* 2005;45:1050–5.
11. Durier S, Fassot C, Laurent S, et al. Physiological genomics of human arteries. *Circulation* 2003;108:1845–51.
12. Bielinski SJ, Lynch AI, Miller MB, et al. Genome-wide linkage analysis for loci affecting pulse-pressure. *Hypertension* 2005;46:1286–93.
13. Jung J, Basile DP, Pratt JH. Sodium reabsorption in the thick ascending limb in relation to blood pressure. *Hypertension* 2011;57:873–9.
14. Kelly TN, He J. Genomic epidemiology of blood pressure salt sensitivity. *J Hypertens* 2012;30:861–73.
15. Bao X, Mills PJ, Rana BK, et al. Interactive effects of common B-2 adrenoceptor haplotypes and age on susceptibility to hypertension and receptor function. *Hypertension* 2005;46:310–7.
16. Lee Y-W, Oh VM, Garcia E, et al. Haplotypes of the B-2 adrenergic receptor gene are associated with essential hypertension in Singaporean Chinese population. *J Hypertens* 2004;22:2111–6.
17. Staessen JA, Wang J-G, Brand E, et al. Effect of three candidate genes on prevalence and incidence of hypertension in a Caucasian population. *J Hypertens* 2001;19:1349–58.
18. Makris TK, Stravroulakis GA, Dafni VG, et al. ACE/DD genotype is associated with hemostasis balance disturbances reflecting hypercoagulability and endothelial dysfunction in patients with untreated hypertension. *Am Heart J* 2000;140:760–5.
19. Lillie EO, O'Connor DT. Early phenotypic changes in hypertension. A role for the autonomic nervous system and heredity. *Hypertension* 2006;47:331–3.
20. Schlaich MP, Lambert E, Kaye DM, et al. Sympathetic augmentation in hypertension. *Hypertension* 2004;43:169–75.
21. Osborn JW, Kuroki MT. Sympathetic signatures of cardiovascular disease. *Hypertension* 2012;59:545–7.
22. Lambert E, Straznicky N, Schlaich M, et al. Differing pattern of sympathoexcitation in normal-weight and obesity-related hypertension. *Hypertension* 2007;50:862–8.
23. Grassi G. Sympathetic neural activity in hypertension and related diseases. *Am J Hypertens* 2010;23:1052–60.
24. Hering D, Kucharska W, Kara T, et al. Resting sympathetic outflow does not predict the morning blood pressure surge in hypertension. *J Hypertens* 2011;29:2381–6.
25. Rao F, Zhang L, Wessel J, et al. Tyrosine hydroxylase: the rate limiting enzyme in catecholamine biosynthesis. *Circulation* 2007;116:993–1006.
26. Johnson AD, Newton-Chek C, Chasman DI, et al. Association of hypertension drug target genes with blood pressure and hypertension in 86,588 individuals. *Hypertension* 2011;57:903–10.
27. Beilin LJ. Hypertension research in the 21st century: where is the gold? *J Hypertens* 2004;22:2243–51.
28. Must A, Spadano J, Coakley EH, et al. The disease burden associated with overweight and obesity. *JAMA* 1999;282:1523–9.

29. Flegal KM, Carroll MD, Ogden CL, et al. Prevalence and trends in obesity among US adults, 1999–2000. *JAMA* 2002;288:1723–7.
30. Tanne JH. As Americans get fatter, the US Institute of Medicine takes action. *BMJ* 2012;344:e3276.
31. Manson TE, Bassuk SS. Obesity in the United States. *JAMA* 2003;289:229–30.
32. Zhang C, Rexrode KM, van Dam RM, et al. Abdominal obesity and the risk of all-cause, cardiovascular and cancer mortality. *Circulation* 2008;117:1658–67.
33. Timpson NJ, Harbord R, Davey-Smith G, et al. Does greater adiposity increase blood pressure and hypertension risk? *Hypertension* 2009;54:84–90.
34. Kotsis V, Stabouli S, Bouldin M, et al. Impact of obesity on 24-hour ambulatory blood pressure and hypertension. *Hypertension* 2005;45:602–7.
35. Foulds HJ, Bredin SS, Warburton DE. The relationship between hypertension and obesity across different ethnicities. *J Hypertens* 2012;30:359–67.
36. Franklin SS, Pio JR, Wong ND, et al. Predictors of new-onset diastolic and systolic hypertension. The Framingham Heart Study. *Circulation* 2005;111:1121–7.
37. Esler M, Straznicky N, Eikelis N, et al. Mechanisms of sympathetic activation in obesity—related hypertension. *Hypertension* 2006;48:787–96.
38. Armitage JA, Burke SL, Prior LJ, et al. Rapid onset of renal sympathetic nerve activation in rabbits fed a high-fat diet. *Hypertension* 2012;60:163–71.
39. Grassi G, Dell'Oro R, Facchini A, et al. Effect of central and peripheral body fat distribution on sympathetic and baroreflex function in obese normotensives. *J Hypertens* 2004;22:236–9.
40. Huggett RJ, Burns J, Mackintosh AF, et al. Sympathetic renal activation in non-diabetic metabolic syndrome and its further augmentation by hypertension. *Hypertension* 2004;44:847–52.
41. Mancia G, Bousquet P, Elghozi JL, et al. The sympathetic nervous system and the metabolic syndrome. *J Hypertens* 2007;25:909–20.
42. Huggett RJ, Scott EM, Gilbey SG, et al. Impact of type 2 diabetes on sympathetic neural mechanisms in hypertension. *Circulation* 2003;108:3097–101.
43. Emdin M, Gastaldelli A, Muscelli E, et al. Hyperinsulinaemia and autonomic nervous system dysfunction in obesity. Effect of weight loss. *Circulation* 2001;103:513–9.
44. Joyner MJ, Charkoudian N, Wallin G. Sympathetic nervous system and blood pressure in humans. *Hypertension* 2010;56:10–16.
45. Druktenis JS, Roman MJ, Fabsitz RR, et al. Cardiac and systemic hemodynamic characteristics of hypertension and prehypertension in adolescents and young adults. The Strong Heart Study. *Circulation* 2007;115:221–7.

46. Coffman TM, Crowley SD. Kidney in hypertension. Guyton redux. *Hypertension* 2008;51:811–6.
47. Johnson RJ, Feig DI, Nagagawa T, et al. Pathogenesis of essential hypertension: historical paradigms and modern insights. *J Hypertens* 2008;26:381–91.
48. Morgan DA, Anderson EA, Mark AL. Renal sympathetic nerve activity is increased in obese Zucker rats. *Hypertension* 1995;25:834–8.
49. Carlson SH, Shelton J, White CR, et al. Elevated sympathetic nerve activity contributes to hypertension and salt sensitivity in diabetic obese Zucker rats. *Hypertension* 2000;35:403–8.
50. Kassab S, Kato T, Wilkins FC, et al. Renal denervation attenuates the sodium retention and hypertension associated with obesity. *Hypertension* 1995;25:893–7.
51. Sonalker PA, Jackson EK. Norepinephrine, via beta-receptors, regulates bumetanide-sensitive contransporter type-1 expression in thick ascending limb cells. *Hypertension* 2007;49:1351–7.
52. Elalouf JM, Buhler JM, Tessiot C, et al. Predominant expression of beta-1 adrenergic receptor in the thick ascending limb of rat kidney. Absolute m RNA quantitation by reverse transcription and polymerase chain reaction. *J Clin Invest* 1993;91:264–72.
53. Orr JS, Gentile CL, Davy BM, et al. Large artery stiffening with weight gain in humans. *Hypertension* 2008;51:1519–24.
54. Kivagyan J, Tabe CE, Xu S, et al. The impact of body mass on pulse-pressure in obesity. *J Hypertens* 2005;23:619–24.
55. Casey DP, Curry TB, Joyner MJ, et al. Relationship between muscle sympathetic nerve activity and aortic wave reflection characteristics in young men and women. *Hypertension* 2011;57:421–7.
56. Julius S, Valentini M, Palatini P. Overweight and hypertension. A two-way street? *Hypertension* 2000;35:807–13.
57. Calhoun DA, Grassi G. Weight gain and hypertension: the chicken—egg question revisited. *J Hypertens* 2004;22:1869–71.
58. Cruickshank JM. Are we misunderstanding beta-blockers? *Int J Cardiol* 2007;120:10–27.
59. Cruickshank JM. *The Modern Role of Beta-Blockers in Cardiovascular Medicine*. Shelton, Connecticut: People's Medical Publishing House; 2011; pp 84–9.
60. Zicardi P, Nappo G, Giugliano G, et al. Reduction in inflammation cytokine concentrations and improvement of endothelial functions in obese women after weight loss over one year. *Circulation* 2002;105:804–9.
61. Dandona P, Aljada A, Chaudhuri A, et al. Metabolic syndrome. A comprehensive perspective based on interactions between obesity, diabetes and inflammation. *Circulation* 2005;111:1448–54.
62. Blake GJ, Rifai N, Buring JE, et al. Blood pressure, C-reactive protein and risk of future cardiovascular events. *Circulation* 2003;108:2993–9.

63. Tack CJ, Smits P, Withelmsen JJ, et al. Effect of insulin on vascular tone and sympathetic nervous system in NIDDM. *Diabetes* 1996;45:15–22.
64. Hespel P, Lijnen P, Vanhees L, et al. Beta-adrenergic receptors and the regulation of blood pressure and plasma renin during exercise. *J Appl Physiol* 1986;60:108–13.
65. Marsh AJ, Fontes AF, Killinger S, et al. Cardiovascular responses evoked by leptin acting on neurones in the ventromedial and dorsomedial hypothalamus. *Hypertension* 2003;42:488–93.
66. Henegar JR, Brower GL, Kabour A, et al. Catecholamine-response to chronic angiotensin II infusion and its role in myocyte and coronary vascular damage. *Am J Physiol* 1995;269:H1564–H1569.
67. Moretti J-L, Burk SL, Davern PJ, et al. Renal sympathetic activation from long-term low-dose angiotensin II infusion in rabbits. *J Hypertens* 2012;30:551–60.
68. Guild S-J, McBryde FD, Malpas SC, et al. High dietary salt and angiotensin II chronically increase renal sympathetic nerve activity: a direct telemetric study. *Hypertension* 2012;59:614–20.
69. Cruickshank JM, Degaute JP, Kuurne T, et al. Reduction of stress/catecholamine-induced cardiac necrosis by beta-1 blockade. *Lancet* 1987;2:585–9.
70. Kramer B, Sautter R, Gulker H, et al. Influence of ISA of beta-blockers on ventricular fibrillation threshold. *Circulation* 1981;64:A461.
71. Helen P, Lorenzen I, Garbarsch C, et al. Arteriosclerosis in the rabbit aorta induced by noradrenaline. *Atherosclerosis* 1970;12:125–32.
72. Strand AH, Gudmundsdottir, Os I, et al. Arterial plasma noradrenaline predicts left ventricular hypertrophy of blood pressure and body build in men who develop hypertension over 20 years. *J Hypertens* 2006;24:905–13.
73. Mark AL, Correia ML, Rahmouni K, et al. Selective leptin resistance: a new concept in leptin physiology with cardiovascular implications. *J Hypertens* 2002;20:1245–50.
74. Eikelis N, Schlaich M, Aggarwal A, et al. Interactions between leptin and human sympathetic nervous system. *Hypertension* 2003;41:1072–9.
75. Ma B, Feitosa MF, Wilk JB, et al. Leptin is associated with blood pressure and hypertension in women from the National heart, Lung and Blood Institute Family Heart Study. *Hypertension* 2009;53:473–9.
76. Ruhl CE, Everhart JE, Ding J, et al. Serum leptin concentrations and body adipose tissue in older black and white adults. *Am J Clin Nutr* 2004;80:576–83.
77. Carlson SH, Wyss JM. Mechanisms underlying hypertension and obesity. A melanocortin linkage in the brain. *Hypertension* 2011;57:375–6.

78. Pischon T, Girman JG, Hotamisligil GS, et al. Plasma adiponectin levels and risk of myocardial infarction. *JAMA* 2004;291:1730–7.
79. Goldfine AB, Kahn CR. Adiponectin: linking the fat cell to insulin sensitivity. *Lancet* 2003:362:1431–2.
80. Lambert M, O'Laughlin J, Delvin E, et al. Association between insulin, leptin, adiponectin and blood pressure in youth. *J Hypertens* 2009;27:1026–32.
81. Hausberg M, Hillebrand V, Kisters K. Addressing the relationship between sympathetic activity and inflammation. *J Hypertens* 2008;26:2276–8.
82. Bu D, Lichtman AH. T-cells and blood vessels. Costimulation turns up the pressure. *Circulation* 2010;122:2495–8.
83. Harrison DG, Guzic, Lob HE, et al. Inflammation, immunity and hypertension. *Hypertension* 2011;57:132–40.
84. Lee Y-C, Chang H-H, Chiang C-L, et al. Role of perivascular adipose tissue-derived methyl palmitate in vascular tone regulation and pathogenesis of hypertension. *Circulation* 2011;124:1160–71.
85. Palatini P, Julius S. The role of cardiac autonomic function in hypertension and cardiovascular disease. *Curr Hypertens Rep* 2009;11:199–205.
86. Simon AC, Safar MA, Levenson JA, et al. Systolic hypertension: hemodynamic mechanism and choice of antihypertensive treatment. *Am J Cardiol* 1979;44:505–11.
87. Tank J. Does aging cause women to be more sympathetic than men? *Hypertension* 2005;45:489–90.
88. Hogarth AJ, Mackintosh AF, Mary DA. The effect of gender on the sympathetic nerve activity in essential hypertension. *J Hum Hypertens* 2007;21:239–45.
89. Yamada Y, Miyajima E, Tochikubo O, et al. Age-related changes in muscle sympathetic nerve activity in essential hypertension. *Hypertension* 1989;13:870–7.
90. Narkiewicz K, Phillips BG, Kato M, et al. Gender-selective interaction between aging, blood pressure and sympathetic nerve activity. *Hypertension* 2005;45:522–5.
91. Hogarth AJ, Graham LN, Corrigan JH, et al. Sympathetic nerve activity and its effect in postmenopausal women. *J Hypertens* 2011;29:167–75.
92. Esler M, Jennings G, Korner P, et al. Measurement of total and organ-specific norepinephrine kinetics in humans. *Am J Physiol* 1984;247:E21–E28.
93. Vestal RE, Wood AJ, Shand DG. Reduced beta-adrenoceptor sensitivity in the elderly. *Clin Pharmacol Ther* 1979;26:181–6.
94. Tenero DM, Bottorf MB, Burlew BS, et al. Altered beta-adrenergic sensitivity and protein binding to I-propranolol in the elderly. *J Cardiovasc Pharmacol* 1990;16:702–7.
95. Feldman RD, Limbird LE, Nadeau J, et al. Alterations in leukocyte beta-receptor affinity with aging. A potential explanation for altered beta-adrenergic sensitivity in the elderly. *N Engl J Med* 1984;310:815–9.

96. Colangelo PM, Blouin RA, Steinmetz JE, et al. Age and beta-adrenergic sensitivity to S (-)- and R,S (+/-)- propranolol in humans. *Clin Pharmacol Ther* 1992;51:549–54.
97. Sowers JR, Lester M. Hypertension, hormones and aging. *J Lab Clin Med* 2000;135:379–86.
98. Gavras I, Gavras H. Volume expanded hypertension; the effect of fluid overload and the role of the sympathetic nervous system in salt-dependent hypertension. *J Hypertens* 2012;30:655–9.
99. Vasan RS. Pathogenesis of elevated peripheral pulse pressure. *Hypertension* 2008;51:33–6.
100. Segers P, Rietzschel ER, De Buyzere ML, et al. Non-invasive input impedance, pulse wave velocity, and wave reflection in healthy middle-aged men and women. *Hypertension* 2007;49:1248–55.
101. Mitchell G, Praise H, Benjamin EJ, et al. Changes in arterial stiffness and wave reflection with advancing age in healthy men and women. *Hypertension* 2004;43:1239–45.
102. Wildman RP, Mackey RH, Bostom A, et al. Measures of obesity are associated with vascular stiffness in young and older adults. *Hypertension* 2003;42:468–73.
103. Swierblewska E, Hering D, Kara T, et al. An independent relationship between muscle sympathetic nerve activity and pulse wave velocity in normal humans. *J Hypertens* 2010;28:979–84.
104. Vlachopoulos C, Dima I, Aznaouridis K, et al. Acute systemic inflammation increases arterial stiffness and decreases wave reflection in healthy individuals. *Circulation* 2005;112:2193–200.
105. Mahmud A, Feely J. Arterial stiffness is related to systemic inflammation in essential hypertension. *Hypertension* 2005;46:1118–22.
106. Mäki-Petäjä KM, Hall F, Booth AD, et al. Rheumatoid arthritis is associated with increased aortic PWV, which is reduced by anti-tumor necrosis factor—alpha therapy. *Circulation* 2006;114:1185–92.
107. Franklin SS. Arterial stiffness and hypertension. *Hypertension* 2005;45:349–51.
108. Safar ME. Systolic hypertension in the elderly: arterial wall mechanical properties and the renin-angiotensin-aldosterone system. *J Hypertens* 2005;23:673–81.
109. Hedley AA, Ogden CL, Johnson CL, et al. Prevalence of overweight and obesity among US children, adolescents and adults, 1999–2002. *JAMA* 2004;291:2847–50.
110. Lobstein T. Obesity in children. *BMJ* 2008;337:a669; doi:10.1136/bmj a 669.
111. Muntner P, He J, Cutler JA, et al. Trends in blood pressure among children and adolescents. *JAMA* 2004;291:2107–13.
112. Genovesi S, Antolini L, Giussani M, et al. Usefulness of waist circumference for the identification of childhood hypertension. *J Hypertens* 2008;26:1563–70.

113. Parades G, Lambert M, O'Louglin J, et al. Blood pressure and adiposity in children and adolescents. *Circulation* 2004;110:1832–8.
114. Mayor S. Childhood obesity increases blood pressure in adolescence "quite substantially" study shows. *BMJ* 2012;344:e3065.
115. Din-Dzietham R, Liu Y, Bielo M-V, et al. High blood pressure trends in children and adolescents in National Surveys, 1963–2002. *Circulation* 2007;116:1488–96.
116. Srinivason S, Myers L, Berenson GS. Changes in metabolic syndrome variables since childhood in prehypertensive and hypertensive subjects. The Bogalusa Heart Study. *Hypertension* 2006;48:33–9.
117. Chen X, Wang Y. Tracking of blood pressure from childhood to adulthood. *Circulation* 2008;117:3171–80.
118. Tirosh A, Afek A, Rudich A, et al. Progression of normotensive adolescents to hypertensive adults. *Hypertension* 2010;56:203–9.
119. Aatola H, Hutri-Kahonen M, Viikari JS, et al. Lifetime risk factors and arterial pulse wave velocity in adulthood. The cardiovascular risk in young Finns Study. *Hypertension* 2010;55:806–11.
120. Juanala M, Magnussen CG, Berenson GS, et al. Childhood adiposity, adult adiposity, and cardiovascular risk factors. *N Engl J Med* 2011;365:1876–85.
121. Tu W, Eckert GJ, DiMeglio LA, et al. Intensified effect of adiposity on blood pressure in overweight and obese children. *Hypertension* 2011;58:818–24.
122. Dasgupta K, O'Loughlin J, Chen S, et al. Emergence of sex difference in prevalence of high SBP. Analysis of a longitudinal adolescent cohort. *Circulation* 2006;114:2663–70.
123. Ruiz JR, Ortega FB, Loit HM, et al. Body fat is associated with blood pressure in school-aged girls with low cardiorespiratory fitness: the European Youth Heart Study. *J Hypertens* 2007;25:2027–34.
124. Sakuragi S, Abhayaratna K, Gravemaker KH, et al. Influence of adiposity and physical activity on arterial stiffness in healthy children. *Hypertension* 2009;52:611–6.
125. Lurbe E, Torro I, Aguilar F, et al. Added impact of obesity and insulin resistance in nocturnal blood pressure elevation in children and adolescents. *Hypertension* 2008;51:635–41.
126. Whaley-Connell A, Sowers JR. Obesity, insulin resistance and nocturnal systolic blood pressure. *Hypertension* 2008;51:620–1.
127. Lambert M, O'Loughlin J, Delvin EE, et al. Association between insulin, leptin and adiponectin and blood pressure in youth. *J Hypetens* 2009;27:1025–32.
128. Flaa A, Mundal HH, Eide I, et al. Sympathetic activity and cardiovascular risk factors in young men in the low, normal and high blood pressure ranges. *Hypertension* 2006;47:396–402.
129. Flaa A, Eide IK, Kjeldsen SE, et al. Sympathoadrenal stress reactivity is a predictor of future blood pressure. *Hypertension* 2008;52: 336–41.

130. Taylor SJ, Whincup PH, Cook DG, et al. Size at birth and blood pressure: a cross sectional study in 8–11 year old children. *BMJ* 1997;314:475–80.
131. Hardy R, Kuk D, Langenberg C, et al. Birthweight, childhood social class, and change in adult blood pressure in the 1946 British birth cohort. *Lancet* 2003;362:1178–83.
132. Johansson SJ, Iliadou A, Bergvall N, et al. Risk of high blood pressure among young men increases with the degree of immaturity at birth. *Circulation* 2005;112:3430–6.
133. Barker DJ, Osmond C, Forsen TJ, et al. Maternal and social origins of hypertension. *Hypertension* 2007;50:565–71.
134. Lawlor DA, Najman JM, Sterne J, et al. Associations of parental, birth, and early life characteristics with systolic blood pressure at 5 years of age. *Circulation* 2004;110:2417–23.
135. Singhal A, Cole TJ, Lucas A. Early nutrition in preterm infants and later blood pressure: two cohorts after randomised trials. *Lancet* 2001;357:413–9.
136. Jarvelin M-R, Sovio U, King V, et al. Early life factors and blood pressure at age 31 years in the 1066 Northern Finland Birth Cohort. *Hypertension* 2004;44:838–46.
137. Halldorsson TI, Gunnarsdottir I, Birgisdottir BE, et al. Childhood growth and adult hypertension in a population of high birth weight. *Hypertension* 2011;58:8–15.
138. Rahmouni K. Sympathetic tone in the young. The mother weighs in. *Hypertension* 2010;55:21–2.
139. Jennings G. Arterial pulse wave forms: deferred at birth or barking up the wrong tree? *J Hypertens* 2005;23:1337–9.
140. Dustan HP. Obesity and hypertension in blacks. *Cardiovasc Drugs Ther* 1990;4:395–402.
141. Calhoun DA, Mutinga ML Wyss JM, et al. Muscle sympathetic nerve activity in black and Caucasian hypertensive subjects. *J Hypertens* 1994;12:1291–6.
142. Attramadal H. Hypertension: are we Barking up the wrong tree? *Hypertension* 2009;54:27–8.
143. Adrogue HJ, Madias NE. Sodium and potassium in the pathogenesis of hypertension. *NEJM* 2007;356:1966–78.
144. Sanders PW. Salt sensitivity. It is not always in the genes. *Hypertension* 2008;51:823–4.
145. Schmidlin O, Forman A, Leone A, et al. Salt sensitivity in blacks. *Hypertension* 2011;58:380–5.
146. Chadola T, Brunner E, Marmot M. Chronic stress at work and the metabolic syndrome. *BMJ* 2006;332:521–5.
147. Steptoe A, Willemsen G. The influence of job control on ambulatory blood pressure and perceived stress over the working day in men and women from the Whitehall Cohort. *J Hypertens* 2004;22:915–20.

148. Poulter NR, Khaw KT, Hopwood BE, et al. The Kenyan Luo migration: observations on the initiation of the rise in blood pressure. *BMJ* 1990;300:967–72.
149. Meng L, Chen D, Yang Y, et al. Depression increases the risk of hypertension incidence: a meta-analysis of prospective cohort studies. *J Hypertens* 2012;30:842–51.
150. Marshall IJ, Wolfe CD, McKevitt C. Lay perspectives on hypertension and drug adherence: Systematic review of quantitative research. *BMJ* 2012;12:e3953.
151. Beilin LJ, Puddey IB. Alcohol and hypertension. *Hypertension* 2006;47:1035–8.
152. Stamler J, Liu K, Ruth KJ, et al. Eight-year blood pressure change in middle-aged men. Relationship to multiple nutrients. *Hypertension* 2002;39:1000–6.
153. Wildman RP, Gu D, Muntner P, et al. Alcohol intake and hypertension in Chinese men. *J Hypertens* 2005;23;737–43.
154. Ohkubo T, Metoki H, Imai Y. Alcohol intake, circadian blood pressure variation and stroke. *Hypertension* 2009;53:4–5.
155. Zilkens RR, Burke V, Hodgson JM, et al. Red wine and beer elevate blood pressure in normotensive men. *Hypertension* 2005;45:874–9.
156. Stranges S, Wu T, Dorn JM, et al. Relationship of alcohol drinking pattern to risk of hypertension. *Hypertension* 2004;44:813–9.
157. Klatsky AL. Alcohol-associated hypertension. *Hypertension* 2004;44:805–6.
158. Niskanen L, Laaksonen DE, Nyyssonen K, et al. Inflammation, abdominal obesity and smoking as predictors of hypertension. *Hypertension* 2004;44:859–65.
159. Jatoi NA, Jerrard-Dunne P, Feely J, et al. Impact of smoking cessation on arterial stiffness and aortic wave reflection in hypertension. *Hypertension* 2007;49:981–5.
160. Winkelmayer WC, Stampfer MK, Willet WC, et al. Habitual caffeine intake and the risk of hypertension in women. *JAMA* 2005;294:2330–5.
161. Mahmud A, Feely J. Acute effect of caffeine on arterial stiffness and aortic pressure waveform. *Hypertension* 2001;38:227–31.
162. McCall DO, McGartland CP, McKinley MC, et al. Dietary intake of fruit and vegetables improves microvascular function in hypertensive subjects in a dose-dependent manner. *Circulation* 2009;119:2153–60.
163. Brown IJ, Stamler J, Van Horn L, et al. Sugar-sweetened beverage, sugar intake of individuals, and their blood pressure. *Hypertension* 2011;57:695–701.
164. Stolarz-Skrzypek K. Sugar and salt in the pathogenesis of elevated blood pressure. *Hypertension* 2011;57:676–8.
165. Gopinath B, Flood VM, Rochtchina E, et al. Influence of high glycemic index and glycemic load diets on blood pressure during adolescence. *Hypertension* 2012;59:1272–7.

166. Ha V, Sievenpiper JL, de Souza RJ, et al. Effect of fructose on blood pressure. A systematic review and meta-analysis of controlled feeding trials. *Hypertension* 2012;59:787–95.
167. Carnethon MR, Evans NS, Church TS, et al. Joint associations of physical activity and aerobic fitness on the development of incident hypertension. *Hypertension* 2010;56:49–55.
168. Rheaume C, Arsenault BJ, Belanger S, et al. Low cardiorespiratory fitness levels and elevated blood pressure. *Hypertension* 2009;54:91–7.
169. Pouliou T, KI M, Law C, et al. Physical activity and sedentary behaviour at different life stages and adult blood pressure in the 1958 British cohort. *J Hypertens* 2012;30:275–83.
170. Williams RB. How does lower education get inside the body to raise blood pressure? *Hypertension* 2010;55:617–8.
171. Reckelhoff JF, Roman RJ. Androgens and hypertension. Role in both males and females? *Hypertension* 2011;57:681–2.
172. Reckelhoff JF, Fortepianni LA. Novel mechanisms responsible for postmenopausal hypertension. *Hypertension* 2004;43:918–23.
173. Coylewright M, Reckelhoff JF, Ouyang P. Menopause and hypertension. *Hypertension* 2008;51:952–9.
174. Faraut B, Touchette E, Gamble H, et al. Short sleep duration and increased risk of hypertension: A primary care medicine investigation. *J Hypertens* 2012;30:1354–63.
175. Grassi G, Facchini A, Trevano FQ, et al. Obstructive sleep apnea-dependent and -independent adrenergic activation in obesity. *Hypertension* 2005;46:321–5.
176. Haas DC, Foster GL, Nieto J, et al. Age-dependent associations between sleep-disordered breathing and hypertension. *Circulation* 2005;111:614–21.
177. Marin JM, Agusti A, Villar I, et al. Association between treated and untreated obstructive sleep apnea and risk of hypertension. *JAMA* 2012;307:2169–76.
178. Barbe F, Duran-Cantolla J, Sanchez-de-la-Torre M, et al. Effect of continuous positive airway pressure on the incidence of hypertension and cardiovascular events in non-sleepy patients with obstructive sleep apnea. *JAMA* 2012;307:2161–8.
179. Perlstein TS, Gumieniak O, Williams GH, et al. Uric acid and the development of hypertension. *Hypertension* 2006;48:1031–6.
180. Loeffler LF, Navas-Acien A, Brady TM, et al. Uric acid level and elevated blood pressure in US adolescents. *Hypertension* 2012;59:811–7.
181. Coogan PF, White LF, Jerrett M, et al. Air pollution and incidence of hypertension and diabetes mellitus in black women living in Los Angeles. *Circulation* 2012;125:767–72.
182. Cosselman KE, Krishnan RM, Oron AP, et al. Blood pressure response to controlled diesel exhaust exposure in human subjects. *Hypertension* 2012;59:943–8.

183. Nash D, Magder L, Lustberg M, et al. Blood lead, blood pressure and hypertension peri-menopausal and post-menopausal women. *JAMA* 2003;289:1523–32.
184. Berthold HK, Michalke B, Krone W, et al. Influence of serum selenium concentrations on hypertension: The Lipid Analytic Cologne cross-sectional study. *J Hypertens* 2012;30:1328–35.
185. Li S, Zhu J, Zhang W. Signature micro RNA expression profile in essential hypertension and it's novel link to human cytomegalovirus infection. *Circulation* 2011;124:175–84.

High Blood Pressure (and the Sympathetic Nervous System) as a Predictor of Premature Death and Cardiovascular Events

CHAPTER 5

GLOBAL BURDEN OF HYPERTENSION

High blood pressure (BP) is number 1 risk factor for premature death all around the world, way ahead of smoking and high cholesterol (**Figure 5-1**) (1); cardiovascular deaths predominate (2). About 54% of stroke and 47% of ischemic heart disease were attributable to high BP (with about 50% of high BP group being so-called prehypertension) (3). About 80% of this burden occurred in low- and middle-income economies (3).

1. Clinic (office) blood pressure as a risk factor for cardiovascular events

The relationship between systolic blood pressure (SBP) and diastolic blood pressure (DBP) in middle-aged men and women, and cardiovascular events over 38 years of observation in the Framingham Survey, is shown in **Figure 5-2** (4). Myocardial infarction and stroke are the major killers; and the relationship between SBP and DBP and these two events is shown in **Figures 5-3** and **5-4**, reflecting the results of a meta-analysis of 61 prospective studies in middle-aged subjects (5). The relationship between SBP and DBP and cardiovascular events is linear down to SBP of 115 mm Hg and DBP of 75 mm Hg, and a difference of 20 mm Hg SBP, or 10 mm Hg DBP, is linked to a twofold difference in the frequency of cardiovascular events (5). In a

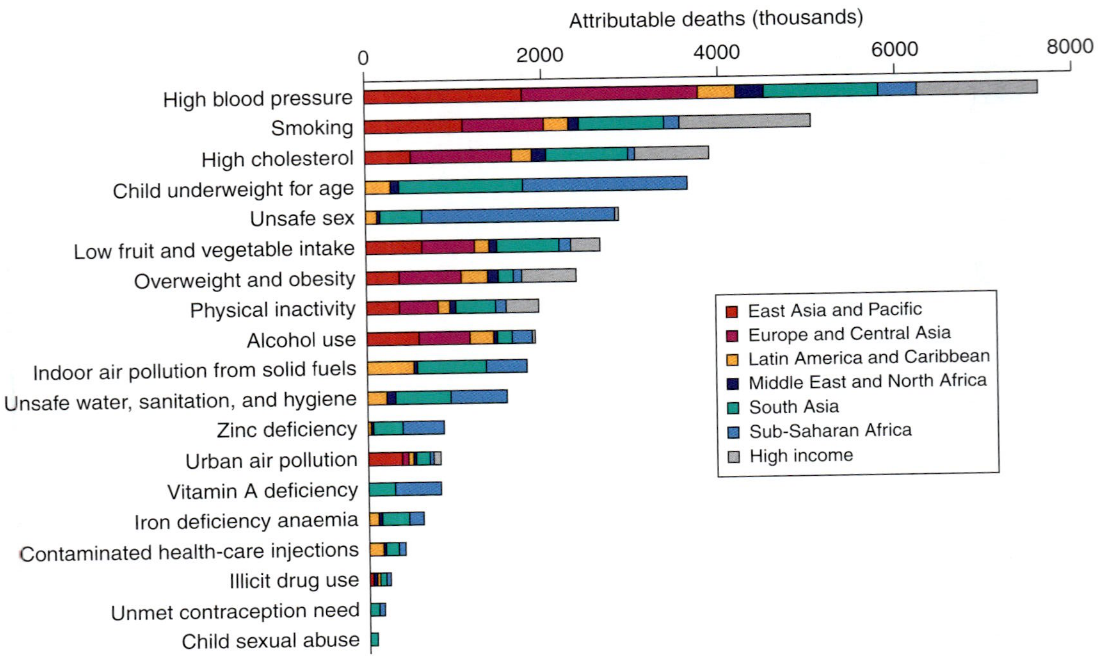

Fig. 5-1 Mortality due to global risk factors in different parts of the world. (From Lopez AD, Mathers CD, Ezzati M, et al. Global and regional burden of disease and risk factors, 2001: systematic analysis of population health data. *Lancet* 2006;367:1747–57.)

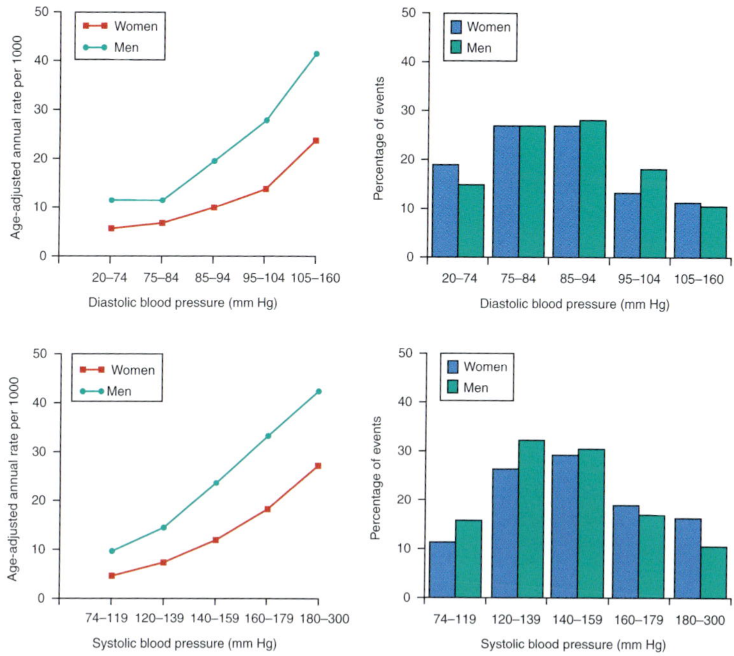

Fig. 5-2 Framingham; risk of cardiovascular events over 38-year follow-up in men and women aged 35–64 years, in relation to diastolic blood pressure (DBP) (upper panels) and systolic blood pressure (SBP). (From Kannel WB. Elevated systolic blood pressure a cardiovascular risk factor. *Am J Cardiol* 2000;85:251–5.)

study involving 61,585 middle-aged/elderly (age 55 years plus) men and women, followed up for 14 years, individuals who maintained, or had a decrease in their BP to normal levels, had a lifetime risk for cardiovascular disease of 22%–41%; whereas those who had, or developed, hypertension by 55 years had a lifetime risk of 42%–69% (6). In the very old, that is, greater than 85 years old, there is no relationship between high BP and mortality; and below 140/70 mm Hg, there is an excess mortality (7).

Some databases indicate that almost 70% of all stroke cases result from raised BP (8), particularly so for hemorrhagic stroke (9). Such a relationship is particularly important in countries where there is a high prevalence of stroke; for example, in Japan stroke is about 6 times more common than myocardial infarction (10). Hypertension is the most common risk factor for congestive heart failure, particularly in the elderly (**Figure 5-5**) (11). Likewise, high BP is a major risk factor for end-stage renal disease (**Figure 5-6**) (12).

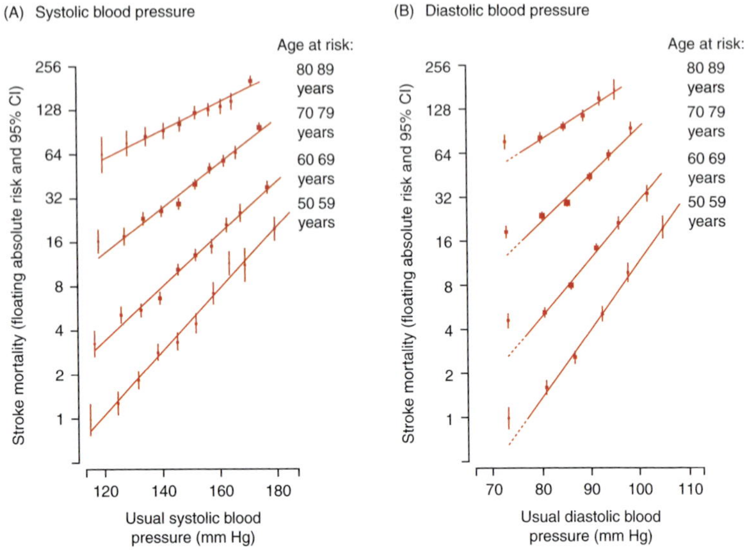

Fig. 5-3 Relationship between systolic blood pressure (SBP), diastolic blood pressure (DBP) and ischemic heart disease (IHD) mortality in different age groups; data from one million subjects from 61 prospective studies. (From Prospective Studies Collaboration. Age-specific relevance of usual blood pressure to vascular mortality: a meta-analysis of individual data for one million adults in 61 prospective studies. *Lancet* 2002;360:1903–13.)

2. Clinic (office) differences in blood pressure between arms and prognosis

A sizable difference in BP readings between arms is normally associated with congenital heart disease, aortic dissection, peripheral vascular disease, and unilateral neuromuscular abnormalities (13). In the absence of these conditions, discrepancies in BP are usually minor (5/4 mm Hg or less). About 20% of patients in primary care have a between-arm BP difference of 10 mm Hg or more, and 4% have a difference of 20 mm Hg or more (13); such differences are believed to be a marker of atherosclerosis.

A study in general practice extending over 10 years (14) showed that patients with an interarm difference of SBP of 10 mm Hg or more had a reduced survival expectation compared with those with an interarm difference of less than 10 mm Hg.

Technique is important. If blood pressure is taken simultaneously in both arms, 80% of the difference noted with non-simultaneous measurements disappears (15).

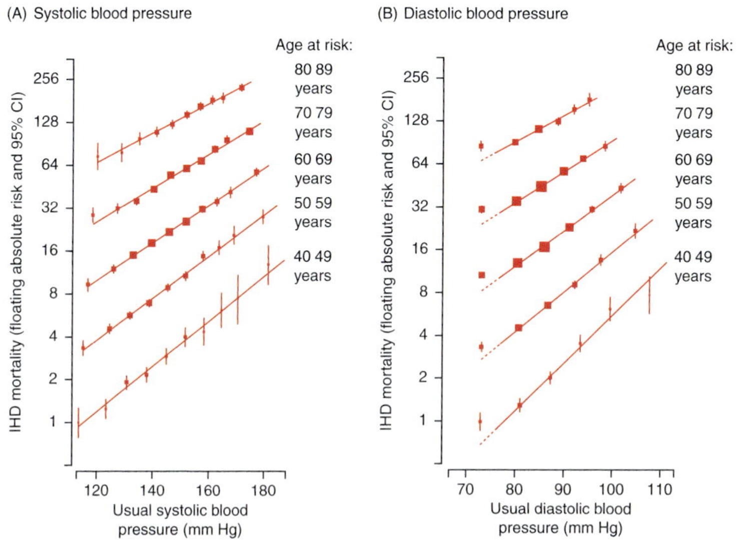

Fig. 5-4 Relationship between systolic blood pressure (SBP), diastolic blood pressure (DBP) and ischemic heart disease (IHD) mortality in different age groups; data from one million subjects from 61 prospective studies. (From Prospective Studies Collaboration. Age-specific relevance of usual blood pressure to vascular mortality: a meta-analysis of individual data for one million adults in 61 prospective studies. *Lancet* 2002;360:1903–13.)

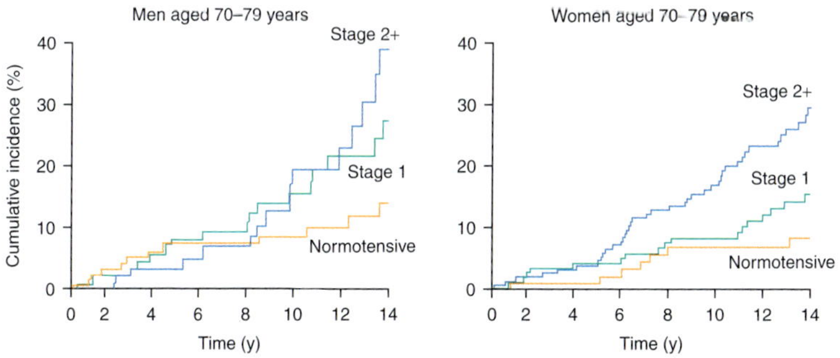

Fig. 5-5 Framingham; risk of congestive heart failure in relation to blood pressure (BP) severity in elderly men and women. (From Levy D, Larson MG, Vasan RS, et al. The progression from hypertension to congestive heart failure. *JAMA* 1996;275:1557–62.)

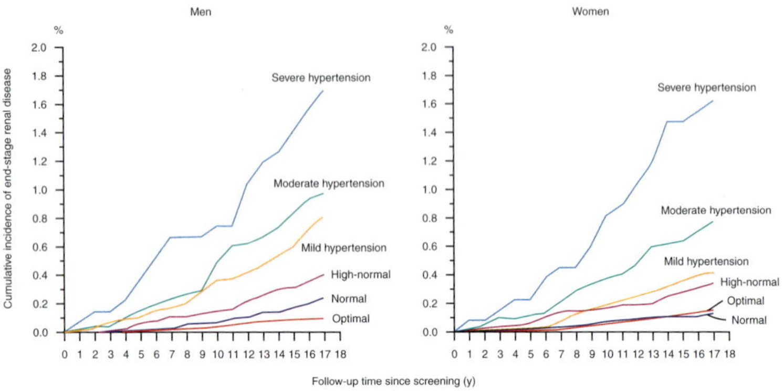

Fig. 5-6 Blood pressure severity predicts end-stage renal failure in middle-aged men and women. (From Tozawa M, Iseki K, Iseki C, et al. Blood pressure predicts risk of developing end-stage renal disease in men and women. *Hypertension* 2003;41:1341–5.)

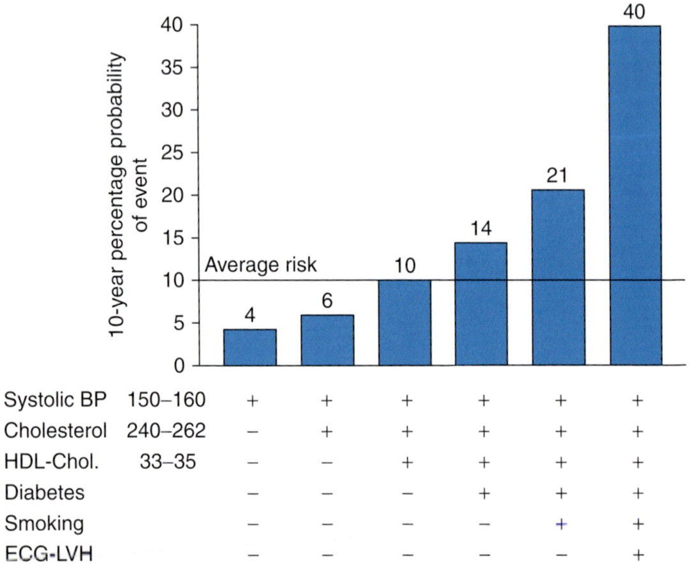

Fig. 5-6a Framingham; risk of coronary heart disease event in middle-aged men with mild hypertension increases as extra risk factors are added. (From Kannel WB. Elevated systolic blood pressure a cardiovascular risk factor. *Am J Cardiol* 2000;85:251–5.)

3. Clinic (office) blood pressure as a part of cardiovascular risk factor spectrum

The Framingham group has shown clearly that hypertension in middle-aged men has to be regarded in the context of multiple risk factors, for the development of coronary heart disease (**Figure 5-6a**) (4). The modest risk of lone systolic hypertension increases progressively with high total cholesterol, low high-density lipoprotein (HDL) cholesterol, diabetes, smoking and, particularly, electrocardiogram-left ventricular hypertrophy (ECG-LVH).

It is possible to derive a risk score, taking into account sex, age, cigarette smoking, SBP, total cholesterol, height, renal function, LVH, diabetes, and a history of myocardial infarction or stroke (16). Risk scores rise steeply with an increasing age (**Figure 5-7**), and scores above 40 are linked to a marked increase in the probability of dying from cardiovascular disease within the next 5 years (**Figure 5-8**). Thus, the total risk needs to be addressed in treating hypertension (17), and many patients will need to be treated with a combination of interventions to lower the risk of atherothrombotic disease (18).

4. Prehypertension as a risk factor

As mentioned earlier, an increased cardiovascular risk is present at BPs as low as 115/75 mm Hg (5). Prehypertension often develops into frank hypertension (19). In a 19-year follow-up of 2634 middle-aged Japanese subjects (20), both lower- and higher-range

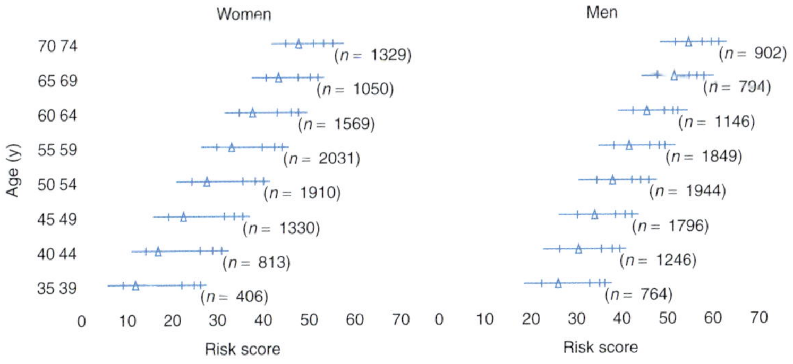

Fig. 5-7 In hypertensive men and women the risk scores for cardiovascular death in the next 5 years increases with age. (From Pocock SJ, McCormack V, Grueuffier F, et al. A score for predicting risk of death from cardiovascular disease in adults with raised blood pressure, based on individual patient data from randomized controlled trials. *BMJ* 2001;323:75–81.)

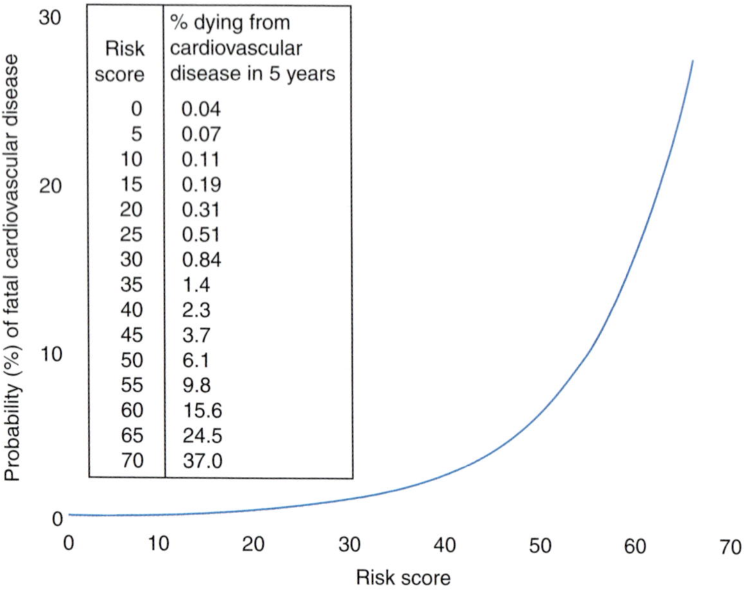

Risk score	% dying from cardiovascular disease in 5 years
0	0.04
5	0.07
10	0.11
15	0.19
20	0.31
25	0.51
30	0.84
35	1.4
40	2.3
45	3.7
50	6.1
55	9.8
60	15.6
65	24.5
70	37.0

Fig. 5-8 Based on eight randomized hypertension trials, the risk of dying of cardiovascular disease over 5 years increases as the risk score increases. (From Pocock SJ, McCormack V, Grueuffier F, et al. A score for predicting risk of death from cardiovascular disease in adults with raised blood pressure, based on individual patient data from randomised controlled trials. *BMJ* 2001;323:75–81.)

prehypertension were associated with increased cardiovascular risk (Figure 5-8a), being responsible for about one-third of all cardiovascular events. Prehypertension is very common in young/middle-aged, often with multiple risk factors (21). Hence, the increased cardiovascular risk associated with prehypertension (Figure 5-9) (20, 22, 23), is exacerbated by additional risk factors such as diabetes (**Figure 5-10**) (24). Although it may not be cost effective to treat simple prehypertension (25), it would be if diabetes was also present (24).

5. Blood pressure during exercise and cardiovascular risk

Regular physical activity is beneficial in reducing mortality in hypertensive patients (26). Subjects with normal BP who have an excessive increase in BP during exercise (greater than 180–215 mm Hg SBP) are at a greater risk of developing resting hypertension in later life (27, 28), and are at increased cardiovascular risk (29). Also, the rate of recovery, 2 minutes postexercise, of the DBP (30)

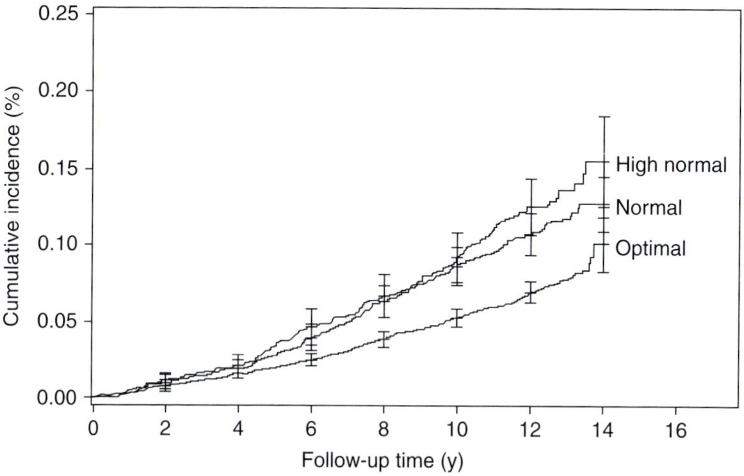

Fig. 5-9 In 8960 middle-aged subjects followed up for 14 years, the risk of cardiovascular disease (CVD) increased in those with high-normal blood pressure (BP) (prehypertension = 130–9/85–9 mm Hg) compared to those with optimal BP (<120/80 mm Hg). (From Kshirsagar AV, Carpenter M, Bang H, et al. Blood pressure usually considered normal is associated with an elevated risk of cardiovascular disease. *Am J Medic* 2006;119:133–41.)

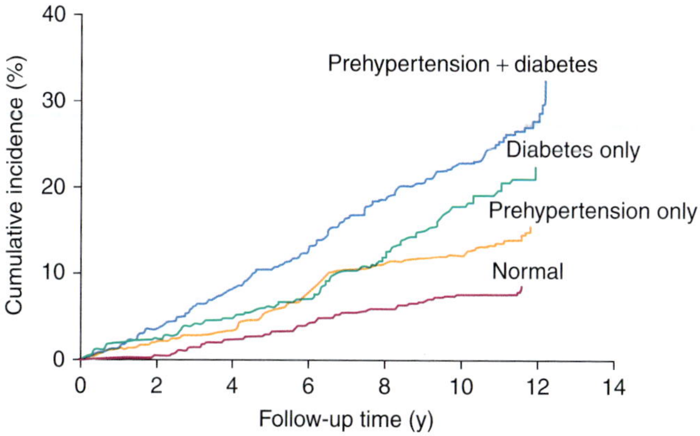

Fig. 5-10 The Strong Heart Study; the cardiovascular risk of subjects with prehypertension is markedly increased in the presence of diabetes. (From Zhang Y, Lee ET, Devereux RB, et al. Prehypertension, diabetes and cardiovascular disease risk in a population-based sample. *Hypertension* 2006;47:410–4.)

and SBP (31), is related to a later risk of cardiovascular events and myocardial infarction; probably a reflection of an ongoing activation of the sympathetic nervous system (32), and the fact that a high post-exercise BP is closely linked to endothelial dysfunction and vascular stiffness (33).

6. "White-coat" hypertension and the benefits of home and ambulatory blood pressure monitoring

A) Is "white-coat" hypertension innocent?

"White-coat" hypertension is common, present in about 25% of people who appear to have hypertension with conventional measurement (34). White-coat hypertension is regarded by some as benign (35, 36), particularly in the elderly with isolated systolic hypertension (37). However, most studies suggest that this condition is not entirely benign (38, 39), though it is clearly less dangerous than sustained hypertension (**Figure 5-11**) (40), falling between normotension and "masked" hypertension, in its predictive powers for cardiovascular events, stroke, and cardiac events (**Figure 5-12**) (41).

Patients with white-coat hypertension, or masked hypertension, are at an increased risk of developing sustained hypertension over a 10-year follow-up period (42).

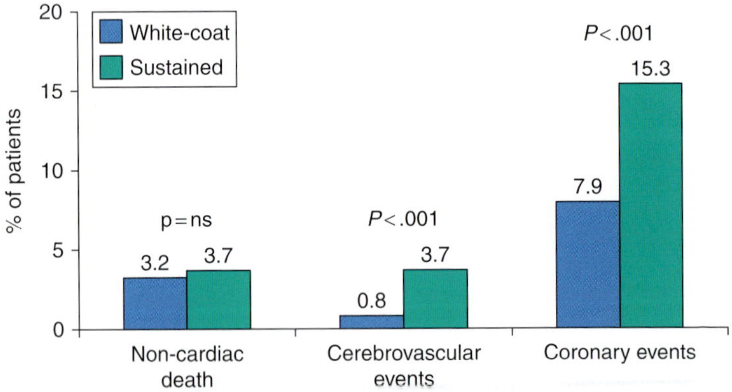

Fig. 5-11 Relatively benign outcome of white-coat versus sustained hypertension. (From Khattar R, Senior R, Lahiri A. Cardiovascular outcome in white-coat versus sustained mild hypertension: a 10-year follow-up study. *Circulation* 1998;98:1992–7.)

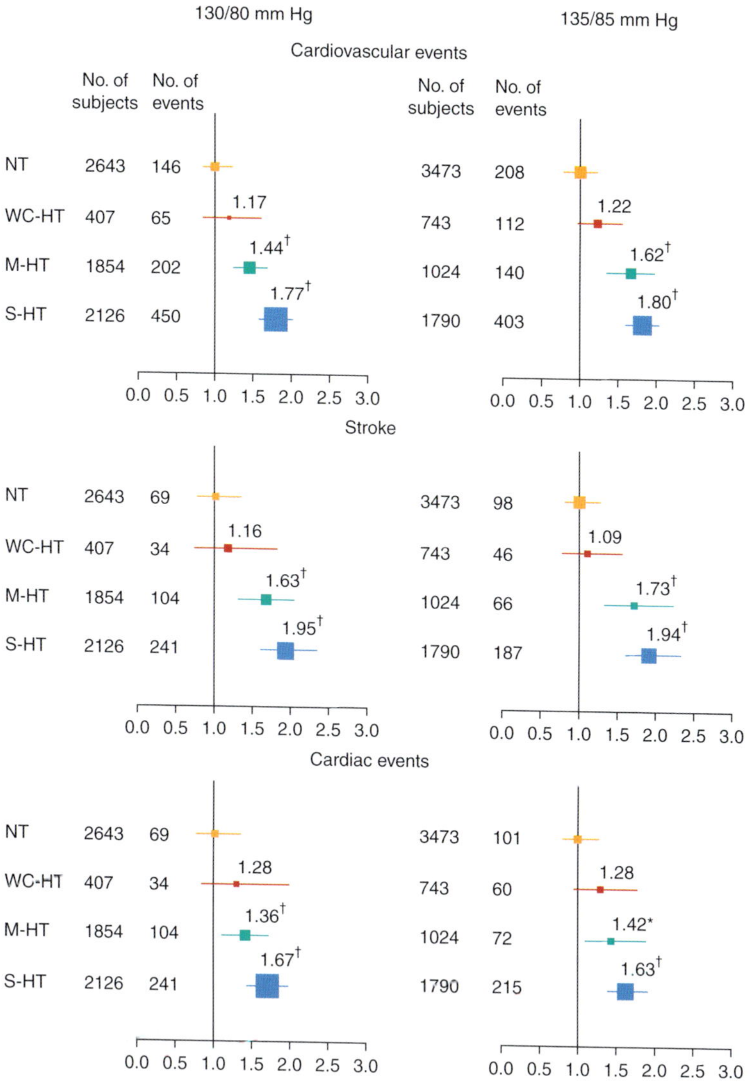

Fig. 5-12 In 7030 middle-aged (mean age of 56 years) subjects followed up for 9.5 years, day-time ambulatory blood pressure (ABP) was superior to clinic blood pressure (BP) as a cardiovascular disease (CVD) predictor; if hypertension diagnosed as 130/80 or 135/85 mm Hg, sustained hypertension (S-HT) was a more powerful predictor of CV, stroke, and cardiac events than white-coat (WCHT) or masked (M-HT). (From Hansen TW, Kikuya M, Thijs L, et al. Prognostic superiority of daytime ambulatory over conventional blood pressure in four populations: a meta-analysis of 7,030 individuals. *J Hypertens* 2007;25:1554–64.)

B) Home blood pressure as a cardiovascular outcome predictor

An early study indicated that home BP readings were superior to clinic values in predicting cardiovascular death (43). However, another study indicated that home BP was no better than office BP as a predictor of cardiovascular risk (44). More recent studies find home BP superior to office BP as a predictor of cardiovascular events (45). Maximum home SBP seems to be a good predictor of end-organ damage relating to the heart, carotid intima-media thickness, and the kidney (**Figure 5-13**) (46). Home BP is also superior to office BP as a predictor of future cardiovascular events due to its lower variability of readings, and its ability to reveal "masked" hypertension (47). Best results will be obtained with multiple readings (48), well illustrated in the Finn-Home Study (49), which suggested that best predictions of future cardiovascular events occurred when 2 BP measurements in the morning, and 2 in the evening, were performed over a 1-week period. The most recent data from the Finn-Home Study (36) show that, after 7.5 years follow-up on 2046 middle-aged subjects, neither "white-coat" nor "masked," hypertension was an independent predictor of cardiovascular risk or all-cause mortality when concomitant factors, such as age, sex, BMI, smoking, alcohol, medication, diabetes, blood cholesterol, medical history, were taken into account. Long-term follow-up with home BP measurement should be highly cost effective (50).

Variability in home-measured systolic and diastolic blood pressure in middle aged, assessed over 7 consecutive days was a good predictor of cardiovascular events over the next 8 years (51).

C) Ambulatory blood pressure monitoring as a cardiovascular outcome predictor

i) Daytime blood pressure and the early morning surge

As already shown (41), in 7030 middle-aged subjects over 9.5 years, daytime ambulatory blood pressure (ABP) is superior to conventional BP as a predictor of cardiovascular events, stroke, and cardiac events (Figure 5-12). This is particularly true for stroke, where daytime BP was superior to nocturnal BP as a predictor (52). Others have shown that in middle-aged hypertensives followed up for 9.5 years, both daytime ambulatory SBP and DBP are superior to office SBP, as predictors of all-cause mortality (**Table 5-1**) (53).

There is an early morning surge in BP (coincident with an increase in sympathetic nerve activity) (54), which, in the elderly,

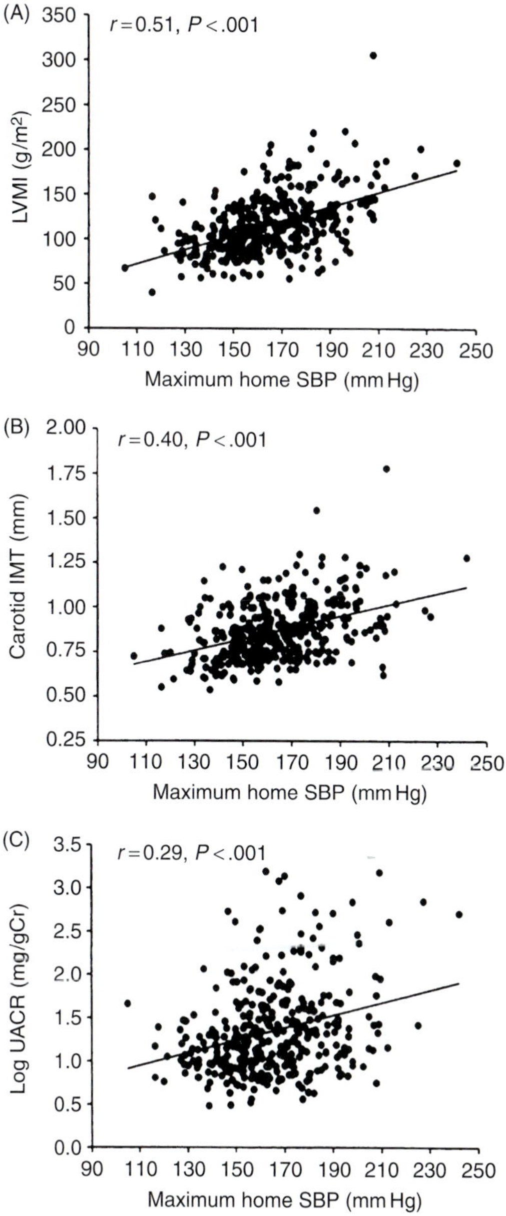

Fig. 5-13 In 356 untreated older (mean age of 66 years) hypertensives, maximum home SBP correlates with LV mass (A), intimal medial thickness (B), and urinary albumin/creatinine ratio (C). (From Matsui Y, Ishikawa J, Eguchi K, et al. Maximum value of home blood pressure: a novel indicator of target organ damage in hypertension. *Hypertension* 2011;57:1087–93.)

TABLE 5-1 In 1700 middle-aged subjects followed up for 9.5 years, 24-hour, daytime and nighttime ambulatory blood pressure (ABP) values were superior to office BP values in predicting all-cause mortality (hazard ratios)

Variables	Univariate	Adjusted
Ambulatory blood pressure		
Systolic 24-h	1.39 (1.26–1.54)‡	1.18 (1.06–1.31)†
Systolic daytime	1.36 (1.23–1.50)‡	1.15 (1.04–1.28)†
Systolic nighttime	1.36 (1.24–1.49)‡	1.19 (1.08–1.30)†
Diastolic 24-h	1.18 (1.09–1.28)‡	1.18 (1.09–1.28)‡
Diastolic daytime	1.16 (1.08–1.25)‡	1.16 (1.08–1.26)‡
Diastolic nighttime	1.18 (1.10–1.27)‡	1.16 (1.08–1.25)‡
Office blood pressure		
Systolic	1.24 (1.15–1.33)‡	1.05 (0.96–1.14)
Diastolic	1.08 (1.01–1.16)*	1.06 (0.99–1.14)

*$P < .05$.
†$P < .01$.
‡$P < .0001$.
In multivariate analysis adjusted for age, smoking status, alcohol consumption, and physical activity.
From Hansen TW, Jeppesen J, Rasmussen S, et al. Ambulatory blood pressure and mortality. *Hypertension* 2005;45:499–504.

is a strong predictor of silent and clinical cerebrovascular events (55). This is particularly relevant to cerebral hemorrhage (56). The morning surge is also associated with an increased risk of myocardial infarction (54). However, there are also data suggesting that a blunted morning surge in BP is a predictor of cardiovascular events (57).

ii) Nocturnal blood pressure and dipping

In the elderly, nocturnal SBP is the best predictor of cardiovascular events (**Figure 5-14**) (58, 59), and all nocturnal measurements are superior to clinic SBP as a predictor. Nocturnal BP is also superior to clinic BP in predicting heart failure (60).

In a large study involving 5292 middle-aged hypertensives followed up for 8.4 years, nocturnal SBP and DBP were superior to daytime and clinic SBP and DBP, as predictors of cardiovascular death (**Figure 5-15**) (61). Although women are at lower cardiovascular risk than men, a large study showed that the relation of all cardiovascular events, stroke, and cardiac events with nocturnal BP were steep in women (62). Thirty to fifty percent of hypertensives

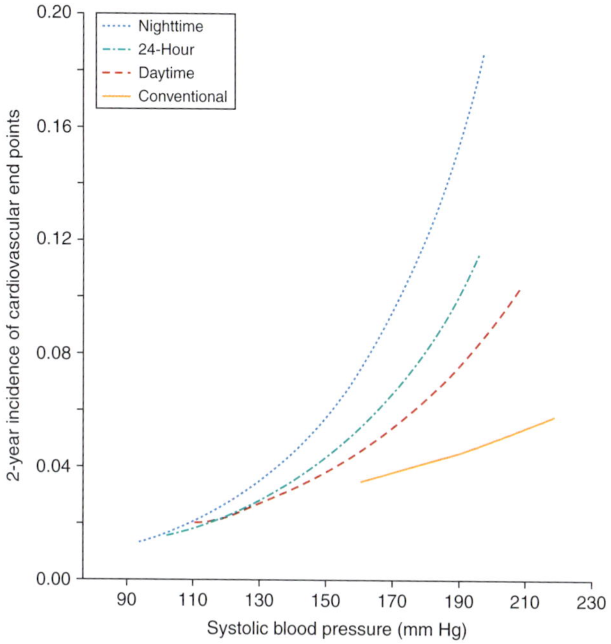

Fig. 5-14 In the older systolic hypertensives, nocturnal SBP is the best predictor of cardiovascular end points. (From Staessen JA, Thijs L, Fagard R, et al. Predicting cardiovascular risk using conventional vs ambulatory blood pressure in older patients with systolic hypertension. *JAMA* 1999;282:539–46.)

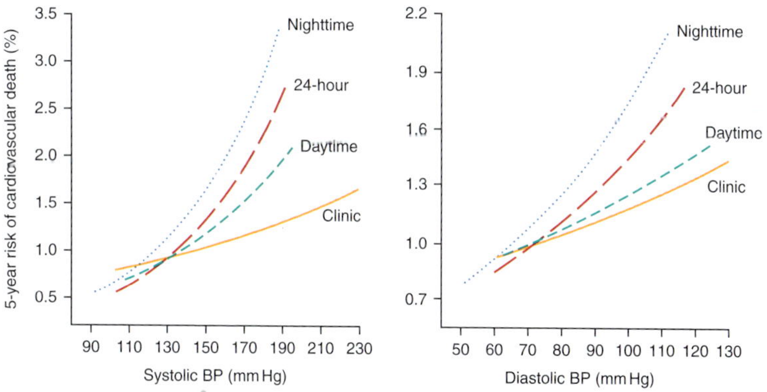

Fig. 5-15 In 5292 untreated middle-aged hypertensives followed up for 8.4 years, nocturnal BP was the best predictor of cardiovascular death (SBP > DBP). (From Dolan E, Stanton A, Thijs L, et al. Superiority of ambulatory over clinic blood pressure measurement in predicting mortality: the Dublin outcome study. *Hypertension* 2005;46:156–61.)

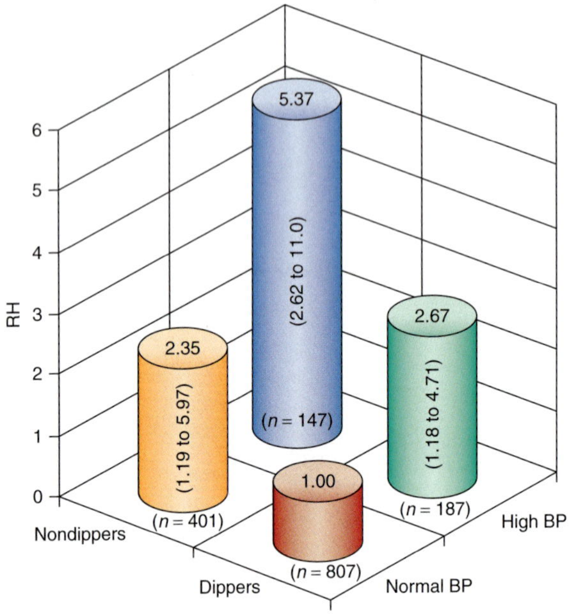

Fig. 5-16 In 1542 subjects aged greater than 40 years, followed up for 9.2 years, nocturnal blood pressure (BP) "nondippers" had the greatest risk of cardiovascular death. (From Ohkubo T, Hozawa A, Yamaguchi J, et al. Prognostic significance of the nocturnal decline in blood pressure in individuals with and without high 24-h blood pressure: the Ohasama Study. *J Hypertens* 2002;20:2183–9.)

are nondippers (fall in nocturnal BP less than 10/5 mm Hg), being more common in the elderly, type 2 diabetics, obese, and renal disease (63). Nondippers, even with a normal BP, have an increased risk of cardiovascular mortality (**Figure 5-16**) (64).

Interestingly, in a large study of middle-aged subjects followed up for 10 years, in untreated subjects daytime BP, adjusted for night-time BP, predicts fatal combined with nonfatal cardiovascular events, but not in treated patients (65).

D) Central blood pressure as a cardiovascular outcome predictor

i) Is central blood pressure superior to brachial BP as a predictor of cardiovascular events?

Some studies suggest that central P-P is superior to brachial P-P in predicting cardiovascular events (66). Certainly, the linear relationship between central SBP and stroke is more persuasive than the

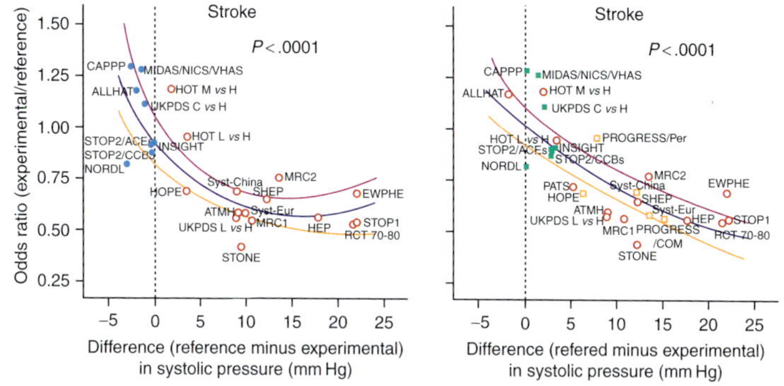

Fig. 5-17 The fall in treated central systolic blood pressure (SBP) (on right) is a better predictor of the reduced risk of stroke (linear relationship) than the fall in brachial SBP (on left) and risk of stroke (curvilinear relationship). (From Agabiti-Rosei E, Mancia G, O'Rourke MF, et al. Central blood pressure measurements and antihypertensive therapy. *Hypertension* 2007; 50:154–60.)

curvilinear relationship with brachial SBP, mainly in elderly subjects (**Figure 5-17**) (67). Other studies, mainly in the elderly, suggest that brachial and central SBP are similar in predicting clinical events, although central P-P might be superior to brachial P-P in this respect (**Figure 5-18**) (68).

In middle-aged subjects, followed up for 15 years, office central BP is better than brachial BP in predicting all-cause and cardiovascular mortalities; but ambulatory SBP, over 24 hours, seems superior to central SBP in predicting cardiovascular mortality (**Figure 5-19**) (69).

However, in elderly female hypertensives (unlike men), brachial is superior to central SBP and P-P in predicting cardiovascular disease outcome (**Figure 5-20**) (70).

ii) Central augmentation index (AIx) as a predictor of outcome

In elderly women, AIx was not a predictor of cardiovascular disease (Figure 5-20) (70). However, in 6057 subjects from the general population, the AIx increased with an increasing risk score for all-cause mortality, based on age, BMI SBP, pulse rate, smoking, diabetes, and myocardial infarction (EPOZ risk score) (**Figure 5-21**) (71). In middle-aged patients, mainly with hypertension, an increasing AIx was linked to a greater likelihood of coronary artery disease (**Figure 5-21a**) (72). Also, in high-risk patients on hemodialysis, a high AIx was related to a reduced

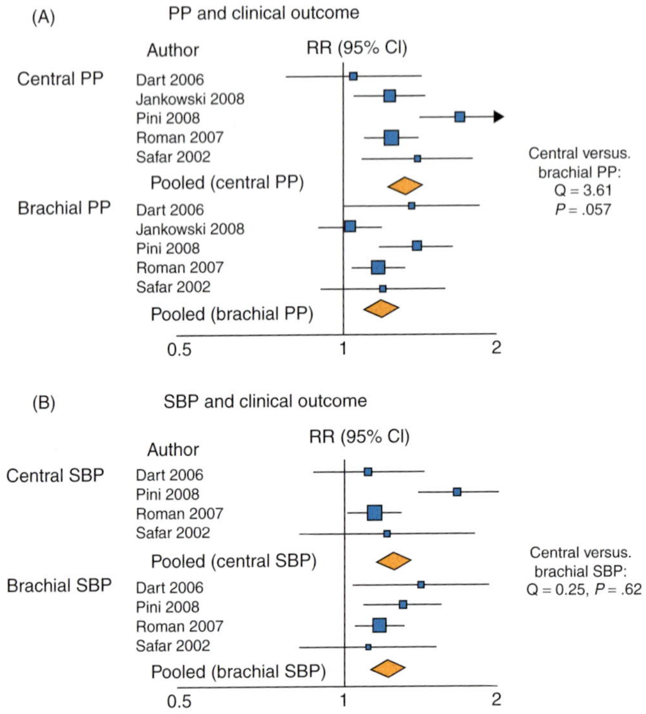

Fig. 5-18 In elderly subjects, central P-P, but not systolic blood pressure (SBP), is a better predictor of outcome than brachial blood pressure (BP) values. (From Vlachopoulos C, Aznaouridis K, O'Rourke MF, et al. Prediction of cardiovascular events and all-cause mortality with central haemodynamis. *Eur Heart J* 2010;31:1865–71.)

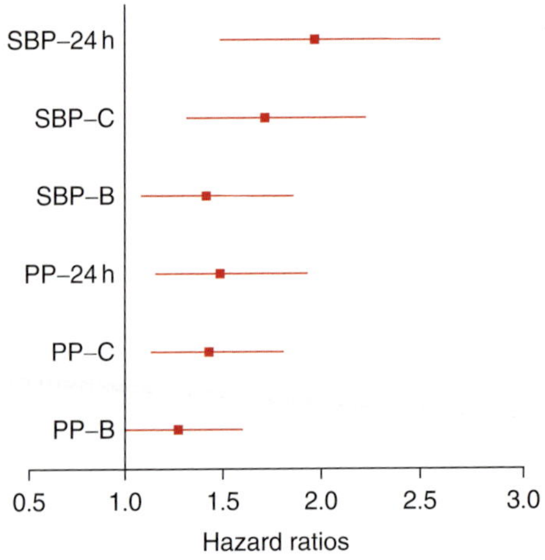

Fig. 5-19 In middle-aged subjects followed up for 15 years, mean ambulatory 24-hour systolic blood pressure (SBP) was better than brachial (B) SBP and P-P, central (C) SBP and P-P, and mean ambulatory 24-hour P-P, in predicting CV death. (From Huang C-M, Wang K-L, Cheng H-M, et al. Central versus ambulatory blood pressure in the prediction of all-cause and cardiovascular mortalities. *J Hypertens* 2011;29:454–9.)

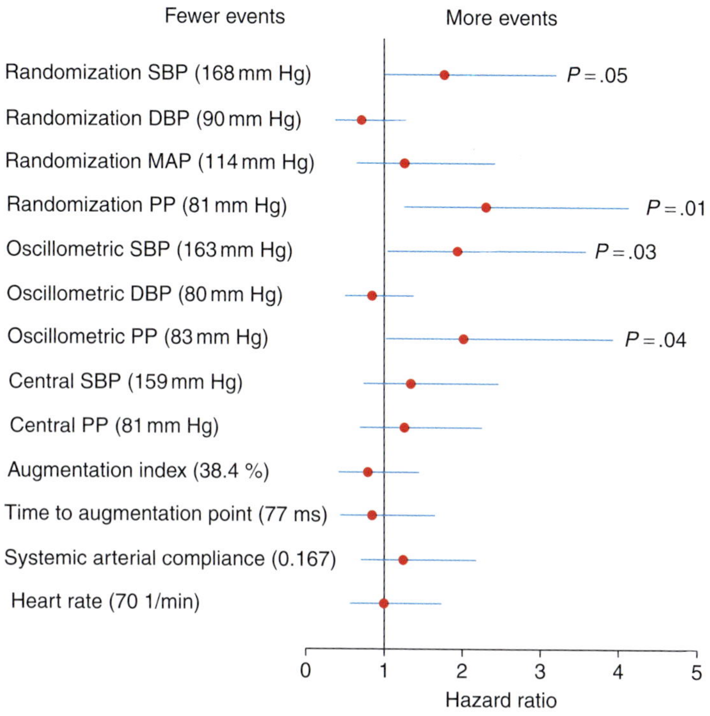

Fig. 5-20 In elderly female hypertensives, clinic (sphygmomanometer at randomization and oscillometric) SBP and P-P were superior to central SBP, P-P, and augmentation index (AIx), in predicting CVD-free interval. (From Dart AM, Gatzka CD, Kingwell BA, et al. Brachial blood pressure but not carotid arterial waveforms predict cardiovascular events in elderly female hypertensives. *Hypertension* 2006;47:785–90.)

risk of cardiovascular survival (**Figure 5-22**) (73). However, the Framingham Heart Study, in an elderly population followed up for 8 years, found that AIx was not a predictor of cardiovascular outcome (74).

iii) Pulse wave velocity as a predictor of outcome

Carotid-femoral pulse wave velocity (PWV) is the golden standard regarding arterial stiffness and is a good predictor of fatal and non-fatal cardiovascular events (75).

Certainly, a high PWV is a marker of cardiovascular disease in the elderly (76), as well as coronary artery calcium score (77), and the severity of coronary artery disease (78). A high PWV predicts

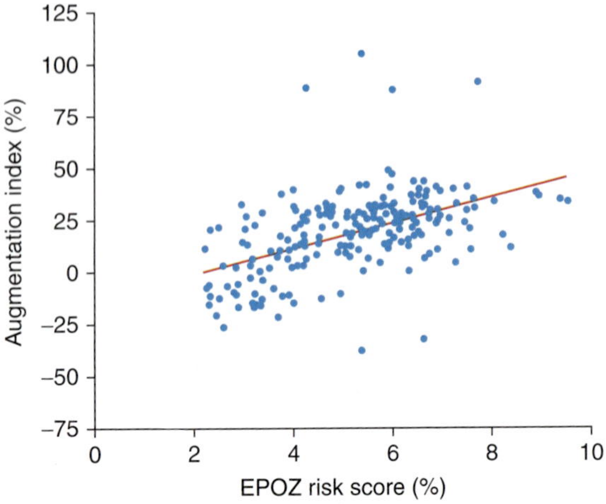

Fig. 5-21 In normal middle-aged subjects increasing cardiovascular (CV) risk (EPOZ score) was linked to increasing central augmentation index. (From Nurnberger J, Keflioglu-Schreiber A, Saez AM, et al. Augmentation index is associated with cardiovascular risk. *J Hypertens* 2002;20:2407–14.)

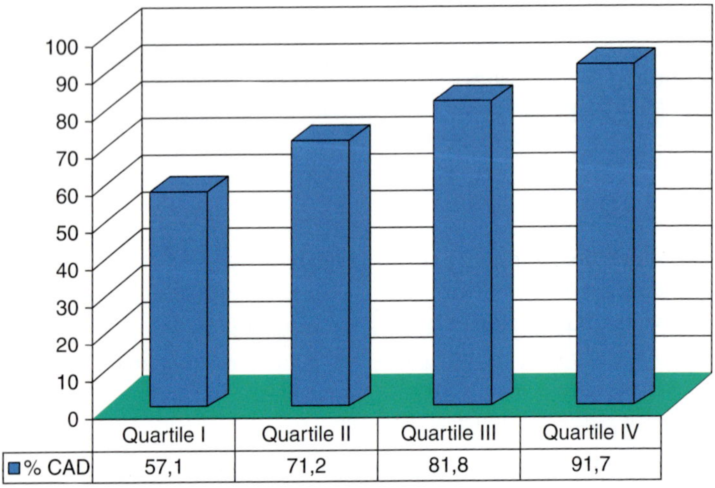

Fig. 5-21a In middle-aged men the level of central augmentation index (AIx) correlated with the degree of coronary artery disease (CAD) (angiography). (From Weber T, Auer J, O'Rourke MF, et al. Arterial stiffness, wave reflections and the risk of coronary artery disease. *Circulation* 2004;109:184–9.)

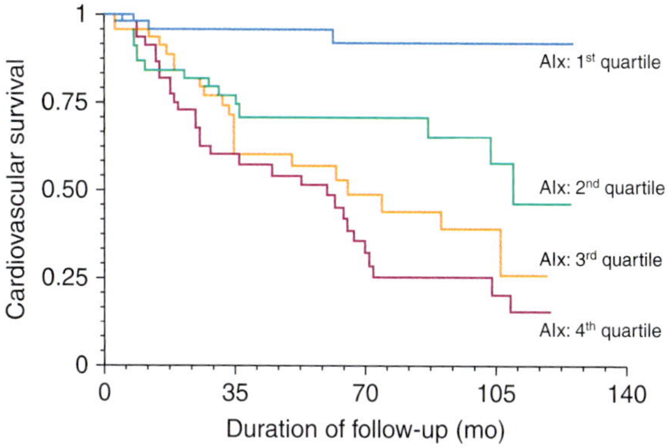

Fig. 5-22 In patients with end-stage renal failure a high augmentation index (AIx) predicted a low cardiovascular (CV) survival. (From O'Rourke MF. From theory into practice: arterial haemodynamics in clinical hypertension. *J Hypertens* 2002;20:1901–15.)

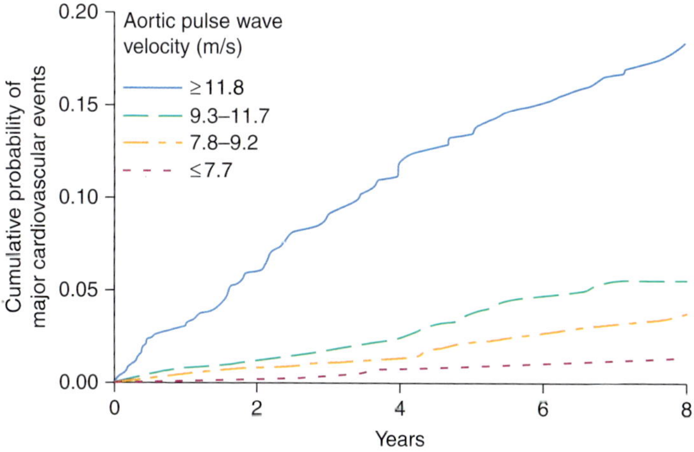

Fig. 5-23 Framingham: in 2232 subjects (mean age of 63 years) followed up for 8 years, a high aortic pulse wave velocity (PWV) predicted a major cardiovascular (CV) event. (From Mitchell GF, Hurang S-J, Vasan RS, et al. Arterial stiffness and cardiovascular events. The Framingham Heart Study. *Circulation* 2010;121:505–11.)

cardiovascular events in the elderly (**Figure 5-23**) (74, 79) and in patients on hemodialysis (Figure 5-22) (73). The relationship between PWV and 10-year risk of composite end points was particularly steep for women (**Figure 5-24**) (80), and related to all-cause death, stroke, and coronary artery disease (81).

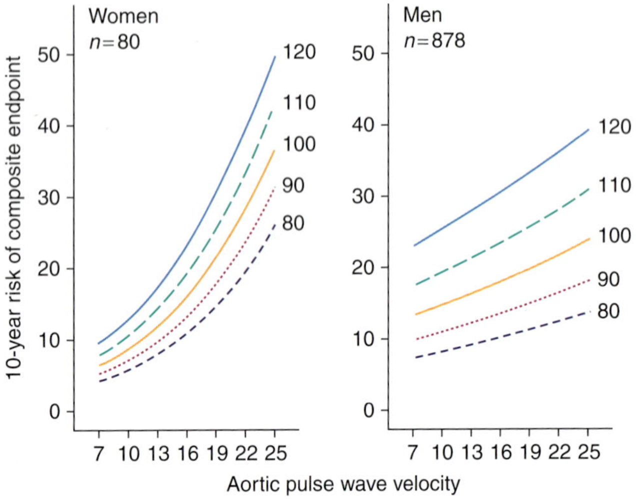

Fig. 5-24 In 1678 normal middle-aged subjects followed up for 9.4 years, pulse wave velocity (PWV) (at different mean BP levels) related to cardiovascular (CV) outcomes were more stronger in women than in men. (From Hansen TW, Staessen JA, Torp-Pedersen C, et al. Prognostic value of aortic pulse wave velocity as index of arterial stiffness in the general population. *Circulation* 2006;113:664–70.)

7. Key blood pressure predictors of cardiovascular disease—DBP, SBP, P-P, or BP variability in relation to age

A) Younger subjects—DBP and plasma noradrenaline/adrenaline/inflammatory factors

i) Blood pressure

The Framingham heart study showed that in younger subjects DBP was the prime predictor of cardiovascular events, shifting to SBP, then P-P, with increasing age (82). In a 21-year follow-up of 49,321 late-adolescent men, DBP was the best predictor of cardiovascular events, being somewhat superior to SBP; P-P was the weakest predictor (83). A similar study in over one million late-adolescent men, followed up for 24 years, showed that DBP was superior to SBP in predicting all-cause mortality with a steep increase above 90 mm Hg (**Figure 5-25**) (84). This effect was particularly evident in overweight/obese subjects (85).

Others have confirmed the importance of DBP as a predictor of death from stroke, congenital heart disease (CHD) or heart failure

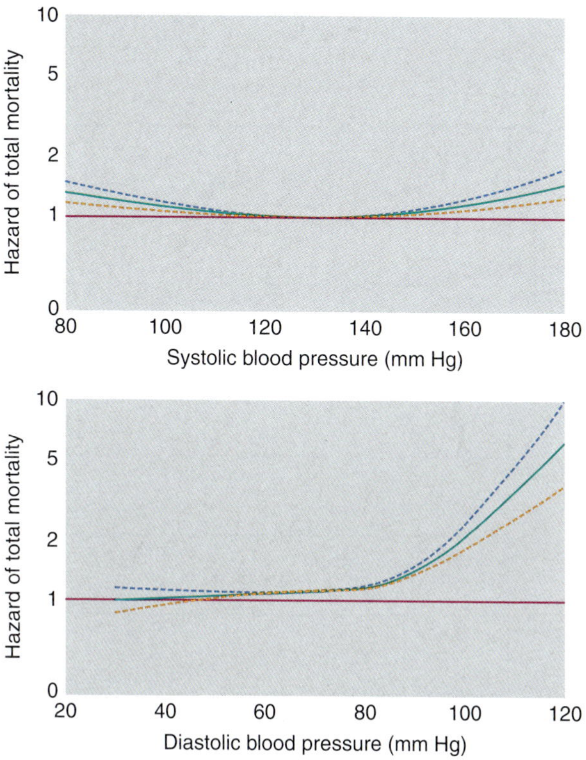

Fig. 5-25 In a 24-year follow-up of 1.2 million late adolescent (mean age of 18.4 years) men, diastolic blood pressure (DBP) [but not systolic blood pressure (SBP)] predicted total mortality. (From Sundstrom J, Neovius M, Tynelius P, et al. Association of blood pressure in late adolescence with subsequent mortality: cohort study of Swedish man conscripts. *BMJ* 2011;342:483.)

in young/middle-aged subjects, in contrast to P-P (**Figure 5-26**) (86). Addition of central BP values in the younger age group could complement the powerful prediction value of brachial DBP (87). Whereas DBP, in the presence of a raised SBP, is a powerful predictor, isolated diastolic hypertension appears to be a relatively benign condition in younger subjects (88, 89).

ii) Blood pressure, inflammatory markers, and sympathetic nerve activity

In the young/middle-aged, a high DBP plus a high c-reactive protein (CRP) level is the most powerful predictor of diminished event-free survival, indicating the importance of an underlying inflammatory

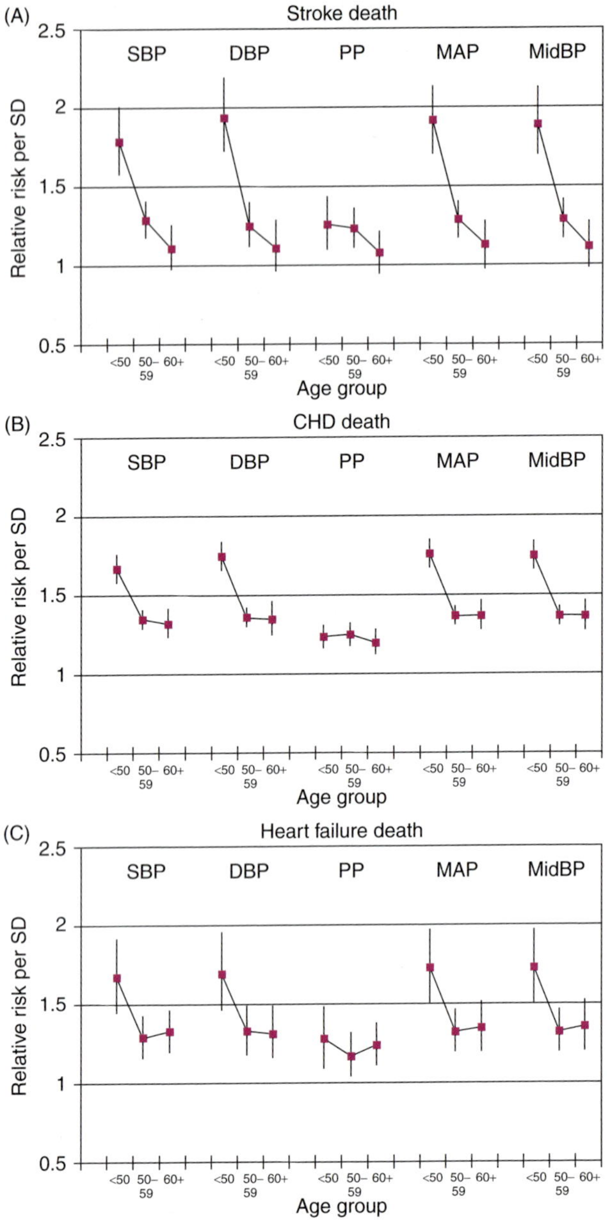

Fig. 5-26 In a 33-year follow-up of 36,314 young/middle-aged (mean age of 39 years) subjects (43% women), in those with mean age of less than 50 years diastolic blood pressure (DBP) and systolic blood pressure (SBP), but not P-P, were strong predictors of deaths from stroke (A), coronary heart disease [CHD] (B), and heart failure (C). (From Mosley II WJ, Greenland P, Garside DB, et al. Predictive utility of pulse-pressure and other blood pressure measures for cardiovascular outcomes. *Hypertension* 2007;49:1256–64.)

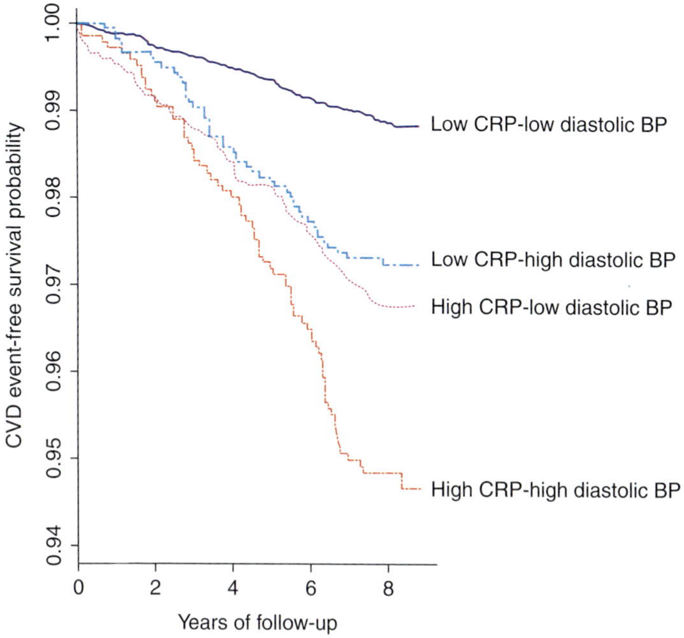

Fig. 5-27 In an 8-year follow-up of 15,215 middle-aged (mean age of 54 years) women, a high (>85 mm Hg) DBP (or SBP) + a high (>3 mg/L) CRP level was a powerful predictor of CVD event-free survival. (From Blake GJ, Rifai N, Buring JE, et al. Blood pressure, C-reactive protein, and risk of future cardiovascular events. *Circulation* 2003;108:2993–9.)

process (**Figure 5-27**) (90). Others have shown that in younger/ middle-aged subjects, a high CRP level predicts cardiovascular events (91), and CHD/MI events (92, 93), and that HIV infection is linked to high CRP levels and an increased risk of myocardial infarction (94).

High sympathetic nerve activity is known to be linked to the inflammatory process in younger women (95), and a high noradrenaline concentration is associated with high CRP and IL-6 levels (96), and closely relates to DBP in younger subjects (**Figure 5-28**) (97). It is thus perhaps not surprising that high plasma noradrenaline levels, independent of smoking and BP, are strong predictors of cardiovascular death and survival in younger/middle-aged hypertensives (**Figure 5-28a**), and high intralymphocyte β-receptor density (B_{max}) and cyclic adenosine monophosphate (AMP) levels predict myocardial infarction, but not stroke (**Figure 5-28b, Table 5-2**) (98). An illustration of the β-1 receptor, and its relationship with intracellular cyclic AMP, is shown in **Figure 5-28c** (99).

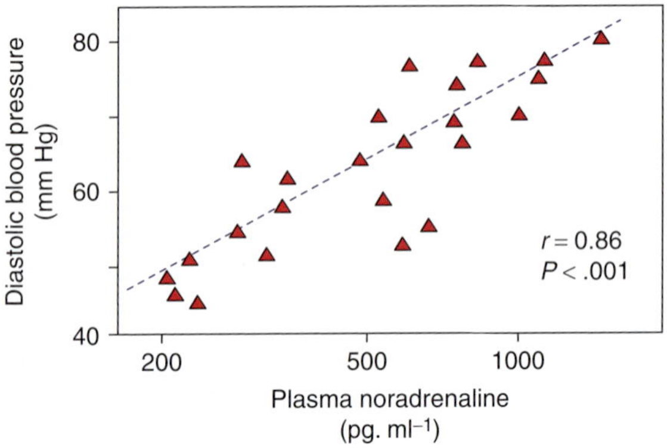

Fig. 5-28 In normal middle-aged men there was a strong relationship between DBP and plasma noradrenaline levels. (From Richards AM, Nicholls MG, Espiner EA, et al. Diurnal patterns of blood pressure, heart rate and vaso-active hormones in normal man. *Clin Exp Hypertens A* 1986;8:153–66.)

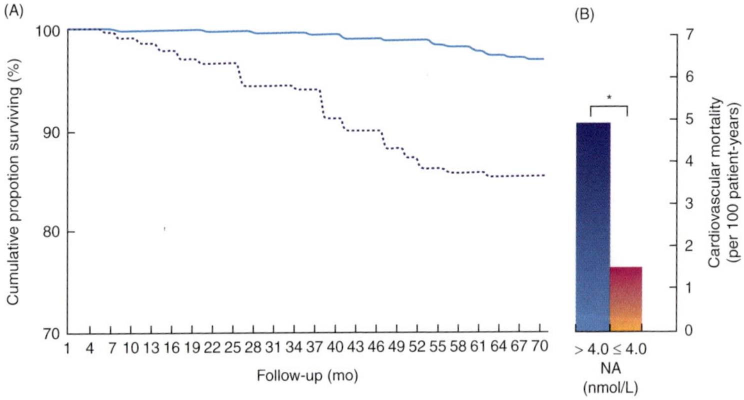

Fig. 5-28a Relationship between high (>4 nmol/L) and low (<4 nmol/L) plasma noradrenaline levels (independent of BP) and (A) survival and (B) cardiovascular mortality, in middle-aged hypertensives. (From Peng Y-X, Shan J, Qi XY, et al. The catecholamine-β-adrenoceptor-cAMP system and prediction of cardiovascular events in hypertension. *Clin Exp Pharmacol Physiol* 2006;33:227–31.)

In young hypertensives, high CRP and noradrenaline concentrations are associated with endothelial dysfunction (early indicator of the atheromatous process) (100). Certainly noradrenaline can induce an atherosclerotic process in the rabbit (101). Stress, accompanied

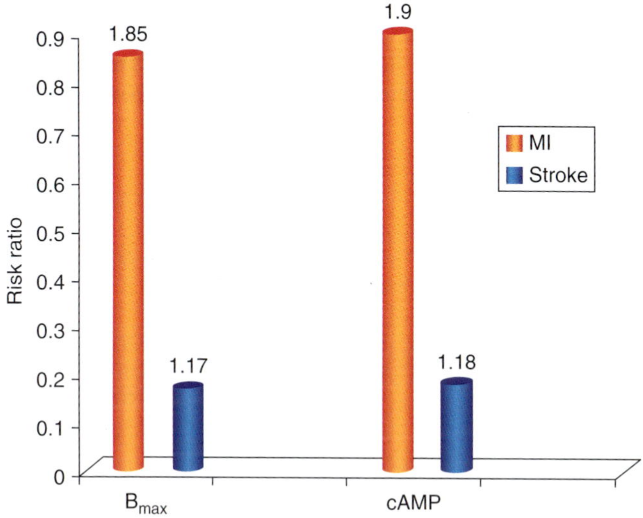

Fig. 5-28b β-Receptor density (B_{max}) and cAMP levels (in lymphocytes) as predictors of MI and stroke in middle-aged hypertensives followed up for 7 years. (From Peng Y-X, Shan J, Qi XY, et al. The catecholamine-β-adrenoceptor-cAMP system and prediction of cardiovascular events in hypertension. *Clin Exp Pharmacol Physiol* 2006;33:227–31.)

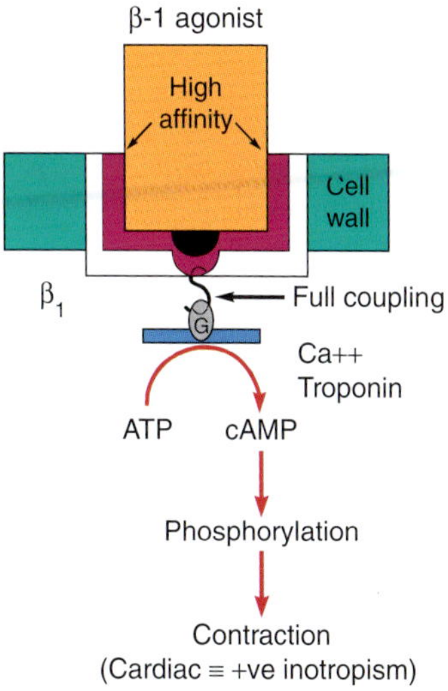

Fig. 5-28c Agonist activity (e.g., noradrenaline) and the β_1-receptor.

TABLE 5-2 Relationship between plasma noradrenaline/adrenaline and lymphocyte β-receptor density (B_{max}) and cAMP (independent of BP), and the hazard ratio (HR) for cardiovascular mortality, myocardial infarction, and stroke

Outcome variable	HR	95% CI	χ^2	*P*
Noradrenaline				
Composite end point	1.21	1.16–1.27	11.72	.0006
Cardiovascular mortality	1.22	1.17–1.28	11.24	.008
Fatal/nonfatal MI	1.25	1.19–1.31	14.81	.001
Fatal/nonfatal stroke	1.28	1.21–1.36	9.53	.002
Adrenaline				
Composite end point	1.33	1.11–1.59	9.55	.002
Cardiovascular mortality	1.53	1.18–2.00	9.99	.002
Fatal/nonfatal MI	1.55	1.19–1.36	8.91	.003
Fatal/nonfatal stroke	1.27	1.09–1.25	8.20	.004
B_{max}				
Composite end point	1.27	1.19–1.36	5.14	.004
Cardiovascular mortality	1.12	1.06–1.178	7.23	.007
Fatal/nonfatal MI	1.85	1.53–2.22	10.42	.002
Fatal/nonfatal stroke	1.17	1.09–1.25	0.80	.367
cAMP				
Composite end point	1.90	1.04–2.47	10.55	.002
Cardiovascular mortality	1.15	1.09–1.21	5.64	.005
Fatal/nonfatal MI	1.76	1.39–2.21	8.91	.003
Fatal/nonfatal stroke	1.18	1.10–1.26	2.30	.131

CI, confidence interval; MI, myocardial infarction.

From Peng Y-X, Shan J, Qi XY, et al. The catecholamine-β-adrenoceptor-cAMP system and prediction of cardiovascular events in hypertension. *Clin Exp Pharmacol Physiol* 2006;33:227–31.

by an increase in BP and blood flow velocity, can induce plaque rupture (102). A high CRP level is associated with a thin atheromatous plaque-cap thickness (103) and an increased risk of plaque-rupture (104).

Thus, in the young subjects, but not in the elderly, (105), there is a close linkage between DBP, high noradrenaline and CRP levels, the atheromatous process, and a poor prognosis. It is noteworthy that β-blockers are the best antihypertensive agents in reducing plasma CRP levels (**Figure 5-29**) (106), and that the action is due to β-1 blockade, as β-1 selective metoprolol succinate reduced the CRP levels by a significant 32% in younger/middle-aged hypertensives (107). Certainly stress-induced inflammation is inhibited by β-blockade (108), as is ischemia-induced increases in CRP (109, 110).

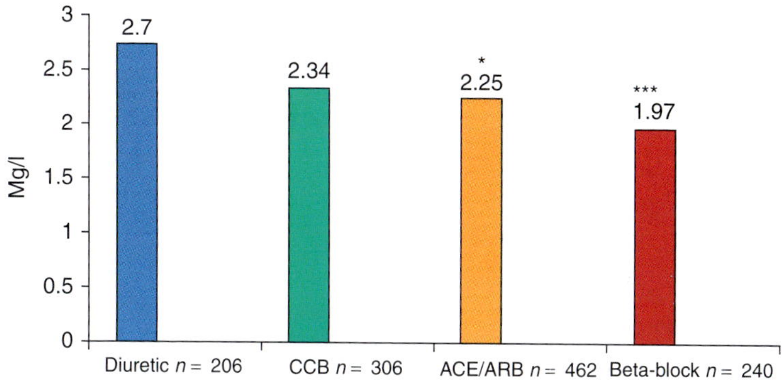

Fig. 5-29 The effect of mono-therapy antihypertensive treatments upon CRP levels(mg/l). (From Palmas W, Ma S, Psaty B, et al. Antihypertensive medications and C-reactive protein in the multi-ethnic study of atherosclerosis. *Am J Hypertens* 2007;20:233–41.)

B) Middle-aged/older subjects and systolic blood pressure/variability

More than 75% of hypertensive patients are over the age of 50 years, and it is this group where SBP becomes a major factor regarding prognosis (111). Diastolic blood pressure falls progressively after the age of 50 years and is no longer a major predictor of cardiovascular events. Indeed, DBP is often normal, or low, in the highest risk middle-aged/older patients. The risk of cardiovascular disease rises continuously as SBP increases from 115 mm Hg (112).

Examples of studies in middle-aged/older patients, followed up for over 20 years, where SBP is the prime predictor of outcome (vs. DBP and P-P), are the Chicago Heart Association Detection Project in Industry Study, where 28,360 men and women were studied (113), and the Dubo Study (114).

It has been shown that visit-to-visit variability in clinic SBP, maximum SBP, and episodic hypertension are strong predictors of cardiovascular events (115), particularly in patients on hemodialysis (116). In patients who had had a recent transient ischemic attack (TIA) or ischemic stroke, the maximum SBP of the first 7 measurements over a 2-year follow-up, was a good predictor of further stroke, as was variability of SBP (assessed in deciles of standard deviation) (**Figure 5-30**). Likewise, in older hypertensives (ASCOT trial), variability of SBP [deciles of standard deviation or variation independent of mean (VIM)], was a good predictor of both stroke and coronary events (**Figure 5-31**) (115). Variability of ambulatory blood pressure monitoring (ABPM) was a weaker predictor (115).

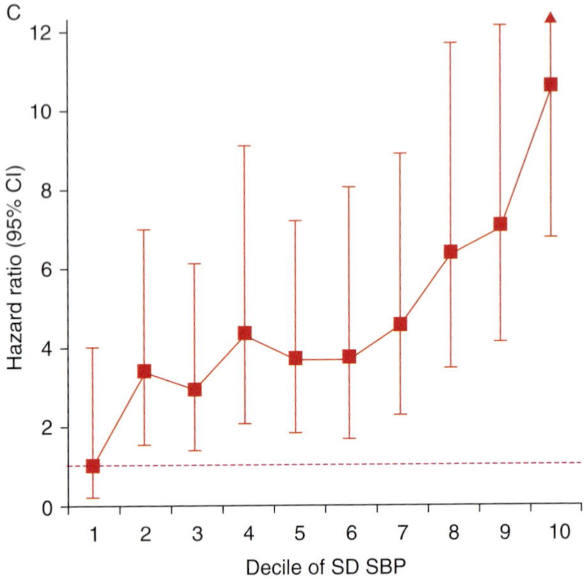

Fig. 5-30 The UK-TIA trial; in those without a previous stroke or cerebral infarct, a high decile of SBP variability (SD of first seven SBP measurements) was related to a high risk of a stroke. (From Rothwell PM, Howard SC, Dolan E, et al. Prognostic significance of visit to visit variability, maximum systolic blood pressure, and episodic hypertension. *Lancet* 2010;375:895–905.)

Others have shown no relationship between 24 hour BP variability and cardiovascular outcome (117).

Variability of home-measured systolic and diastolic blood pressures in middle aged, assessed over 7 consecutive days, was a good predictor of cardiovascular events over the next 8 years (51).

C) Elderly systolic hypertensives and P-P

The relationship between office or central P-P and outcome in the elderly has been discussed earlier. In addition, the Framingham group, in a 50-year follow-up, showed that the combination of P-P and mean arterial (MAP) is perhaps the best predictor of cardiovascular events in older subjects (**Figure 5-32**) (118). P-P is also a good predictor of degree of coronary atheroma severity in elderly with diabetes (119). The Framingham group have also shown that in older subjects, CHD risk increased with a lower DBP (**Figure 5-33**) (120), as is the case for CV risk in patients with isolated systolic hypertension (121). In elderly hypertensives with coronary artery disease, P-P was a weaker predictor of cardiovascular outcome than either SBP or DBP (122).

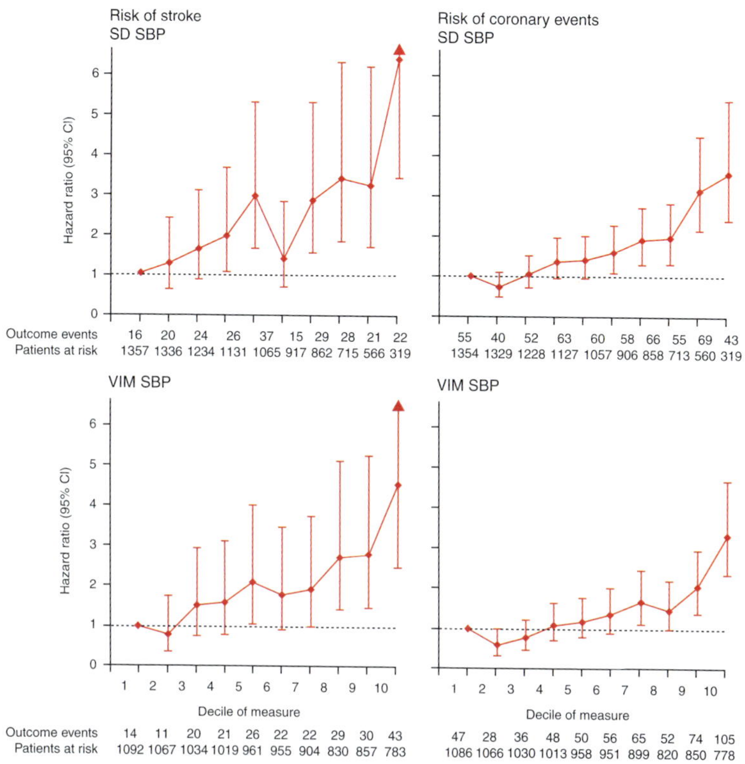

Fig. 5-31 The ASCOT Study; in older hypertensives a high variability of SBP [SD of first seven readings or variation independent of mean (VIM)] was a strong predictor of both stroke (left) and coronary events (right). (From Rothwell PM, Howard SC, Dolan E, et al. Prognostic significance of visit to visit variability, maximum systolic blood pressure, and episodic hypertension. *Lancet* 2010;375:895–905.)

8. Some final thoughts

A) Plasma renin as a risk factor

It was in 1972 that Brunner and Laragh addressed the issue of renin as a predictor of cardiovascular disease in hypertensives (123). They indicated that normal and high-renin subjects, compared with low-renin subjects, experienced an excess of myocardial infarction and stroke events. In middle-aged (mean age of 53 years) hypertensives, high renin levels were particularly powerful in predicting myocardial infarction, especially in the presence of other risk factors such as smoking, LVH, high cholesterol, and blood sugar levels (**Figure 5-34**)

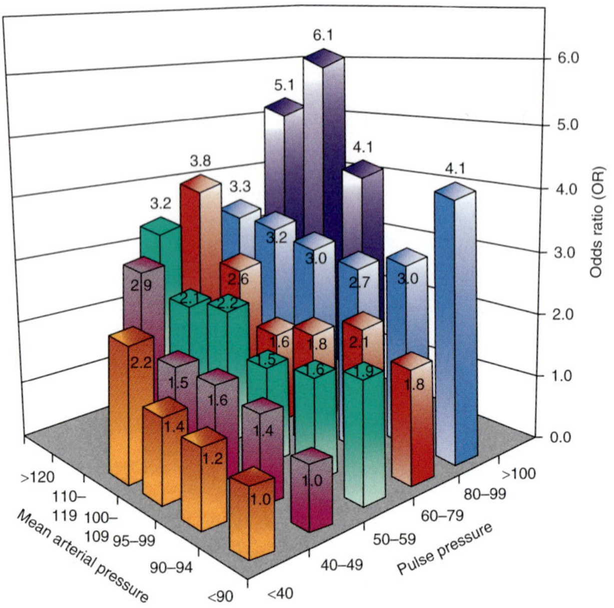

Fig. 5-32 Framingham: in a 50-year follow-up of 9657 subjects, the best predictor of CV events was a combination of mean BP and P-P. (From Franklin SS, Lopex VA, Wong DD, et al. Single versus combined blood pressure components and risk of cardiovascular disease: the Framingham Heart Study. *Circulation* 2009;119:243–50.)

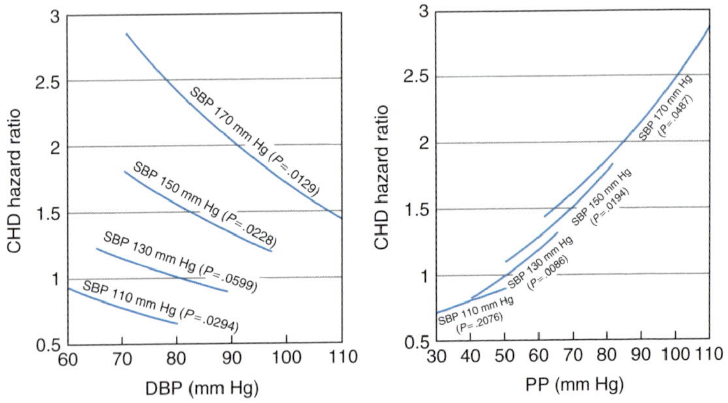

Fig. 5-33 Framingham: in 1924 older (mean age of 62 years) subjects who were followed up for 20 years, the risk of CHD increased with a decreasing DBP (left) and an increasing P-P (right). (From Franklin SS, Khan SA, Wong ND, et al. Is pulse pressure useful in predicting risk for coronary heart disease? The Framingham Study. *Circulation* 1999;100:354–60.)

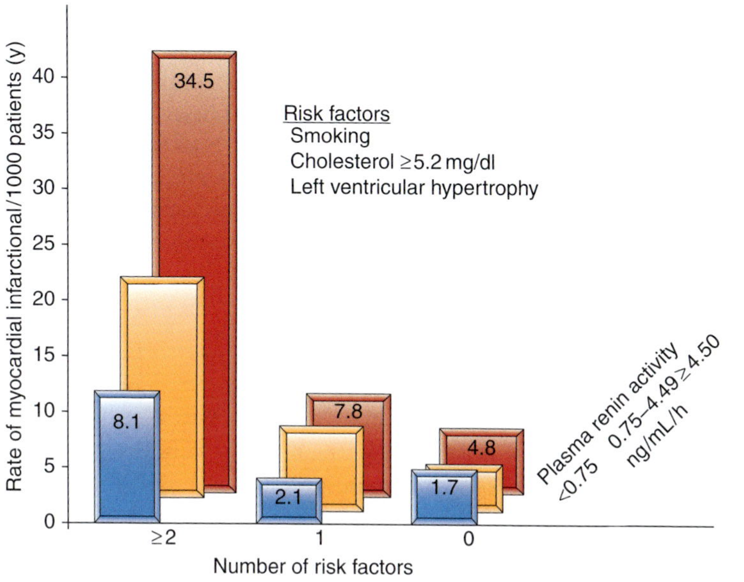

Fig. 5-34 Plasma renin is a good predictor of MI in middle-aged hypertensive patients, particularly when other risk factors are present. (From Alderman MH, Laragh JH, Sealey JE. More about plasma renin and cardiovascular mortality. *Eur Heart J* 2011;32:2610–2.)

(124, 125). In middle-aged subjects, high plasma renin levels are also a powerful predictor of sudden death and heart failure (126). Several other studies, but not all, confirmed these findings (127). The HOPE study, involving high-risk subjects, showed that high plasma renin activity predicted major vascular events and mortality (128).

The Framingham group studied 3408 subjects, having a mean age of 59 years, (with a 1413 subset of hypertensives) for 7.2 years (129). They showed that a higher plasma renin level was associated with a greater short-term mortality, but not with cardiovascular end points.

However, plasma renin activity may just be a surrogate marker for sympathetic nerve activity (plasma noradrenaline), as the predictive value of renin in heart failure disappears, when corrected for plasma noradrenaline levels (130).

B) Blood pressure and pregnancy

In pregnant women with no history of hypertension (131), 24-hour BP measurements were able to rule out white-coat hypertension and showed that true hypertension in the third trimester was linked to a shorter duration of pregnancy, increased risk of preeclampsia, increased risk of cesarean delivery, a lower neonatal weight, and a longer hospital stay. In a large study of 210,814 first singleton births from mothers with no hypertension before 20 weeks gestation (132), both low and high DBP were associated with small babies and high perinatal mortality. Interestingly, the onset of preeclampsia was a predictor of later onset (postpregnancy) of cardiovascular disease (133).

C) Blood pressure and postischemic stroke

A high BP postischemic stroke is self-limiting over a 10-day period (134). Poststroke hypertension occurs in 70%–80% of cases and is associated with a poor prognosis (134), the best outcome being associated with a low/normal BP in the first 24–48 hours (135). No benefit accrues from lowering acute poststroke, high BP (136). In the sub-acute poststroke period, bendrofluazide may limit the BP rise seen during stroke recovery (137). A large study, $n = 20{,}330$, of postischemic stroke cases showed that over a period of 2.5 years, an increasing SBP from low-normal, through high to very high, was associated with an increasing risk of further stroke and myocardial infarction or vascular death (138).

D) Blood pressure and dementia

The Framingham group have shown that raised mid-life BP is closely linked to cognitive impairment in later life (139). Certainly, this was the case for middle-aged women followed up for 37 years (140). In middle-aged men followed up for 20 years, a combination of high middle-aged DBP and low plasma β-amyloid levels, predicted Alzheimer disease later in life (141). In hypertensive mice there is brain parenchymal beta-amyloid deposition, accompanied by cognitive deterioration (142).

E) Resistant hypertension

Resistant hypertension is defined as high BP that remains uncontrolled in spite of receiving at least 3 different classes (1 being a diuretic) of antihypertensive medications (143). On the basis of 3 large studies, the prevalence of resistant hypertension appeared to be between 12% and 15% (143). However, a 4-year follow-up of 205,750 hypertensives revealed that only 2% developed resistant hypertension, and they were more likely to be men, older, and had higher rates of diabetes than nonresistant patients (144). The prognosis of these resistant hypertensives was not good; such cases had a significant 47% increased risk of experiencing a cardiovascular event—mainly related to the kidney (144).

SUMMARY AND CONCLUSIONS

1. High BP is number 1 risk factor for premature death around the world, with about 80% of this burden falling in low- and middle-income economies.
2. Most risk factor outcome studies have been based on clinic/office BP values and show that myocardial infarction and stroke are the major killers, followed by heart failure and renal failure, and that the risk is linear down to 115 mm Hg SBP and 75 mm Hg; at age greater than 85 years, there is no relationship between high BP and mortality.
3. Hypertension and prehypertension have to be viewed in the context of multiple risk factors, that is, total cholesterol, HDL cholesterol, diabetes, smoking, renal function, LVH and BP during exercise and the rate of recovery; so that the decision to treat will depend on total risk to make the intervention optimally cost effective.
4. Home BP readings avoid white-coat hypertension, often seen in office/clinic readings, and reveal masked hypertension; home BP is accordingly a better predictor of premature death and cardiovascular end points than clinic BP and is cost effective.
5. ABPM provides a 24-hour picture of BP and, like home BP, is superior to clinic/office BP as a predictor of outcome; additional information of the early morning BP "surge," nocturnal BP, and "dipping" status, add to ABPM's power as a predictor of outcome.
6. Central BP, particularly P-P, has proved to be superior to clinic (but maybe not ABPM) P-P, as a predictor of cardiovascular outcome in elderly men, but maybe not women; central augmentation index (AIx) and pulse wave velocity (PWV) can add to the predictive powers of central BP in the elderly, but not all agree.
7. In younger/middle-aged subjects, DBP (but not isolated diastolic hypertension) is the most powerful predictor of outcome, undoubtedly due to its close link to high sympathetic nerve activity and the resultant underlying inflammatory process (high CRP and IL-6); certainly, β-blockade is highly effective in suppressing raised CRP levels associated with stress, hypertension,

and ischemia: importantly, high plasma noradrenaline levels predict CV mortality (independent of BP and smoking), and high levels of intralymphocyte β-receptor density and cyclic AMP levels strongly predict myocardial infarction (but not stroke), again independent of BP.

8. In middle-aged/older subjects, SBP becomes the major determinant of outcome; variability (SD) of clinic and home, but not 24 hour, BPs has been shown to be a powerful predictor of cardiovascular outcome; an interarm difference of SBP of 10 mm Hg or more is predictive of reduced cumulative survival.
9. In elderly systolic hypertensives (in the absence of coronary heart disease), P-P, particularly if combined with mean arterial pressure, is the most powerful predictor of outcome; in this group, a low DBP is linked to a worse prognosis.
10. High plasma renin levels (probably reflecting high sympathetic nerve activity) in middle aged, are associated with a higher short-term mortality, particularly myocardial infarction.
11. True hypertension, in the third trimester of pregnancy, is linked to a shorter duration of pregnancy, an increased risk of preeclampsia, an increased risk of cesarean delivery, a lower neonatal weight, and a longer hospital stay: both a high and low DBP increases the risk of small babies and perinatal mortality.
12. A high BP immediately postischemic stroke is self-limiting, should not be treated, but is nevertheless linked to a poor prognosis: a low- normal through to a very high SBP in the subacute period, over a 2.5-year period, is linked to an increased risk of a further cardiovascular event.
13. A high, mid-life BP is predictive of cognitive impairment and dementia in later life.
14. Resistant hypertension occurs in about 12%–15% of cases, more likely in men, older patients, and those with diabetes; patients with resistant hypertension have a significant 47% increased risk of experiencing a cardiovascular event.

REFERENCES

1. Lopez AD, Mathers CD, Ezzati M, et al. Global and regional burden of disease and risk factors, 2001: systematic analysis of population health data. *Lancet* 2006;367:1747–57.
2. Yang Q, Cogswell ME, Flanders WD, et al. Trends in cardiovascular health metrics and associations with all-cause and CVD mortality among US adults. *JAMA* 2012;307:1273–83.

3. Lawes CM, Hoorn SV, Rodgers A, et al. Global burden of blood pressure-related disease, 2001. *Lancet* 2008;371:1513–18.
4. Kannel WB. Elevated systolic blood pressure a cardiovascular risk factor. *Am J Cardiol* 2000;85:251–5.
5. Prospective Studies Collaboration. Age-specific relevance of usual blood pressure to vascular mortality: a meta-analysis of individual data for one million adults in 61 prospective studies. *Lancet* 2002;360:1903–13.
6. Allen N, Berry JD, Ning H, et al. Impact of blood pressure and blood pressure change during middle-age on the remaining lifetime risk foe cardiovascular disease. *Circulation* 2012;125:37–44.
7. Van Bemmel T, Gussekl J, Westendorp R, et al. In a population-based prospective study, no association between high blood pressure and mortality after age 85 years. *J Hypertens* 2006;24:287–92.
8. Staessen JA, Kuznetsova T, Stolarz K. Hypertension prevalence and stroke mortality across populations. *JAMA* 2003;289:2420–2.
9. Song Y-M, Sung J, Lawlor DA, et al. Blood pressure, haemorrhagic stroke and ischaemic stroke: the Korean national prospective occupational cohort study. *BMJ* 2004;328:324–5.
10. Miura K, Nakagawa H, Ohashi Y, et al. Four blood pressure indexes and the risk of stroke and myocardial infarction in Japanese men and women. *Circulation* 2009;119:1892–8.
11. Levy D, Larson MG, Vasan RS, et al. The progression from hypertension to congestive heart failure. *JAMA* 1996;275:1557–62.
12. Tozawa M, Iseki K, Iseki C, et al. Blood pressure predicts risk of developing end-stage renal disease in men and women. *Hypertension* 2003;41:1341–5.
13. Kim DH. Differences in blood pressure between arms. *BMJ* 2012; 344:9.
14. Clark CE, Taylor RS, Shore AC, et al. The difference in blood pressure readings between arms and survival: a primary care cohort study. *BMJ* 2012;344:19.
15. Kleefstra N, Houweling ST, Bilo HJ. Interarm blood pressure differences and vascular disease. *BMJ* 2012;380:23.
16. Pocock SJ, McCormack V, Grueuffier F, et al. A score for predicting risk of death from cardiovascular disease in adults with raised blood pressure, based on individual patient data from randomised controlled trials. *BMJ* 2001;323:75–81.
17. Tozawa M, Oshiro S, Iseki C, et al. Multiple risk factor clustering of hypertension in a screened cohort. *J Hypertens* 2000;18:1379–85.
18. Nash IS. Reassessing normal blood pressure. *BMJ* 2007;335:408–9.
19. Wu K, Xie L, Chen D, et al. The natural history of borderline hypotension in a Chinese population. *J Hum Hypertens* 1997;11:95–100.
20. Fukuhara M, Arima H, Ninomiya T, et al. Impact of lower range of prehypertension on cardiovascular events in a general population: the Hisayama Study. *J Hypertens* 2012;30:893–900.

21. Grotto I, Grossman E, Huerta M, et al. Prevalence of pre-hypertension and associated cardiovascular risk profiles among young Israeli adults. *Hypertension* 2006;48:254–9.
22. Conen D, Ridker PM, Buring JE, et al. Risk of cardiovascular events among women with high, normal blood pressure or blood pressure progression: prospective cohort study. *BMJ* 2007;335:432–6.
23. Kshirsagar AV, Carpenter M, Bang H, et al. Blood pressure usually considered normal is associated with an elevated risk of cardiovascular disease. *Am J Medic* 2006;119:133–41.
24. Zhang Y, Lee ET, Devereux RB, et al. Prehypertension, diabetes and cardiovascular disease risk in a population-based sample. *Hypertension* 2006;47:410–4.
25. Ventura HO, Lavie CJ. Antihypertensive therapy for pre-hypertension. *JAMA* 2011;305:940–1.
26. Rossi A, Dikareva A, Bacon SL, et al. The impact of physical activity on mortality in patients with high blood pressure: a systematic review. *J Hypertens* 2012;30:1277–88.
27. Singh JP, Larson MG, Manolio TA, et al. Blood pressure response during treadmill testing as a risk factor for new-onset hypertension. The Framingham heart study. *Circulation* 1999;99:1831–6.
28. Weiss SA, Blumenthal RS, Sharatt AR, et al. Exercise blood pressure and future cardiovascular death in asymptomatic individuals. *Circulation* 2010;121:2109–16.
29. Allison TG, Cordeiro MA, Miller TD, et al. Prognostic significance of exercise-induced systemic hypertension in healthy subjects. *Am J Cardiol* 1999;83:371–5.
30. Lewis GD, Gona P, Larson MG, et al. Exercise blood pressure and the risk of incident cardiovascular disease (from the Framingham Heart Study). *Am J Cardiol* 2008;101:1614–20.
31. Laukkanen JA, Kurl S, Salonen R, et al. Systolic blood pressure during recovery from exercise and the risk of myocardial infarction in middle-aged men. *Hypertension* 2004;44:820–5.
32. Madias JE. Blunted decline in systolic blood pressure after exercise predicts future acute myocardial infarction. *Hypertension* 2004; 44:807–8.
33. Thanassoulis G, Lyass A, Benjamin EJ, et al. Relations of exercise blood pressure responce to cardiovascular risk factors and vascular function in the Framingham Heart Study. *Circulation* 2012;125: 2836–43.
34. Pickering TG, James GD, Bodie C, et al. How common is white-coat hypertension. *JAMA* 1988;259:225–8.
35. Gosse P, Promax H, Durandet P, et al. White-coat hypertension. No harm to the heart. *Hypertension* 1993;22:766–70.
36. Hänninen MR, Niiranen TJ, Puukka PJ, et al. Prognostic significance of masked and white-coat hypertension in the general population: the Finn-Home Study. *J Hypertens* 2012;30:705–12.

37. Franklin SS, Thijs L, Hansen TW, et al. Significance of white-coat hypertension in older persons with isolated systolic hypertension. *Hypertension* 2012;59:564–71.
38. O'Brien E. Blood pressure measurement is changing. *Heart* 2001; 85:3–5.
39. Glen SK, Elliot HL, Curzio JL, et al. White-coat hypertension is a cause of cardiovascular dysfunction. *Lancet* 1996;348:654–7.
40. Khattar RS, Senior R, Lahiri A. Cardiovascular outcome in white-coat versus sustained mild hypertension: a 10-year follow-up study. *Circulation* 1998;98:1892–7.
41. Hansen TW, Kikuya M, Thijs L, et al. Prognostic superiority of daytime ambulatory over conventional blood pressure in four populations: a meta-analysis of 7,030 individuals. *J Hypertens* 2007;25:1554–64.
42. Mancia G, Bombelli M, Facchetti R, et al. Long-term risk of sustained hypertension in white-coat or masked hypertension. *Hypertension* 2009;54:226–32.
43. Ohkubo T, Imai Y, Tsuji I, et al. Home blood pressure measurement has a stronger predictive power for mortality than does screening blood pressure measurement: a population-based observation in Ohasama, Japan. *J Hypertens* 1998;16:971–5.
44. Stergiou GS, Baibas NM, Kalogeropoulos PG. Cardiovascular risk prediction based on home blood pressure measurement: the Didima study. *J Hypertens* 2007;25:1590–6.
45. Ward AM, Takahashi O, Stevens R, et al. Home measurement of blood pressure and cardiovascular disease: systematic review and meta-analysis of prospective studies. *J Hypertens* 2012;30:449–56.
46. Matsui Y, Ishikawa J, Eguchi K, et al. Maximum value of home blood pressure. A novel indicator of target organ damage in hypertension. *Hypertension* 2011;57:1087–93.
47. Bobrie G, Chatellier G, Genes N, et al. Cardiovascular prognosis of masked hypertension detected by blood pressure self-measurement in elderly treated hypertensive patients. *JAMA* 2004;291:1342–9.
48. Stergiou G, Mengden T, Padfield P, et al. Self monitoring of blood pressure at home. *BMJ* 2004;329:870–1.
49. Niiranen TJ, Johansson JK, Reunanen A, et al. Optimal schedule for home blood measurement based on prognostic data: the Finn-Home Study. *Hypertension* 2011;57:1081–6.
50. Stergiou GS, Siontis KC, Ioannidis JP. Home blood pressure as a cardiovascular outcome predictor: it's time to take it seriously. *Hypertension* 2010;55:1301–3.
51. Johansson JK, Niiranen TJ, Puukka PJ, et al. Prognostic value of the variability in home-measured blood pressure and heart rate: the Finn-Home Study. *Hypertension* 2012;59:212–18.
52. Ohkubo T, Hozawa A, Nagai K, et al. Prediction of stroke by ambulatory blood pressure monitoring versus screening blood pressure

measurements in a general population: the Ohasama study. *J Hypertens* 2000;18:847–54.
53. Hansen TW, Jeppesen J, Rasmussen S, et al. Ambulatory blood pressure and mortality. *Hypertension* 2005;45:499–504.
54. White WB. The risk of waking up. Impact of the morning surge in blood pressure. *Hypertension* 2010;55:835–7.
55. Kario K, Pickering TG, Umeda Y, et al. Morning surge in blood pressure as a predictor of silent and clinical cerebrovascular disease in elderly hypertensives. *Circulation* 2003;107:1401–6.
56. Metoki H, Ohkubo T, Kikuya M, et al. Prognostic significance for stroke of a morning pressure surge and nocturnal blood pressure decline: the Ohasama study. *Hypertension* 2006;47:149–54.
57. Verdecchia P, Angeli F, Mazzotta G, et al. Day-night dip and early-morning surge in blood pressure in hypertension. Prognostic implications. *Hypertension* 2012;60:34–42.
58. Staessen JA, Thijs L, Fagard R, et al. Predicting cardiovascular risk using conventional vs ambulatory blood pressure in older patients with systolic hypertension. *JAMA* 1999;282:539–46.
59. de la Sierra A, Banegas JR, Segura J, et al. Ambulatory blood pressure monitoring and development of cardiovascular events in high-risk patients included in the Spanish ABPM registry. *J Hypertens* 2012;30:713–9.
60. Ingelsson E, Björklund-Bodegård K, Lind L, et al. Diurnal blood pressure pattern and risk of congestive heart failure. *JAMA* 2006;295:2859–66.
61. Dolan E, Stanton A, Thijs L, et al. Superiority of ambulatory over clinic blood pressure measurement in predicting mortality: the Dublin outcome study. *Hypertension* 2005;46:156–61.
62. Boggia J, Thijs L, Hansen TW, et al. Ambulatory blood pressure monitoring in 9,357 subjects from 11 populations highlights missed opportunities for cardiovascular prevention in women. *Hypertension* 2011;57:397–405.
63. O'Brien E. Dipping comes of age: the importance of nocturnal blood pressure. *Hypertension* 209;53:446–7.
64. Ohkubo T, Hozawa A, Yamaguchi J, et al. Prognostic significance of the nocturnal decline in blood pressure in individuals with and without high 24-h blood pressure: the Ohasama study. *J Hypertens* 2002;20:2183–9.
65. Boggia J, Thijs L, Hansen TW, et al. Prognostic accuracy of day versus night ambulatory blood pressure: a cohort study. *Lancet* 2007;370:1219–29.
66. Roman MJ, Devereux RB, Kizer JR, et al. Central pressure more strongly relates to vascular disease and outcome than does brachial pressure. *Hypertension* 2007;50:197–203.
67. Agabiti-Rosei E, Mancia G, O'Rourke MF, et al. Central blood pressure measurements and antihypertensive therapy. *Hypertension* 2007;50:154–60.

68. Vlachopoulos C, Aznaouridis K, O'Rourke MF, et al. Prediction of cardiovascular events and all-cause mortality with central haemodynamis. *Eur Heart J* 2010;31:1865–71.
69. Huang C-M, Wang K-L, Cheng H-M, et al. Central versus ambulatory blood pressure in the prediction of all-cause and cardiovascular mortalities. *J Hypertens* 2011;29:454–9.
70. Dart AM, Gatzka CD, Kingwell BA, et al. Brachial blood pressure but not carotid arterial waveforms predict cardiovascular events in elderly female hypertensives. *Hypertension* 2006;47:785–90.
71. Nürnberger J, Keflioglu-Scheiber A, Saez AM, et al. Augmentation index is associated with cardiovascular risk. *J Hypertens* 2002;20:2407–14.
72. Weber T, Auer J, O'Rourke MF, et al. Arterial stiffness, wave reflections and the risk of coronary artery disease. *Circulation* 2004;109:184–9.
73. O'Rourke MF. From theory into practice: arterial haemodynamics in clinical hypertension. *J Hypertens* 2002;20:1901–15.
74. Mitchell GF, Hwang SJ, Vasan RS, et al. Arterial stiffness and cardiovascular events: the Framingham Heart Study. *Circulation* 2010;121:505–11.
75. Laurent S, Cockcroft J, Van Bortel L, et al. Expert consensus document on arterial stiffness methodological issues and clinical applications. *Eur Heart J* 2006;27:2588–605.
76. Meaume S, Rudnichi A, Lynch A, et al. Aortic pulse wave velocity as a marker of cardiovascular disease in subjects over 70 years old. *J Hypertens* 2001;19:871–7.
77. van Popele NM, Mattace-Raso FV, Vliegenthart R, et al. Aortic stiffness is associated with atherosclerosis of the coronary arteries in older adults: the Rotterdam Study. *J Hypertens* 2006;24:2371–6.
78. Hope SA, Antonis P, Adam D, et al. Arterial pulse wave velocity but not augmentation index is associated with coronary artery disease extent and severity: implications for arterial transfer function applicability. *J Hypertens* 2007;25:2105–9.
79. Sutton-Tyrell K, Najjar SS, Boudreau RM, et al. Elevated pulse wave velocity, a marker of arterial stiffness, predicts cardiovascular events in well-functioning older adults. *Circulation* 2005;111:3384–90.
80. Hansen TW, Staessen JA, Torp-Pedersen C, et al. Prognostic value of aortic pulse wave velocity as index of arterial stiffness in the general population. *Circulation* 2006;113:664–70.
81. Lebrun CE, van der Schouw YT, Bak AA, et al. Arterial stiffness in postmenopausal women: determinants of pulse wave velocity. *J Hypertens* 2002;20:2165–72.
82. Franklin SS, Larson MG, Khan SA, et al. Does the relation of blood pressure to coronary heart disease risk change with aging? The Framingham Heart Study. *Circulation* 2001;103:1245–9.

83. Falkstedt D, Koupil L, Hemmingsson T. Blood pressure in late adolescence and early incidence of coronary artery disease and stroke in the Swedish 1969 conscription cohort. *J Hypertens* 2008;26:1313–20.
84. Sundstrom J, Neovius M, Tynelius P, et al. Association of blood pressure in late adolescence with subsequent mortality: cohort study of Swedish man conscripts. *BMJ* 2011;342:483.
85. Silventoinen K, Magnasson PK, Neovius M, et al. Does obesity modify the effect of blood pressure on the risk of cardiovascular disease? *Circulation* 2008;118:1637–42.
86. Mosley II WJ, Greenland P, Garside DB, et al. Predictive utility of pulse-pressure and other blood pressure measures for cardiovascular outcomes. *Hypertension* 2007;49:1256–64.
87. Wilkinson IB, Franklin SS, Hall I, et al. Pressure amplification explains why pulse pressure is unrelated to risk in young subjects. *Hypertension* 2001;38:1461–6.
88. Strandberg TE, Salomaa VV, Vanhanen HT, et al. Isolated diastolic hypertension, pulse-pressure, and mean arterial pressure as predictors of mortality during a follow-up of up to 32 years. *J Hypertens* 2002;20:399–404.
89. Verdecchia P, Angeli F. Natural history of hypertension subtypes. *Circulation* 2005;111:1094–6.
90. Blake GJ, Rifai N, Buring JE, et al. Blood pressure, C-reactive protein, and risk of future cardiovascular events. *Circulation* 2003;108:2993–9.
91. Hamer M, Chida Y, Stamatakis E. Utility of C-reactive protein for cardiovascular risk stratification across three age groups in subjects without existing cardiovascular diseases. *Am J Cardiol* 2009;104:538–42.
92. Koenig W, Khuseyinova N, Baumert J, et al. Increased concentration of C-reactive protein and IL-6, but not IL-8, are independently associated with increased coronary events in middle-aged men and women. *Atheroscler Thromb Vasc Biol* 2006;26:2745–51.
93. Ridker PM, Glynn RJ, Henneken CH. C-reactive protein adds to the predictive value of total and HDL cholesterol in determining risk of first myocardial infarction. *Circulation* 1998;97:2007–11.
94. Triant VA, Meigs JB, Grinspoon SK. Association of C-reactive protein and HIV infection with acute myocardial infarction. *J Acquir Immune Defic Syndr* 2009;51:268–73.
95. Bernstein IM, Damron D, Schonberg AL, et al. The relationship of plasma volume, sympathetic tone, and inflammatory cytokines in young healthy non-pregnant women. *Reprod Sci* 2009;16:980–5.
96. Kop WJ, Weissman NJ, Zhu J, et al. Effects of acute mental stress and exercise on inflammatory markers in patients with coronary artery disease and healthy controls. *Am J Cardiol* 2008;101: 767–73.

97. Richards AM, Nicholls MG, Espiner EA, et al. Diurnal patterns of blood pressure, heart rate and vasoactive hormones in normal man. *Clin Exp Hypertens A* 1986;8:153–66.
98. Peng Y-X, Shan J, Qi XY, et al. The catecholamine-beta-adrenoceptor-cAMP system and prediction of cardiovascular events in hypertension. *Clin Exp Pharmacol Physiol* 2006;33:227–31.
99. Cruickshank JM, Prichard BNC. *Beta-Blockers in Clinical Practice.* Edinburgh: Churchill Livingstone; 1994, p95.
100. Kaklinska AM, Mroczko B, Musial WJ, et al. Endothelial dysfunction and sympathetic nervous system activation in young patients with essential arterial hypertension and without hypercholesterolaemia. *Acta Cardiol* 2010;65:535–40.
101. Helin P, Lorenzen I, Garbarsh C, et al. Atherosclerosis in rabbit aorta induced by noradrenaline. The importance of the duration of noradrenaline action. *Atherosclerosis* 1970;12:125–32.
102. Ni M, Wang Y, Zhang M, et al. Atherosclerotic plaque disruption induced by stress and lipopolysaccharide in apolipoprotein E knockout mice. *Am J Physiol Heart Circ Physiol* 2009;296:HI598–606.
103. Li QX, Fu QQ, Shi SV, et al. Relationship between plasma inflammatory markers and plaque fibrous cap thickness determined by intravascular optical coherence tomography. *Heart* 2010;96:196–201.
104. Hong YJ, Mintz GS, Kim SW, et al. Impact of plaque rupture and elevated C-reactive protein on clinical outcome in patients with acute myocardial infarction: an intravascular ultrasound study. *J Invasive Cardiol* 2008;20:428–35.
105. Sattar N, Murray HM, McConnachie A, et al. C-reactive protein and prediction of coronary artery disease and global vascular events in the Prospective Study of Pravastatin in the Elderly at Risk (PROSPER). *Circulation* 2007;115:981–9.
106. Palmas W, Ma S, Psaty B, et al. Antihypertensive medications and C-reactive protein in the multi-ethnic study of atherosclerosis. *Am J Hypertens* 2007;20:233–41.
107. King DE, Egan BM, Mainous AG, et al. The effect of extended release metoprolol succinate on C-reactive protein levels in persons with hypertension. *J Clin Hypertens* 2006;8:257–60.
108. Woiciechowsky C, Asadullah K, Nestler D, et al. Sympathetic activation triggers systemic interleaukin-10 to release in immunodepression induced brain injury. *Nat Med* 1998;4:808–13.
109. Jenkins NP, Keevil BG, Hutchinson LV, et al. Beta-blockers are associated with lower C-reactive protein concentrations in patients with coronary artery disease. *Am J Med* 2002;112:269–74.
110. Beattie MS, Shlipak MG, Liu H, et al. C-reactive protein and ischemia in users and non-users of beta-blockers and statins. *Circulation* 2003;107:245–50.
111. Williams B, Lindholm LH, Sever P. Systolic pressure is all that matters. *Lancet* 2008;371:2219–21.

112. Vasan RS, Larson MG, Leip EP, et al. Impact of high-normal blood pressure on the risk of cardiovascular disease. *N Engl J Med* 2001;345:1291–7.
113. Miura K, Dyer AR, Greenland P, et al. Pulse-pressure compared with other blood pressure indexes in the prediction of 25 year cardiovascular and all-cause mortality rates. *Hypertension* 2001;38:232–7.
114. Palaniappan L, Simons LA, Simons J, et al. Comparison of usefulness of systolic, diastolic and mean blood pressure and pulse-pressure as predictors of cardiovascular death in patients > 60 years of age. *Am J Cardiol* 2002;90:1398–401.
115. Rothwell PM, Howard SC, Dolan E, et al. Prognostic significance of visit to visit variability, maximum systolic blood pressure, and episodic hypertension. *Lancet* 2010;375:895–905.
116. Rossignol P, Cridlig J, Lehert P, et al. Visit-to-visit blood pressure variability is a strong predictor of cardiovascular events in hemodialysis. *Hypertension* 2012;60:339–46.
117. Mancia G, Facchetti R, Parati G, et al. Visit-to-visit blood pressure variability, carotid atherosclerosis, and cardiovascular events in the European Lacidipine Study on Atherosclerosis. *Circulation* 2012;126:569–78.
118. Franklin SS, Lopex VA, Wong DD, et al. Single versus combined blood pressure components and risk of cardiovascular disease: the Framingham Heart Study. *Circulation* 2009;119:243–50.
119. Halon DA, Dobrecky-Mery I, Gaspar T, et al. Pulse-pressure and coronary atherosclerosis in asymptomatic type 2 diabetes mellitus. *Int J Cardiol* 2010;143:63–71.
120. Franklin SS, Khan SA, Wong ND, et al. Is pulse pressure useful in predicting risk for coronary heart disease? The Framingham heart study. *Circulation* 1999;100:354–60.
121. Franklin SS, Chow VH, Mon AD, et al. The significance of low DBP in US adults with isolated systolic hypertension. *J Hypertens* 2011;29:1101–8.
122. Bangalore S, Messerli FH, Franklin SS, et al. Pulse pressure and risk of cardiovascular outcomes in patients with hypertension and coronary artery disease: an INVEST Study. *Eur Heart J* 2009;30:1395–401.
123. Brunner HR, Laragh JH, Baer L, et al. Essential hypertension: renin and aldosterone, heart attack, stroke. *N Engl J Med* 1972;286:441–8.
124. Alderman MH, Madhaven S, Ooi WL, et al. Association of the renin-sodium profile with the risk of myocardial infarction in patients with hypertension. *N Engl J Med* 1991;324:1098–104.
125. Alderman MH, Laragh JH, Sealey JE. More about plasma renin and cardiovascular mortality. *Eur Heart J* 2011;32:2610–2.
126. Tomaschitz A, Pilz S, Ritz E, et al. Associations of plasma renin with 10-year cardiovascular mortality, sudden cardiac death, and due to heart failure. *Eur Heart J* 2011;32:2642–9.
127. Adiyaman A, Staessen JA. Renin turning full circle as cardiovascular risk factor. *Eur Heart J* 2007;28:2557–8.

128. Verma S, Gupta M, Holmes DT, et al. Plasma renin activity predicts cardiovascular mortality in the Heart Outcomes Prevention Evaluation (HOPE) study. *Eur Heart J* 2011;32:2135–42.
129. Parikh NI, Gona P, Larson MG, et al. Plasma renin and risk of cardiovascular disease and mortality: the Framingham Heart Study. *Eur Heart J* 2007;28:2644–52.
130. Cohn JN. Is activation of the renin-angiotensin system hazardous to your health? *Eur Heart J* 2011;32:2096–7.
131. Bellomo G, Narducci PL, Rondoni F, et al. Prognostic value of 24-hour blood pressure in pregnancy. *JAMA* 1999;282:1447–52.
132. Steer PJ, Little MP, Kold-Jensen T, et al. Maternal blood pressure in pregnancy, birth weight, and perinatal mortality: prospective study. *BMJ* 2004;329:1312–4.
133. Magee LA. Pre-eclampsia and increased cardiovascular risk. *BMJ* 2007;335:945–6.
134. Qureshi AI. Acute hypertensive response in patients with stroke. *Circulation* 2008;118:176–87.
135. Ntaios G, Lambrou D, Michel P. Blood pressure change and outcome in acute ischemic stroke. *J Hypertens* 2011;29:1583–9.
136. Brege E. Should high blood pressure be lowered in the acute stroke? *J Hypertens* 2011;29:1478–9.
137. Eames PJ, Robinson TG, Panerai RB, et al. The systemic haemodynamic and cerebral autoregulatory effects of bendrofluazide in the subacute post-stroke period. *J Hypertens* 2004;22:2017–24.
138. Ovbiagele B, Diener HC, Yusuf S, et al. Level of systolic blood pressure within the normal range and risk of recurrent stroke. *JAMA* 2011;306:2137–44.
139. Elias MF, Wolf PA, D'Agostino RB, et al. Untreated blood pressure level is inversely related to cognitive functioning: the Framingham Study. *Am J Epidemiol* 1993;138:353–64.
140. Joas E, Backman K, Gustafson D, et al. Blood pressure trajectories from midlife to late life in relation to dementia in women followed for 37 years. *Hypertension* 2012;59:796–801.
141. Shar NS, Vidal J-S, Masaki K, et al. Midlife blood pressure, plasma beta-amyloid, and the risk for Alzeimer disease: the Honolulu Asia Aging Study. *Hypertension* 2012;59:780–6.
142. Carnevale D, Mascio G, D'Andrea I, et al. Hypertension induces brain beta-amyloid accumulation, cognitive impairment, and memory deterioration through activation of receptor for advance glycation end products in brain vasculature. *Hypertension* 2012;60:188–97.
143. Pimenta E, Calhoun DA. Resistant hypertension: incidence, prevalence, and prognosis. *Circulation* 2012;125:1594–6.
144. Daugherty SL, Powers JD, Magid DJ, et al. Incidence and prognosis of resistant hypertension in hypertensive patients. *Circulation* 2012;125:1635–42.

CHAPTER 6

Ways to Lower Blood Pressure

LIFESTYLE

An overview of nondrug ways to lower blood pressure (BP) is shown in **Table 6-1** (1).

1. Weight loss and blood pressure

In obese subjects who lost 13 kg on average, not only was there a fall in plasma insulin, metabolic rate, plasma renin, cardiac output, and heart rate, but also a marked fall in BP (2). A 2-kg loss of weight over 6 months resulted in a fall in BP of 3.7/2.7 mm Hg, and there was a 42% decline in the frequency of hypertension (3). A meta analysis showed that a fall in BP was of the order of 5/5 mm Hg for varying degrees of weight reduction (3).

In younger subjects, weight loss was associated with decreased stiffness of arteries as shown by a significant fall in pulse wave velocity (PWV) (**Figure 6-1**) (4).

2. Exercise and blood pressure

Exercise-induced increases in blood flow result in an increased shear stress on the endothelium, resulting in a release of the vasodilator nitric oxide (NO) (5). The postexercise fall in BP can last until 22 hours, and the degree of fall is similar after a moderate

TABLE 6-1 Overview of nondrug interventions in the treatment of hypertension

Intervention	Treatment effect	Type of evidence available
Lifestyle modification		
DASH diet	↓SBP 5.5 mm Hg (↓SBP 11.4 mm Hg in hypertensive patients)	R, O
Low-salt DASH diet	↓SBP 7.1 mm Hg (↓SBP 11.5 mm Hg in hypertensive patients)	R, O
Dietary supplements		
Potassium	↓SBP 3–12 mm Hg	R, B, P, M
Calcium	↓SBP 1.4–1.7 mm Hg	R, B, P, M
Vitamin D	↓SBP 1.9–3.6 mm Hg[a]	R, B, P, M
Folate	↓SBP 4 mm Hg	R, B, P, C
Coenzyme Q10	↓SBP 16 mm Hg	R, B, P, M
Fish oil	↓SBP 2–3 mm Hg	R, B, P, M
Garlic	↓SBP 10–16 mm Hg[b]	R, P, M
Fruits and vegetables	↓SBP 2.8 mm Hg	R, O
Soy protein	↓SBP 7.8 mm Hg	R, B, P
Flavonoids	↓SBP 3–5 mm Hg	R, P, M
Vegetarian diet	↓SBP 5 mm Hg	R, O
High-fiber diet	↓SBP 1–2 mm Hg	R, B, P, M
Herbal/alternative approaches		
Hawthorn	↓SBP 3.6 mm Hg[a]	R, B, P
Coleus forskohlii	↓Cardiac filling pressures	Comp
Mistletoe	↓BP in rats	Comp, A
Rauwolfia	↓SBP and DBP	Comp
Acupuncture	↓SBP 5 mm Hg[a]	R, B, P, M
Meditation	↓SBP 4.7 mm Hg	R, B, P, M
Devices/interventions		
Rheos implantable baroreflex stimulator	↓SBP 22 mm Hg, >10 mm Hg reduction in SBP in 54% of patients[c]	R, B, P
Symplicity renal sympathetic denervation	↓SBP 32 mm Hg[c]	R, O

TABLE 6-1 Overview of nondrug interventions in the treatment of hypertension (*Continued*)

Intervention	Treatment effect	Type of evidence available
RESPeRATE paced breathing	↓SBP 5–15 mm Hg	R, O
Zona Plus isometric handgrip exercises	↓SBP 5.7 mm Hg	R, O, M

Abbreviations: ↓, decreased; A, animal model; B, blinded; C, cross-sectional; Comp, comparative; DASH, Dietary Approaches to Stop Hypertension; O, open label; P, placebo controlled; M, meta-analysis; R, randomized; SBP, systolic blood pressure.

[a] Nonsignificant.

[b] Study design/blinding issues are present.

[c] Refractory hypertension.

From Woolf KJ (2011).

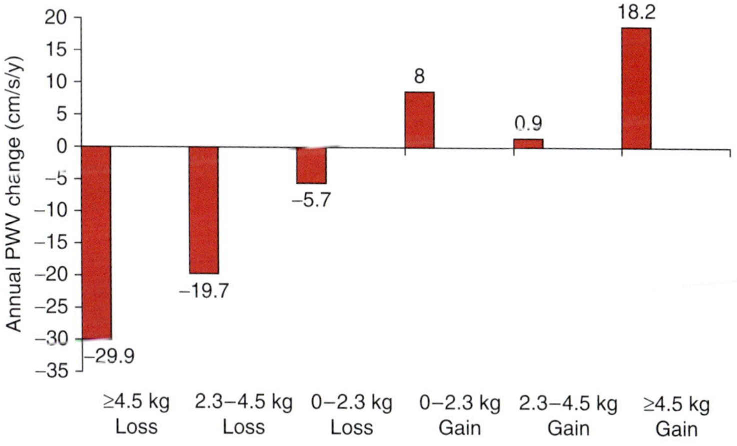

Fig. 6-1 In healthy young adults weight loss was associated with improved vascular compliance (fall in PWV). (From Wildman RP, Farhat GN, Patel AS, et al. Weight change is associated with change in arterial stiffness among healthy young adults. *Hypertension* 2005;45:187–92.)

or light exercise (e.g. brisk walking) (6). Large artery distensibility improves in athletes (7), but this improved vascular compliance observed in the young/middle-aged does not extend to the elderly patients with isolated systolic hypertension (8).

A meta-analysis of randomized, controlled trials showed that aerobic endurance training lowered BP by decreasing the systemic vascular resistance, with no change in cardiac output; plasma, noradrenaline fell by 29%, and plasma renin activity by 20% (**Figure 6-2**) (9). The fall in BP from lifestyle intervention programs was greatest in subjects whose baseline aerobic fitness (vO_2max) was high (**Figure 6-3**) (10). Not all subjects experience a fall in BP with increasing energy expenditure, as no fall in BP occurs with certain genetic variants, for example, GPR1O (G-protein coupled receptor) (11).

The exercise-induced fall in BP is greater in subjects with hypertension, being on average a fall of 7.5/5.8 mm Hg, compared with 2.6/1.8 mm Hg in normotensives (12). High physical activity levels accordingly reduced the risk of developing hypertension, particularly if overweight, in both men (**Figure 6-4**) and women (**Figure 6-5**) (13).

Anaerobic or resistance training also lowers BP by 3.2/3.5 mm Hg (14).

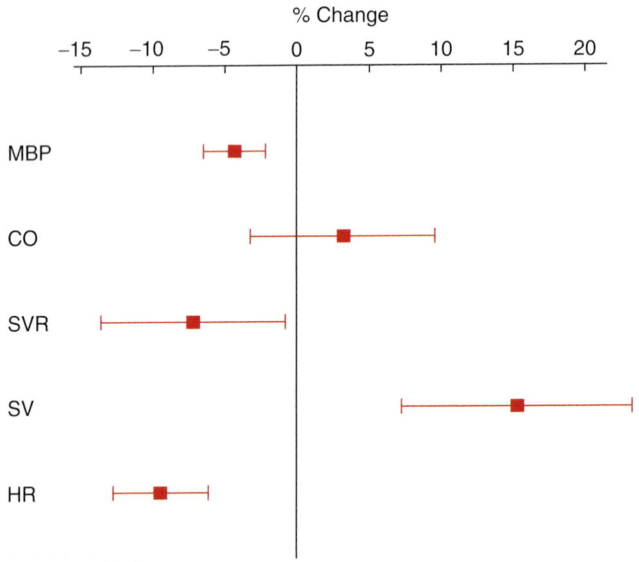

Fig. 6-2 A meta-analysis of 72 trials; aerobic training is linked to a fall in BP, HR and vascular resistance (SVR). (From Cornelissen VA, Fagard RH. Effects of endurance training on blood pressure, blood pressure-regulating mechanisms, and cardiovascular risk factors. *Hypertension* 2005;46:667–75.)

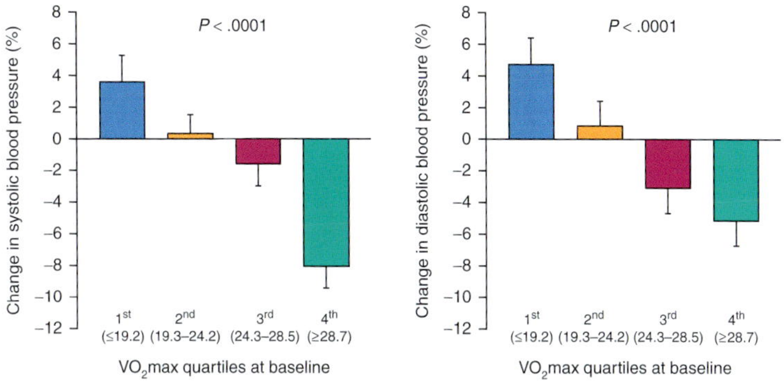

Fig. 6-3 In high-risk middle-aged subjects high cardiorespiratory fitness (vO_2max) is linked to a marked reduction in BP. (From Totsikas C, Rohm J, Kantartzis K, et al. Cardiorespiratory fitness determines the reduction in blood pressure and insulin resistance during lifestyle intervention. *J Hypertens* 2011;29:1220–7.)

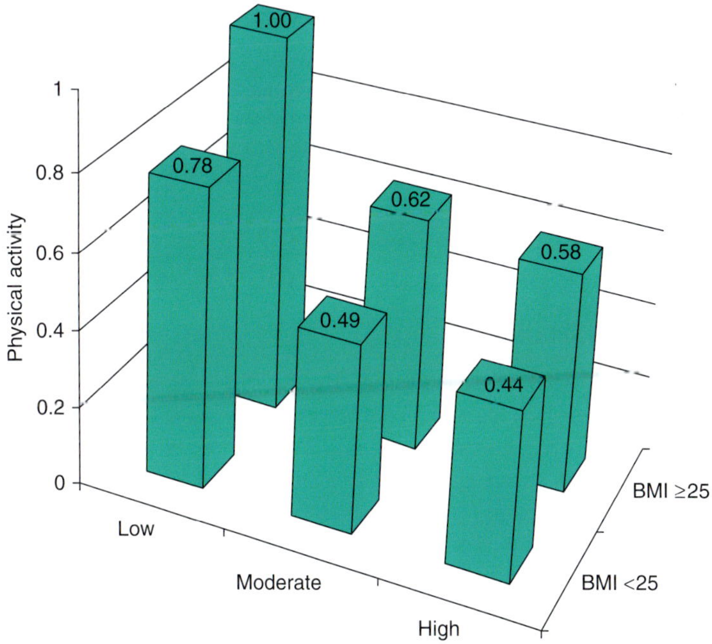

Fig. 6-4 In 8302 middle-aged men followed up for 11 years a low BMI plus a high physical activity level led to a marked reduced risk of developing hypertension. (From Hu G, Barengo NC, Tuomilehto J, et al. Relationship of physical activity and body mass index to the risk of hypertension: a Prospective Study in Finland. *Hypertension* 2004;43:25–30.)

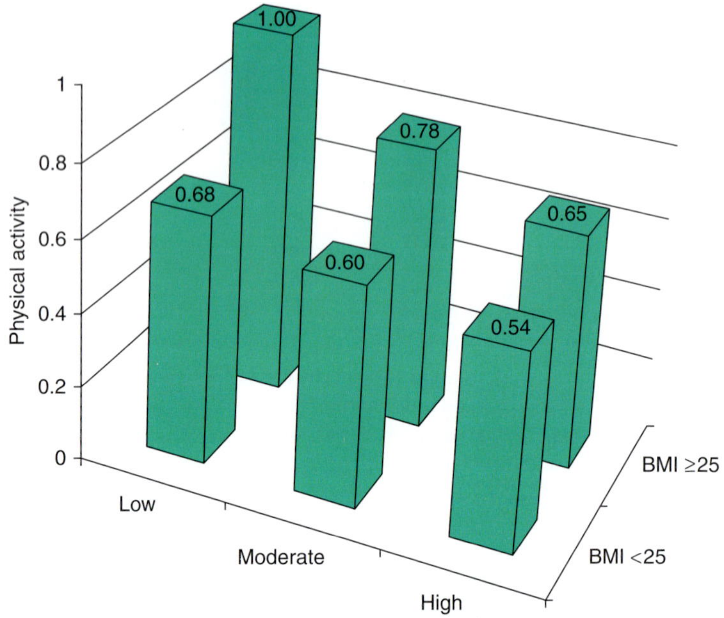

Fig. 6-5 In 9139 middle-aged women followed up for 11 years, a low BMI plus a high physical activity level markedly reduced the risk of developing hypertension. (From Hu G, Barengo NC, Tuomilehto J, et al. Relationship of physical activity and body mass index to the risk of hypertension: a Prospective Study in Finland. *Hypertension* 2004;43:25–30.)

3. Dietary patterns and blood pressure

A) The DASH diet

The classic DASH study examined the BP-lowering effects of a randomized diet rich in fruit and vegetables versus a diet rich in fruit and vegetables plus reduced saturated and total fat versus a control group in 459 subjects, mean age 44 years, and mean BP 131/85 mm Hg, over an 8-week period (15). The results are shown in **Figure 6-6**. The combination diet lowered BP by 5.5/3.0 mm Hg versus control diet and by 11.4/5.5 mm Hg in the 133 subjects with hypertension. This impressive lowering of raised BP is similar to that from drug monotherapy. A further examination of 72 subjects with stage 1 isolated systolic hypertension showed that the combination diet in DASH lowered BP by 12/3 mm Hg (16). In obese subjects (mean age of 35 years) with stage 1 hypertension, the DASH diet lowered BP by 8.1/7.4 mm

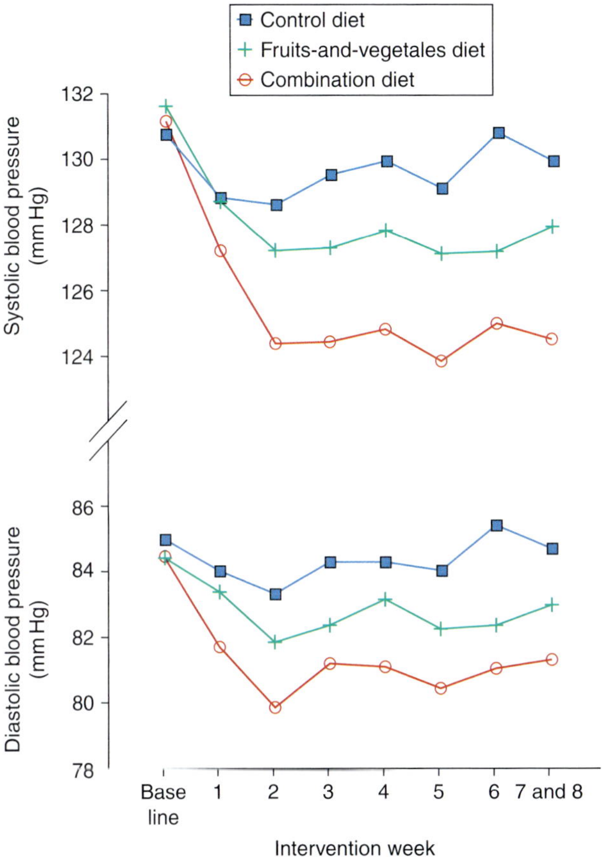

Fig. 6-6 DASH diet; effect of fruit/vegetable or fruit/vegetable/low-fat diet on BP in 459 mild hypertensives. (From Appel LJ, Moore TJ, Obarzanek E, et al. A clinical trial of the effects of dietary patterns on blood pressure. *N Engl J Med* 1997;336:1117–24.)

Hg (**Figure 6-7**) (17). The fall in BP on the DASH diet was found to be linked to a marked naturetic effect (18). The DASH diet was clearly high in potassium content, and increased dietary potassium is known to lower BP (19), as is ascorbic acid (**Figure 6-8**) (20, 21).

B) Carbohydrate diets and chocolate

Reducing the consumption of sugar-sweetened beverages results in a fall in BP (22). In a prospective, randomized, crossover study in patients with prehypertension, or mild hypertension, BP was lower during the

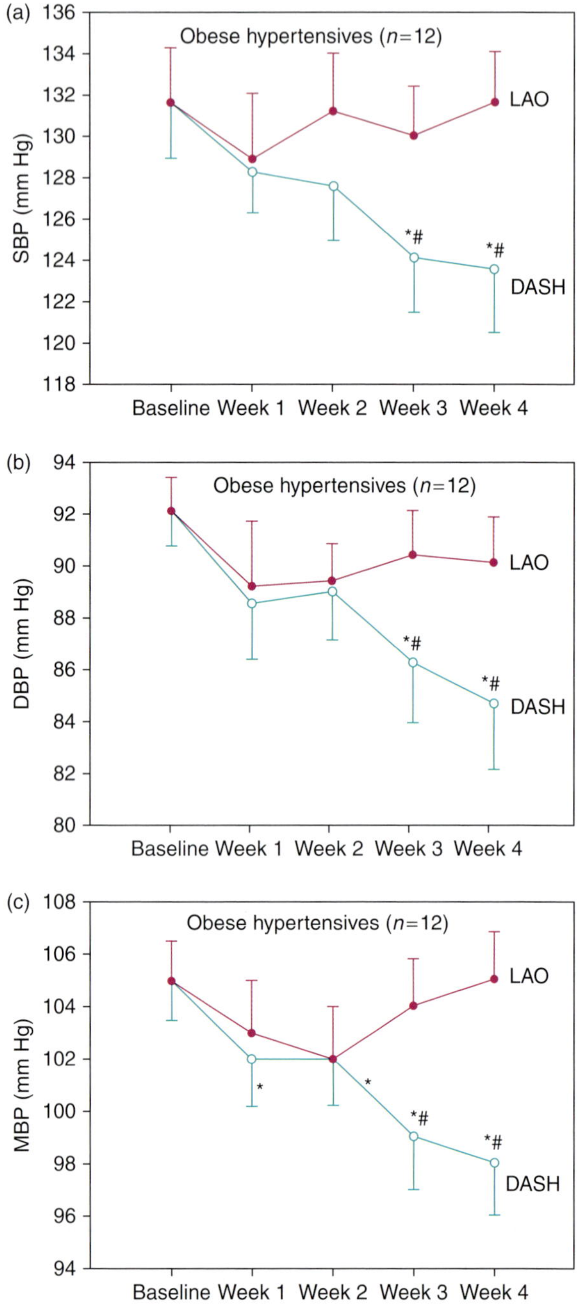

Fig. 6-7 Effect of DASH versus low-antioxidant (LAO) diets on BP in obese hypertensives. (From Lopez HF, Martin KL, Nashar K, et al. DASH diet lowers blood pressure and lipid-induced oxidative stress in obesity. *Hypertension* 2003;41:422–30.)

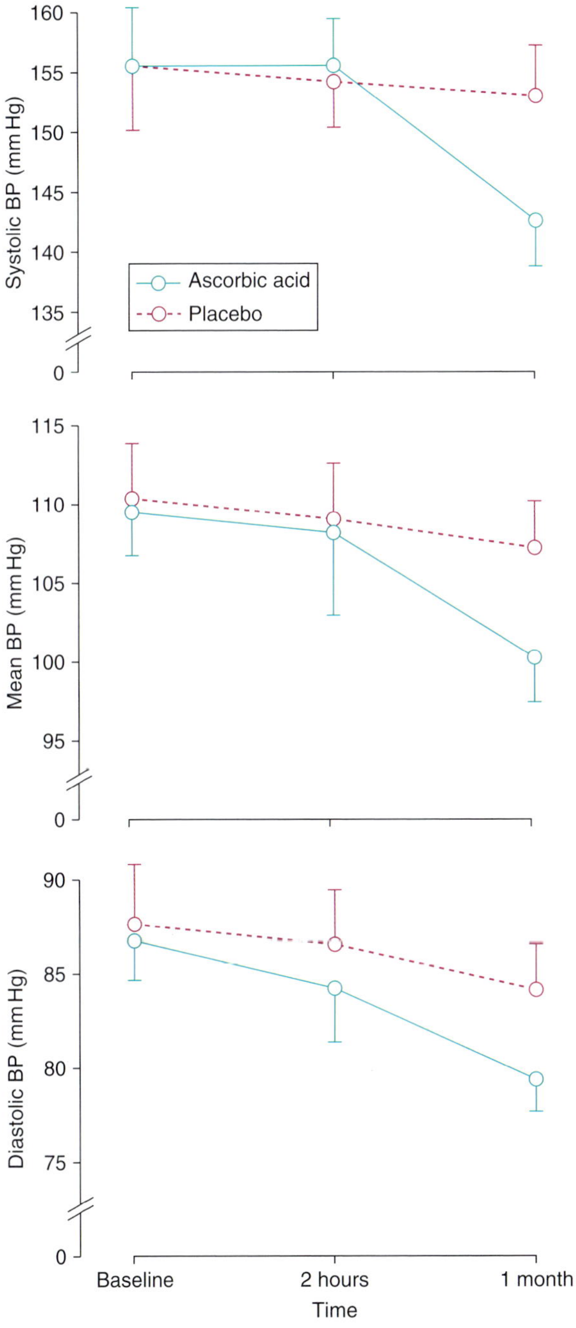

Fig. 6-8 In hypertensive patients, ascorbic acid was more effective than placebo in lowering BP. (From Duffy SJ, Gokce N, Holbrook M, et al. Treatment of hypertension with ascorbic acid. *Lancet* 1999;354:2048–9.)

6-week high protein or high unsaturated fat dietary periods compared with a high carbohydrate 6-week dietary period (**Figure 6-9**) (23).

Cocoa-containing foods improve endothelial function through NO release and lower BP (24). Dark brown, but not white, chocolate was shown to lower BP of mild hypertensives by 3/2 mm Hg (24).

C) Nuts

In the large Nurses Health Study (25), women who consumed > 2 servings of nuts per week had an 18% reduction in cardiac death compared to women who did not eat nuts regularly. Nuts (pistashios) have been noted to lower blood pressure via a reduction in peripheral resistance (26).

D) Beverages

The effect of coffee drinking on BP differs in habitual and nonhabitual drinkers (27). Although habitual coffee drinkers experience an increase in muscle sympathetic nerve activity, there is little or no change in BP (**Figure 6-10**). This contrast with nonhabitual drinkers who experience a similar increase in sympathetic nerve activity

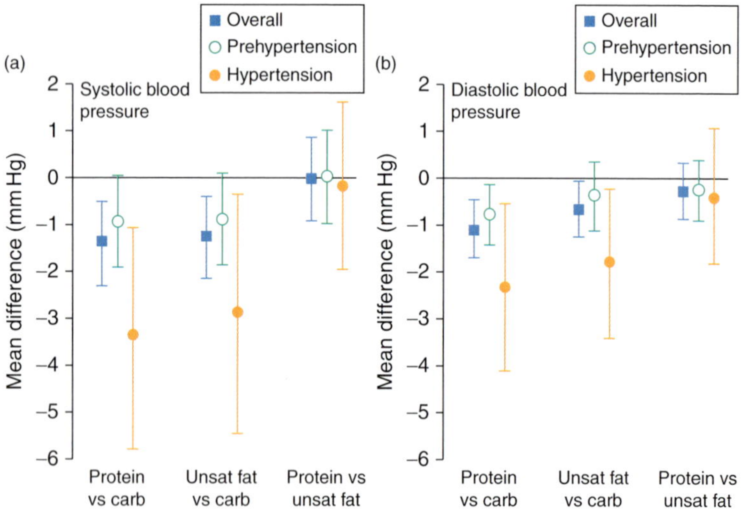

Fig. 6-9 Effect of high protein versus high carbohydrate versus high monounsaturated diets over 6 weeks on BP of hypertensive patients. (From Appel LJ, Sacks FM, Carey VJ, et al. Effects of protein, monosaturated fat, and carbohydrate intake on blood pressure and serum lipids. *JAMA* 2005;294:2455–64.)

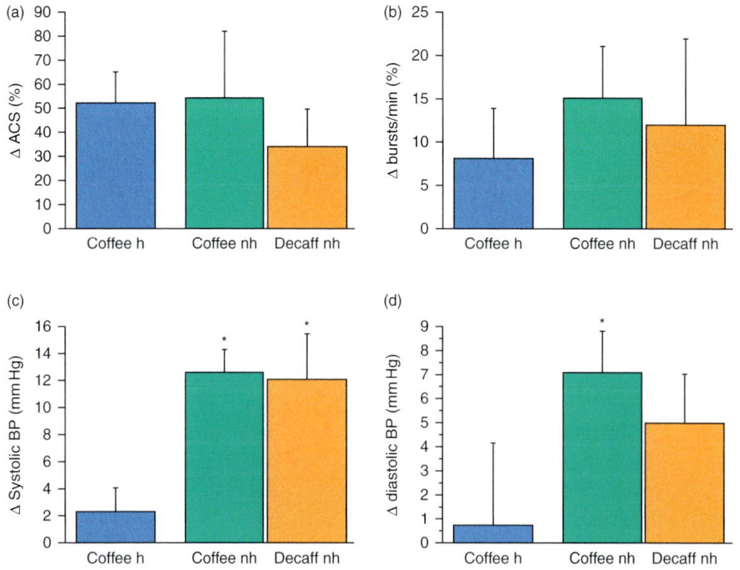

Fig. 6-10 Both coffee and decaffeinated coffee increase sympathetic nerve activity in habitual (h) and non-habitual (nh) drinkers—A and B, but increase BP only in nh-drinkers—C and D. (From Corti R, Binggeli C, Sudano I, et al. Coffee acutely increases sympathetic nerve activity and blood pressure independently of caffeine content. *Circulation* 2002;106:2935–40.)

but also a marked increase in BP, not only with caffeinated, but also with decaffeinated coffee! (Figure 6-10). This implies that ingredients other than caffeine must be responsible for cardiovascular activation.

E) Alcohol

The initial effect of alcohol is to lower both peripheral and central BP within the first few hours of ingestion (28). Both red and white wine were equally effective (28). Although switching from high to low alcohol intake is linked to a modest fall in BP (29), BP is closely linked to the number of drinks per day, particularly in men (**Figure 6-11**) (30). Heavy drinking is linked to an increased arterial stiffening (31).

F) Sodium intake and blood pressure

The classic study to address the issue of dietary sodium and BP was the DASH diet with variable sodium content (32). This study of 412 subjects, mean age of 48 years, with 57 black subjects, compared the DASH diet with a control diet, and within each group were 3 levels of sodium intake—low, intermediate, and high. The

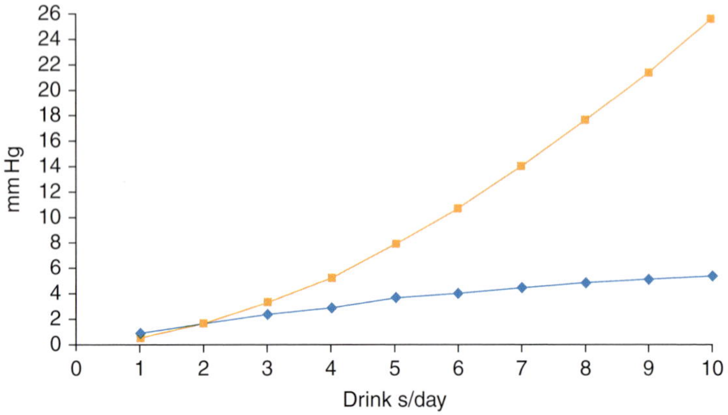

Fig. 6-11 SBP rises in accordance with the number of drinks per day, particularly in men (squares). (From Moreira LB, Fuchs FD, Moraes RS, et al. Alcohol intake and blood pressure: the importance of time since the last drink. *J Hypertens* 1998;16:175–80.)

effects of the various diets on BP are shown in **Figure 6-12**. In the normotensives, the mean fall in SBP was 7.1 mm Hg, and in the hypertensives, the fall was 11.5 mm Hg.

Not all subjects on a low-sodium diet experienced a fall in BP; 38% experience a small (up to 5 mm Hg) increase in systolic blood pressure (SBP) (33). The effect of the low-sodium diet was similar in subjects of African or non-African descent (34). The best results were in the elderly (**Figure 6-13**) (35). Chinese patients with the metabolic syndrome are particularly salt sensitive and have the best fall in BP to low-sodium diets (**Figure 6-14**) (36). The results of an overview indicated that over a 1-year follow-up, the fall in BP to a low-sodium diet in hypertensives was 3.6–8.0 mm Hg SBP and 1.9–2.8 mm Hg diastolic blood pressure (DBP) (37).

Salt reduction improves vascular compliance in white, black, and Asian hypertensives, but the reduction in PWV was significant in black subjects only (38). The improvement in vascular compliance from low-sodium diets in the elderly systolic hypertensives is accompanied by a fall in carotid SBP, pulse pressure, and augmentation index (AIx) (**Table 6-1a**) (39).

One big concern with low-sodium diets is their effect on plasma renin/aldosterone and noradrenaline levels, and the possible detrimental effects on morbidity and survival. A meta-analysis of 58 trials

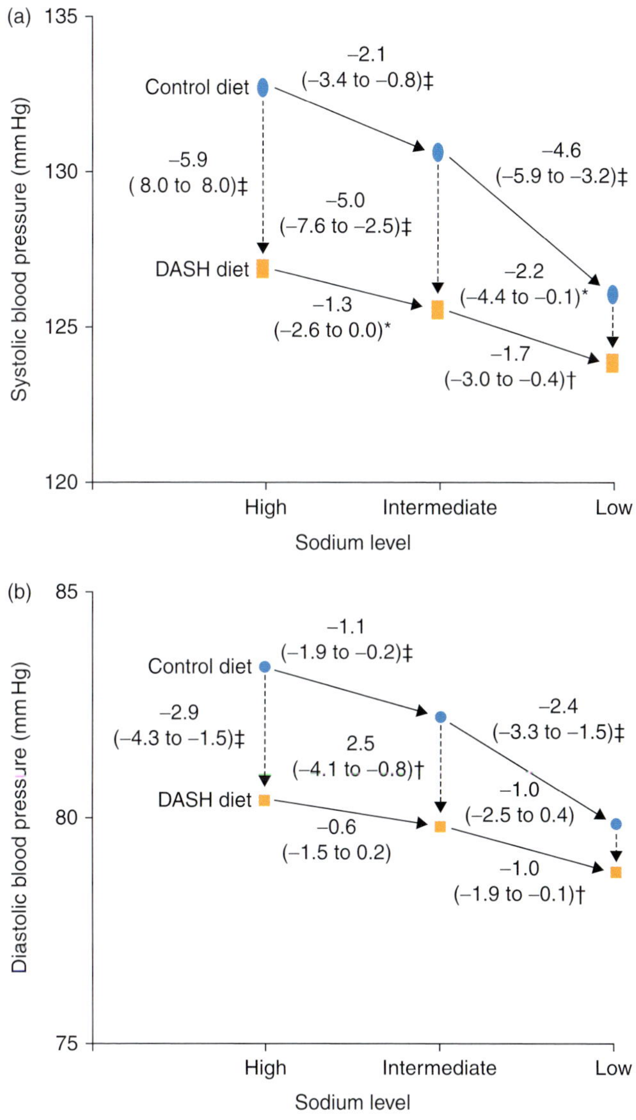

Fig. 6-12 In middle-aged subjects (575 black), a DASH diet plus low sodium intake versus control is highly effective in reducing BP. (From Sacks FM, Svetkey LP, Vollmer WM, et al. Effects on blood pressure of reduced dietary sodium and the dietary approaches to stop hypertension (DASH) diet. *N Engl J Med* 2001;344:3–10.)

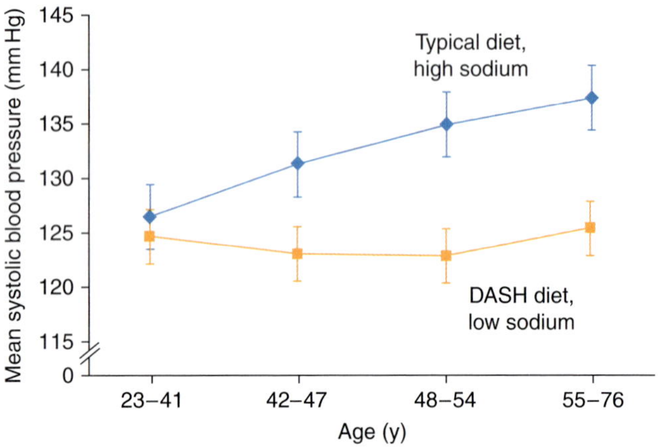

Fig. 6-13 Antihypertensive effect of "low-sodium DASH Diet" is greatest in the middle-aged/elderly patients. (From Sacks FM, Campos H. Dietary therapy in hypertension. *N Engl J Med* 2010;362:2102–12.)

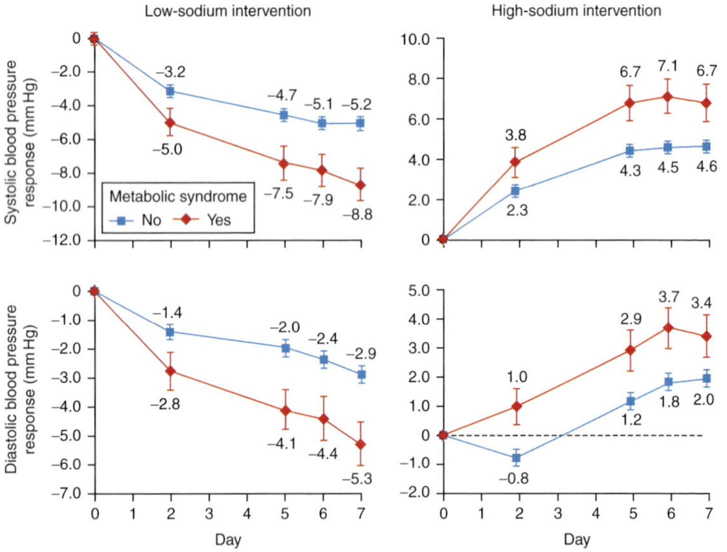

Fig. 6-14 Chinese patients with the metabolic syndrome are highly sensitive to high-/low-sodium diets in terms of change in BP. (From Chen J, Gu D, Huang J, et al. Metabolic syndrome and salt-sensitivity of blood pressure in non-diabetic people in China. *Lancet* 2009;373:829–35.)

TABLE 6-1A In the elderly, central (carotid) pressures are more responsive than brachial BP to low-sodium diets

	Condition		
Variable	Baseline	Low sodium	Normal sodium
Heart rate (bpm)	61 ± 3	60 ± 3	60 ± 3
Augmentation index (%)	40 ± 2	29 ± 2†‡	37 ± 2
Carotid artery systolic pressure (mm Hg)	134 ± 5	119 ± 5†‡	127 ± 4§
Carotid artery pulse pressure (mm Hg)	50 ± 6	40 ± 6†‡	46 ± 5
Brachial artery pulse pressure (mm Hg)	66 ± 3	58 ± 4†‡	62 ± 3§

From Gates PE, Tanaka H, Hiatt WR, et al. Dietary sodium restriction rapidly improves large elastic artery compliance in older adults with systolic hypertension. *Hypertension* 2004;44:35–41.

†‡ high statistical significance

§ lesser statistical significance

in hypertensives showed that low sodium intake (low urinary sodium excretion) was linked to marked and significant increases in plasma renin, aldosterone, and noradrenaline levels (a 3.6-fold increase in renin, a 3.2-fold increase in aldosterone, and a 32% increase in noradrenaline) (40). Such changes in mice on low-sodium diets are linked to increased atherogenesis (41). Only a large prospective, randomized, controlled, hard end-point trial will settle this controversy.

G) Antistress yoga techniques

Yoga, meditation, and music decrease sympathetic nervous activity, and reduce BP variability and resting values (217). Slow breathing can achieve the same results (217). This system requires 2 15-minute sessions daily, aiming for at least 45 minutes slow breathing per week. The system coaches patients to coordinate their breathing with music. Such a technique is lacking in adverse reactions, but does require a fair amount of discipline. Poor hearing (frequent in the elderly) complicates the use of this device. Also, a persistent lowering of BP by this method seems unlikely. Studies on this technique require randomized controls, such as meditative relaxation, to estimate the contributions of the placebo effect to the BP response.

H) Lifestyle and governmental initiatives around the world

The first randomized, controlled study assessing the effects of a comprehensive lifestyle intervention (weight loss, diet, and exercise) in obese hypertensives showed that over 2 months, the intervention group lost 4.9 kg in weight and experienced impressive lowering of BP over 24 hours (particular daytime) (**Figure 6-15**) (42). Other prospective controlled lifestyle trials, extending up to 2 years, have had good results on BP control (43–45).

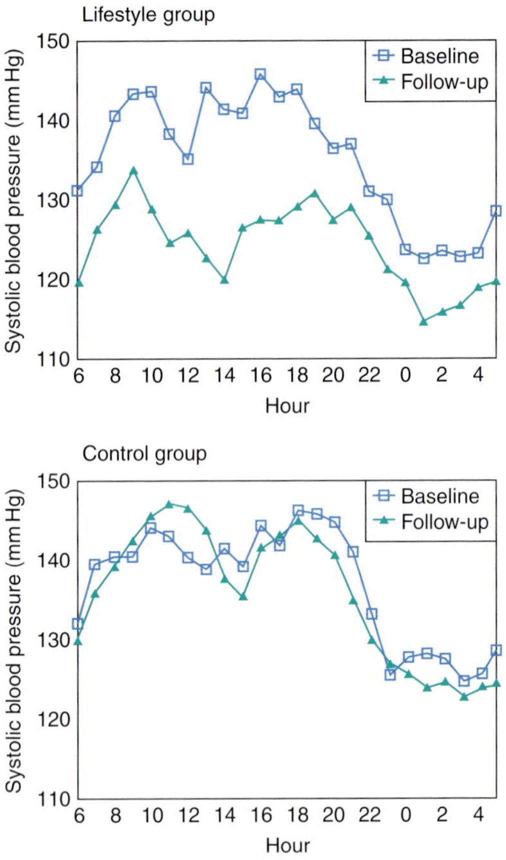

Fig. 6-15 Obese hypertensives respond well to a "lifestyle" regimen (diet, exercise, low salt) versus control over 9 weeks with weight loss and a fall in BP. (From Miller 3rd ER, Erlinger TP, Young DR, et al. Results of Diet, Exercise and Weight Loss Intervention Trial (DEW-IT). *Hypertension* 2002;40:612–8.)

There is clearly a need for educational and governmental programs to influence lifestyle and BP at the national level. It is known that subject-educational level is inversely correlated with BP (46). A public health approach could lead to a small change in BP in the population, which could lead to impressive declines in the number of cardiovascular (CV) events (**Figure 6-16**) (47). Such an approach would be highly cost effective (48), particularly in countries like Japan and China that have very high salt levels in their diet. In Japan, a government-led health plan has greatly reduced salt intake, and as a result of this, stroke rates have fallen by more than 70% (49). Other countries have health strategies, but no such a health campaign has been carried out in China yet (**Table 6-2**) (50). In China, public health services are concentrated in urban areas; for poor rural areas, there is a need for low-cost intervention strategies that include low-cost antihypertensive drugs (51).

The food industry clearly has a role to play, particularly in food labeling. This would be especially relevant to salt levels, with the possible use of a traffic-light device, with red for salt at 2.5 gm per 100 gm or more (52). Statements from the Heart or Hypertension Associations might also be useful, particularly in assessing the strength of the evidence supporting certain approaches (**Table 6-3**) (53).

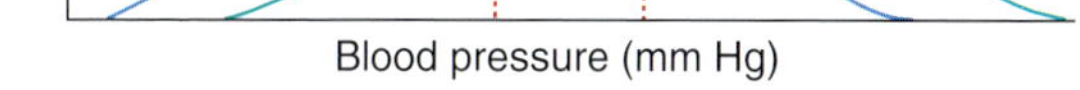

Reduction in BP (mm Hg)	% Reduction in mortality Stroke	CHD	Total
2	−6	−4	−3
3	−8	−5	−4
5	−14	−9	−7

Fig. 6-16 Public health strategies involving regular exercise, loss of weight, alcohol consumption, sodium and potassium intake, fresh fruit and vegetables and sodium intake could prevent hypertension in the population and reduce morbidity. (From Whelton PK, He J, Appel LJ. Primary prevention of hypertension. Clinical and public health advisory from the National High Blood Pressure Education Program. *JAMA* 2002;288:1882–8.)

TABLE 6-2 National salt-reduction initiatives around the world

	Food reformulation	Consumer education	Front-of-back labeling
Argentina	Mandatory (planned)	–	–
Australia	Voluntary	NGO	%DI/Logo (Vol)
Barbados	Voluntary	Government	–
Belgium	Voluntary	Government	–
Brazil	Voluntary	–	–
Bulgaria	Voluntary	–	–
Canada	Voluntary	NGO	Logo (Vol)
Chile	Planned	Government	W (Man)
China	None	Government	–
Cyprus	Voluntary	Government	–
Denmark	Voluntary	Government	Logo (Man)
Fiji	Voluntary	Government	–
Finland	**Voluntary**	**NGO**	**W (Man)**
France	**Voluntary**	**Government**	**–**
Hungary	Voluntary	Planned	–
Ireland	**Voluntary**	**Government**	**%DI (Vol)**
Italy	Voluntary	–	–
Japan	**None**	**NGO**	–
Latvia	Voluntary	Planned	–
Lithuania	Voluntary	Planned	–
Malaysia	Voluntary	NGO	–
Netherlands	Voluntary	NGO	%DI/Logo (Vol)
New Zealand	Voluntary	NGO	%DI/Logo (Vol)
Norway	Voluntary	Planned	–
Poland	Voluntary	Planned	–
Portugal	Mandatory (planned)	Government	–
Singapore	Voluntary	Government	Logo (Vol)
Slovenia	Voluntary	Planned	–
Spain	Voluntary (bread)	Government	–
Switzerland	Planned	Planned	–
UK	**Voluntary**	**Government**	**TL/%DI (Vol)**
USA	Voluntary	NGO	–

Abbreviations: %DI, percentage daily intake labeling (or guideline daily amount in some countries); Man, mandatory; NGO, nongovernment organization; dashes indicate not aware of program in place; TL, traffic light labeling; Vol, voluntary

Countries in bold are countries with evidence of program efficacy.

From Webster JL, Dunford EK, Hawkes C, et al. Salt reduction initiatives around the world. *J Hypertens* 2011;29:1043–50.

TABLE 6-3 Dietary approaches to prevent and treat hypertension; strength of evidence

	Hypothesized effect	Evidence
Weight	Direct	++
Sodium chloride (salt)	Direct	++
Potassium	Inverse	++
Magnesium	Inverse	+/–
Calcium	Inverse	+/–
Alcohol	Direct	++
Fat		
Saturated fat	Direct	+/–
Omega-3 polyunsaturated fat	Inverse	++
Omega-6 polyunsaturated fat	Inverse	+/–
Monounsaturated fat	Inverse	+
Protein		
Total protein	Uncertain	+
Vegetable protein	Inverse	+
Animal protein	Uncertain	+/–
Carbohydrate	Direct	+
Fiber	Inverse	+
Cholesterol	Direct	+/–
Dietary patterns		
Vegetarian diets	Inverse	++
DASH-type dietary patterns	Inverse	++

+/– indicates limited or equivocal evidence; +, suggestive evidence, typically from observational studies and some clinical trials; and ++, persuasive evidence, typically from clinical trials.

From Appel LJ, Brands MW, Daniels SR, et al. Dietary approaches to prevent and treat hypertension. A Scientific Statement from the American Heart Association. *Hypertension* 2006;47:296–308.

DRUG THERAPY

1. Diuretics—thiazide-type and spironolactone

A) Efficacy in lowering brachial BP

i) Effect of age/renin status/race

As indicated in Chapter 5, with increasing age there is desensitization of β-receptors, so that β-1-stimulation-induced increases in plasma renin activity (from the juxtaglomerular apparatus in kidney) are blunted, resulting in low plasma renin activity in the older hypertensives. Low renin, salt-sensitive hypertension responds well to diuretics (and poorly to β-blockers) (**Figure 6-17**) (54).

Like elderly white subjects, black young/middle-aged hypertensives tend to have low renin levels and respond well to diuretics, but not to propranolol (**Figure 6-18**) (55).

ii) Are all diuretics equally effective in lowering BP?

Retrospective analysis of the MRFIT study (56) suggests that chlorthalidone lowers SBP more effectively than hydrochlorthiazide (**Figure 6-19**), and this has been confirmed in a formal randomized, crossover study using 24-hour ambulatory monitoring (57). This advantage of chlorthalidone over hydrochlorthiazide is particularly apparent at night (58). Spironolactone is an aldosterone antagonist as well as a diuretic and appears to be superior to thiazide diuretics in lowering BP (59).

ii) Diuretics compared to other antihypertensive drug classes

In young/middle-aged hypertensives, under double-blind, randomized, crossover conditions (6 weeks on each drug), bendrofluazide

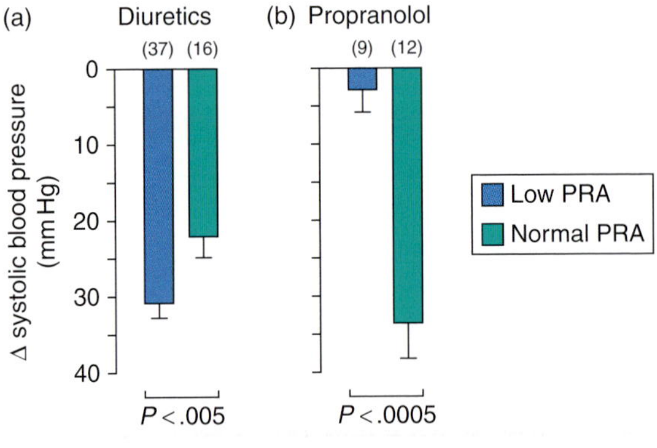

Fig. 6-17 The effect of renin status on response to diuretics and β-blockers in elderly systolic hypertensives. (From Niarchos AP. Pathophysiology, diagnosis and treatment of hypertension in the elderly. *Cardiovasc Rev Rep* 1980;1:621–7.)

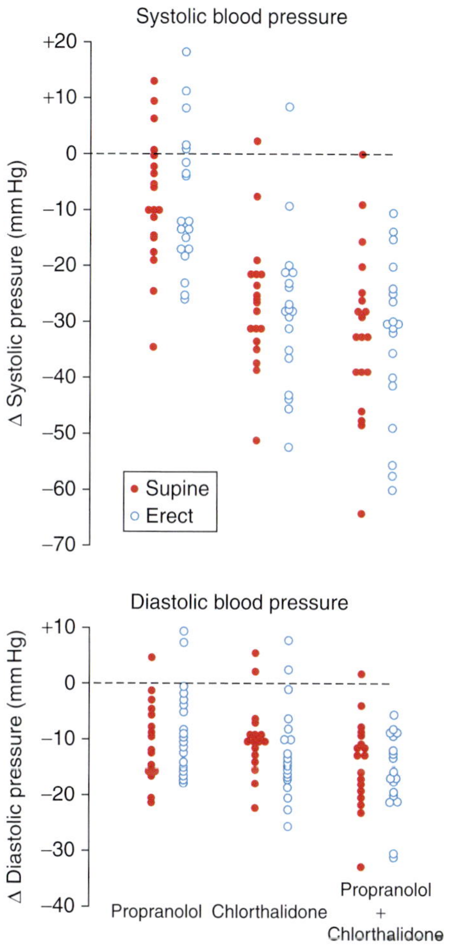

Fig. 6-18 The efficacy of propranolol, diuretics and their combination in black hypertensive patients. (From Richardson DW, Freund J, Gear AS, et al. Effect of propranolol on elevated arterial blood pressure. *Circulation* 1968;37:534–42.)

was the least effective antihypertensive compared with amlodipine, doxazosin, lisinopril, and bisoprolol (**Figure 6-20**) (60).

The so-called HANE study, involving 868 hypertensives, confirmed the poor efficacy of a thiazide diuretic in younger patients (**Figure 6-21**) (61). In subjects aged less than 54 years, atenolol was the best antihypertensive, while the calcium blocker nitrendipine, and the diuretic hydrochlorthiazide the least effective at lowering BP. In contrast, in subjects older than 54 years, the diuretics performed well.

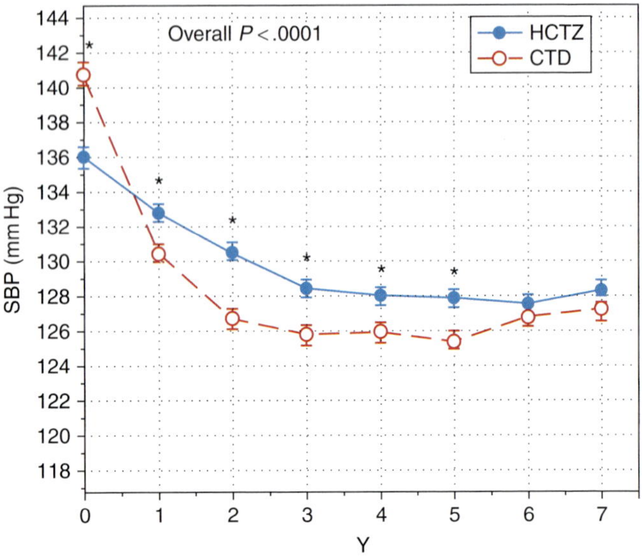

Fig. 6-19 In MRFIT database, chlorthalidone (CTD) was a more effective antihypertensive agent than hydrochlorthiazide (HCTZ). (From Dorsch MP, Gilespie BW, Erickson SR, et al. Chorthalidone reduces cardiovascular events compared with hydrochlorthiazide. *Hypertension* 2011;57:689–94.)

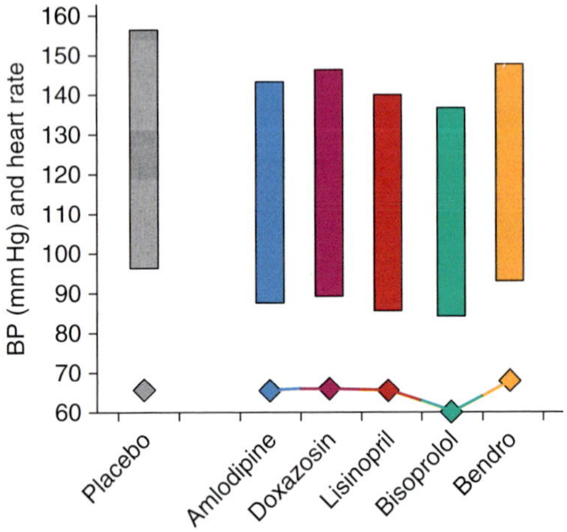

Fig. 6-20 In 34 young/middle-aged (28–55 y) hypertensives, Bisoprolol 5 mg was more effective than Amlodipine 5 mg, Doxazosin 104 mg, Bendrofluazide 2.5 mg, Lisinopril 2.5–10 mg (double-blind, crossover, 1 mo each). (From Deary AJ, Schumann AL, Murfeet H, et al. Double-blind, placebo controlled crossover comparison of 5 classes of drugs. *J Hypertens* 2002;20:771–7.)

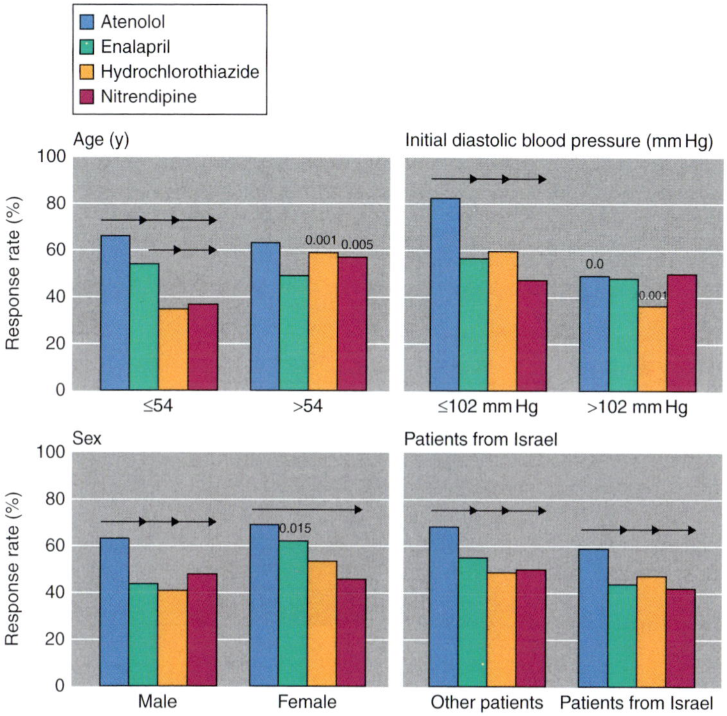

Fig. 6-21 Hane study; In 868 middle-aged hypertensives, under randomized conditions atenolol was the most effective agent, irrespective of age, sex, and severity of hypertension. (From Philipp T, Anlauf M, Distler A, et al. Randomised, double-blind, multicentre comparison of hydrochlorthiazide, atenolol, nitrendipine and enalapril in antihypertensive treatment: results of the HANE study. *BMJ* 1997;315:154–9.)

B) Efficacy in lowering central BP and improving vascular compliance

i) Vascular compliance

Large artery distensibility decreases with age, particularly in elderly subjects with hypertension (**Figure 6-22**) (62). As described in Chapter 2, with stiffening of the large arteries, the reflected wave from the periphery speeds up and arrives centrally during systole, to increase the central SBP, P-P, and AIx. Treatment can improve distensibility (compliance) by improving either structural or functional factors.

Diuretics improve vascular compliance in hypertensives, but this effect reflects only the fall in BP (63, 64); unlike vasodilators such as angiotensin-converting enzyme inhibitors (ACEIs) and calcium

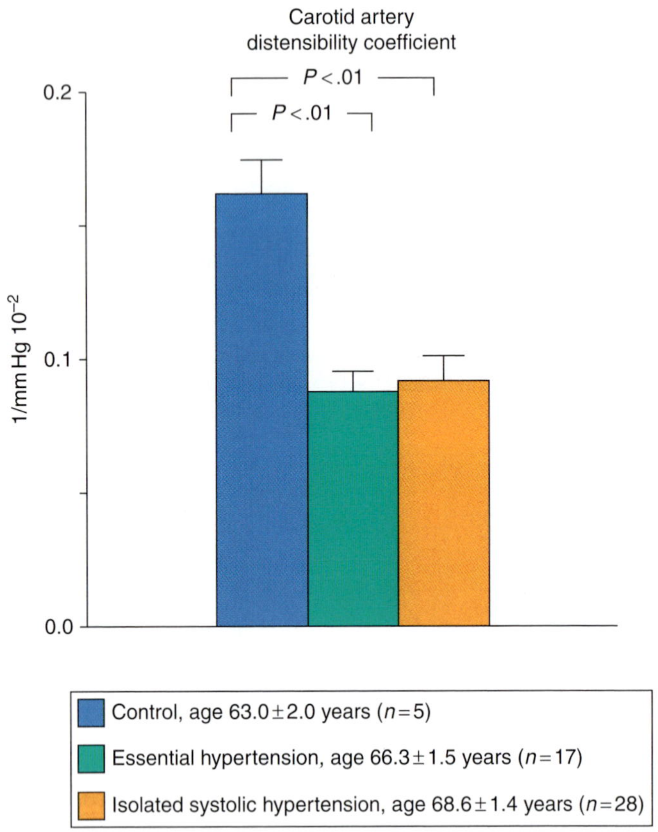

Fig. 6-22 Carotid artery distensibility is reduced in elderly isolated systolic hypertensives. (From Giannattasio C, Mancia G. Arterial distensibility in humans. Modulating mechanisms, alterations in diseases and effects of treatment. *J Hypertens* 2002;20:1889–99.)

blockers (which also improve vascular compliance), diuretics do not slow the speed of the reflected wave; hence, it arrives in the carotid artery during systole (and not diastole as with ACEIs and calcium blockers) (65).

Pulse wave velocity also reflects arterial compliance, with a high PWV indicating poor compliance. Diuretics have been reported to be less effective than calcium blockers in slowing PWV (66), but others disagree (**Figure 6-23**) (67).

ii) Central BP

Diuretics are effective in lowering the central SBP and P-P, compared with placebo, in elderly hypertensives (**Figure 6-24**) (68),

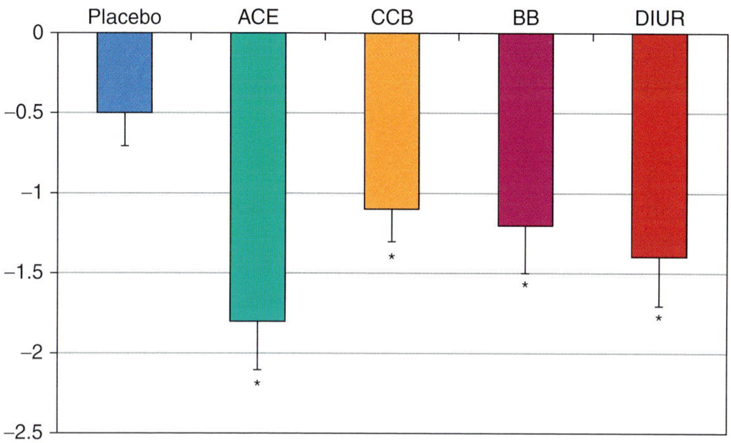

Fig. 6-23 In middle-aged hypertensives, ACE inhibitors, calcium blockers, β-blockers (bisoprolol), and diuretics reduce pulse wave velocity (PWV). (From Ong K-T, Delerme S, Pannier B, et al. Aortic stiffness is reduced beyond blood pressure lowering by short-term and long-term antihypertensive treatment. *J Hypertens* 2011;29:1034–42.)

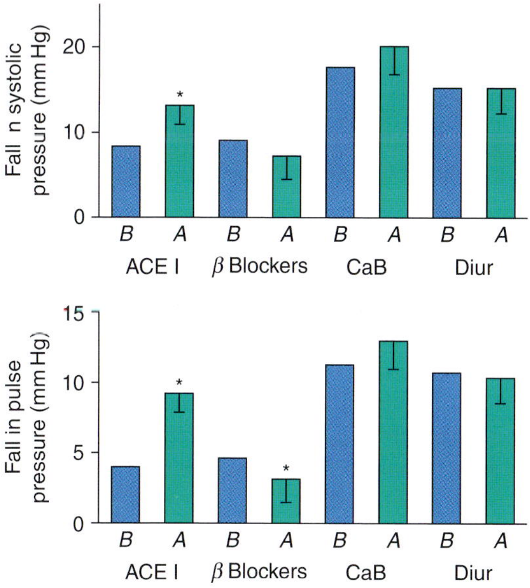

Fig. 6-24 Under randomized, double-blind, crossover conditions, in elderly systolic hypertensives the β-blocker atenolol was the least effective in reducing central aortic (*A*) and brachial (*B*) pressures. (From Morgan T, Lauri J, Bertram D, et al. Effect of different antihypertensive drug classes on central aortic pressure. *Am J Hypertens* 2004;17:118–23.)

and decrease AIx, but unlike ACE-I and calcium blockers, they did not lower central BP to a greater extent than brachial did, that is, did not increase brachial/central BP amplification (**Table 6-4**) (69).

C) Adverse reactions

Thiazide diuretics can cause adverse reactions that require withdrawal from therapy, as illustrated in the Medical Research Council (MRC) mild hypertension study (**Table 6-5**) (70). Of particular note, are impaired glucose tolerance, gout, impotence, lethargy, nausea, and headache.

Other than an increase in uric acid, the metabolic disturbances observed with hydrochlorthiazide may be less with chlorthalidone (56).

The thiazide-induced insulin resistance may be due to increased visceral and hepatic fat accumulation (with an increase in liver enzymes and C-reactive protein (CRP)) (71). There may be a case for regarding chlorthalidone as "nonthiazide-like!" (72). The dysglycemic problems of thiazide-like diuretics are linked to hypokalemia (73). Avoidance of hypokalemia is associated with an increased insulin secretion and a fall in blood sugar (73).

The aldosterone antagonist spironolactone, though a diuretic, avoids many of the aforementioned problems; however, spironolactone has the disadvantage of inducing side effects relating to gynecomastia, sexual dysfunction, and hyperkalemia in about 10% of patients (59). A similar agent, eplerenone, may be less invasive in this respect (59).

Another important, often unrecognized, problem with thiazide-like diuretics is the fact that they increase sympathetic nerve activity in hypertensives, in contrast to spironolactone that does not (Figure 6-24a) (74); indeed, spironolactone may even lower the sympathetic nerve activity (75), and prevent the increase in sympathetic nerve activity which occurs with chlorthalidone (76). The significance of an increase in sympathetic nerve activity in young/middle-aged hypertensives is discussed in Chapters 8 and 9.

2. β-Blockers

As mentioned earlier, β-blockers are most effective in hypertensives with normal/high plasma renin levels (Figure 6-17) (54), that is, in young/middle-aged diastolic hypertensives (**Figure 6-25**) (77). As the elderly, or black, systolic hypertensives tend to have low plasma renin levels, β-blockers (propranolol) are accordingly less effective

TABLE 6-4 Studies evaluating the effect of diuretics on central blood pressure (CBP) beyond peripheral blood pressure (PBP)

Author	Drug	Type of study	Duration[a]	Assessment of CBP	Age (Y)	Number of subjects	Disease/ Risk factor	Evidence of reduction of CBP beyond PBP
Deary AJ et al., Cli Sci 2002 (ADLIP study)	Bendro-fluazide 2.5 mg × 1	Double-blind, crossover, placebo/active controlled	Midterm (6 wk)	Noninvasive[b]	47	30 (22 M)	Untreated eHTN	NEGATIVE Signwificant reduction of PBP but not of CBP versus placebo
Morgan T et al., Am J Hypertens 2004	Hydro-chlorothiazide 50 mg × 1	Randomized, crossover placebo/active controlled	Midterm (2 mo)	Noninvasive[b]	77	32	Never treated eHTN	NEUTRAL Change in SBP amplification: -0.2/-0.7 mm Hg[d]
Dart AM et al., Hypertension 2007 (ANBPT2 vascular sub study)	Diuretics (hydro-chlorothiazide 64%)	Randomized, open label design, blinded assessment of end point	Long term (4 y)	Noninvasive[c]	72 (65–84)	221 (92 M)	Treated/ untreated HTN	NEGATIVE Change in SBP/PP amplification: -2/-3 mm Hg[d]

TABLE 6-4 Studies evaluating the effect of diuretics on central blood pressure (CBP) beyond peripheral blood pressure (PBP) (*Continued*)

Author	Drug	Type of study	Duration[a]	Assessment of CBP	Age (Y)	Number of subjects	Disease/ Risk factor	Evidence of reduction of CBP beyond PBP
Jiang XG et al., J Hypertens 2007	Indapamide 2.5 mg × 1	Randomized, double-blind, active controlled	Midterm (2 mo)	Noninvasive[b]	53	50(26 M)	Wash out or never treated uncom-plicated eHTN	NEUTRAL Chance in SBP/PP amplification: +0.3/+0.1 mm Hg (ns)

Abbreviations: SBP, systolic blood pressure; M, males; eHTN, essential hypertension.

[a]Of the observation period after the administration of the active drug.

[b]Sphygmocor apparatus (radial artery tonometry and application of generalized transfer functions for the assessment of aortic blood pressure).

[c]Direct carotid tonometry (Fitchet–Kelly method).

[d]Post-hoc calculation of the change of SBP amplification—the level of statistical significance was not assessed.

From Protogerou AD, Stergiou GS, Vlachopoulos C, et al. The effect of antihypertensive drugs on central blood pressure beyond peripheral blood pressure: evidence for specific class-effects on antihypertensive drugs on pressure amplification. *Curr Pharmac Design* 2009;15:272–89.

TABLE 6-5 Principal reasons for withdrawal in the MRC Mild Hypertension Study

	Men						Women					
	Bendrofluazide		Propranolol		Placebos		Bendrofluazide		Propranolol		Placebos	
	N	Rate	*N*	Rate	*N*	Rate	*N*	Rate	*N*	Rate	*N*	Rate
Impaired glucose tolerance	60	7.7**	27	3.4	53	3.3	46	5.9**	16	2.1	31	2.0
Gout[b]	100	12.8**	12	1.5	14	0.9	12	1.5**	–		–	
Impotence	98	12.6**	50	6.3**	20	1.3	–		–		–	
Raynaud's phenomenon	–		41	5.1**	3	0.2	2	0.3	34	4.5**	4	0.3
Skin disorder	6	0.8	12	1.5*	5	0.3	3	0.4	9	1.2*	2	0.1
Dyspnea	1	0.1	57	7.1**	7	0.4	2	0.3	53	7.1**	3	0.2
Lethargy	28	3.6**	42	5.3**	8	0.5	13	1.7**	62	8.3**	4	0.3
Nausea, dizziness, or headache	33	4.2**	33	4.1*	22	1.4	58	7.4**	70	9.4**	27	1.8
Pressure at or above levels requiring change of treatment	8	1.0	33	4.1	611	38.2	11	1.4	24	3.2	400	26.0

[a]Patient-years of observation relates here only to years accrued before withdrawal of randomized treatment and while on primary drug alone.
[b]Defined as symptoms plus serum uric acid in excess of 500 μmol/L in men, 450 μmol/L in women.

P < .01 *P* < .01 } Significantly different from rate in controls.
P < .001 *P* < .001 } Miall WE, Greenberg G. *Mild Hypertension – Is There Pressure to Treat?* Cambridge: Cambridge University Press; 1987, pp 70.

* low statistical significance
** high statistical significance

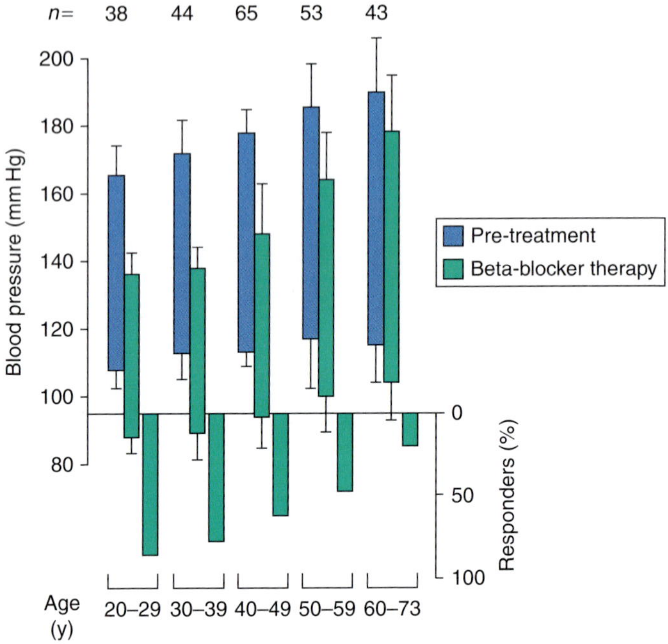

Fig. 6-25 Age-dependent antihypertensive efficacy of β-blockers. (From Buhler FR. Age and cardiovascular response adaptation. *Hypertension* 1983;5:94–100.)

in lowering BP in these groups (Figures 6-18 and 6-25) (55, 77). Asian (India) hypertensive subjects respond well to beta-1 blockade (bisoprolol), with equal benefit in both young and elderly (78).

A) Are all β-blockers equally effective in lowering blood pressure?

Pure β-2 blockade (BB) (ICI 118,551) actually increases BP by about 7.5 mm Hg (79). Thus, nonselective BBs, like propranolol, are less effective in lowering BP than moderately β-1 selective BBs like atenolol (**Figure 6-26**) (80). However, when moderately selective atenolol is compared with highly β-1 selective bisoprolol over a 24-hour period, bisoprolol is clearly the superior antihypertensive agent (**Figure 6-27**) (81). The superiority of bisoprolol over atenolol is particularly evident in smokers (82). This topic, involving comparisons between β-blockers, is covered in some detail elsewhere (83).

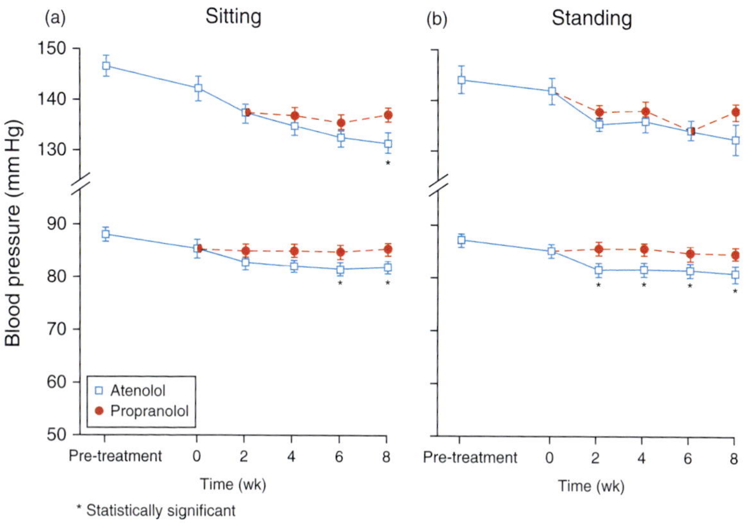

Fig. 6-26 Under randomized, double-blind, crossover conditions, atenolol was a more effective antihypertensive agent than propranolol. (From Zacharias FJ, Cowen KJ. Comparison of propranolol and atenolol in hypertension. *Postgrad Med J* 1977;53:111–3.)

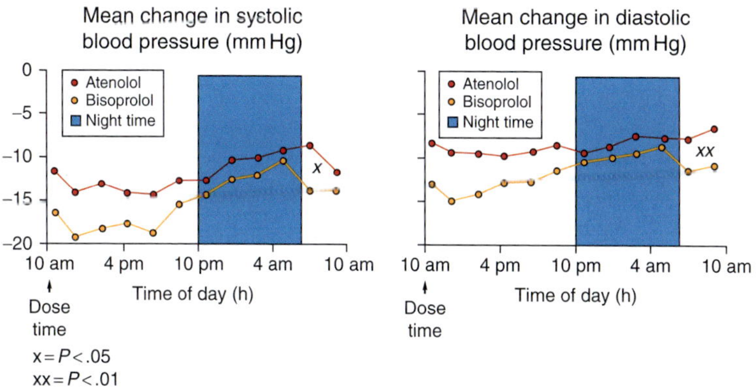

Fig. 6-27 Atenolol (50–100 mg od) versus. bisoprolol (10–20 mg od): effect on 24 hour BP in 659 hypertensives—bisoprolol is the superior antihypertensive agent. (From Neutel JM, Smith DH, Ram CV, et al. Application of ambulatory blood pressure monitoring in differentiating between antihypertensive agents. *Am J Med* 1993;94:181–7.)

The presence of nonselective intrinsic sympathomimetic activity (ISA) tends to diminish efficacy; thus, propranolol was superior to oxprenolol in lowering BP (83, 84). Pindolol, with a very high-level nonselective ISA, is significantly less effective than propranolol in lowering nocturnal BP (83). However, nebivolol, with β-3 ISA (111), was as effective as atenolol in reducing brachial BP in elderly hypertensives (85). It is of interest to note that both β-2 (86, 87) and β-3 ISA (88) are associated with NO release.

Additional α-blocking properties, for example, carvedilol and labetalol, may be more effective in controlling standing/erect BP (89), but at a price, that is, postural hypotension (see later) (111).

B) β-Blockers compared to other antihypertensive drug classes

As mentioned earlier, in younger/middle-aged hypertensives, highly β-1 selective bisoprolol was superior to diuretics, calcium antagonists, α-blockers, and ACE inhibition in lowering 24-hour BP (Figure 6-20) (54). In the HANE study (Figure 6-21) (61), atenolol was the most effective antihypertensive in younger (less than 54 years) hypertensives, and (surprisingly) as effective as enalapril, hydrochlorthiazide, and nitrendipine in older subjects.

Bisoprolol is also a superior antihypertensive agent, in young/middle-aged hypertensives, to angiotensin receptor blockers (ARBs). In a randomized comparison between bisoprolol, losartan amlodipine, and hydrochlorthiazide, bisoprolol was the most effective in reducing both daytime and nocturnal BP (**Figure 6-28**) (90) and was also shown to be at least as renoprotective as losartan over a 1-year period (**Figure 6-29**) (91). In the elderly hypertensives, bisoprolol, like atenolol (Figure 6-21) (61), was as effective as the calcium blocker nifedipine-SR (92).

C) β-Blockers and vascular compliance and central blood pressure

i) Vascular compliance

Reduction in vessel diameter increases wall stiffness. Thus, β-2 stimulation improves (93), and α-1 stimulation reduces (94) vascular compliance. It thus comes as no surprise that nonselective propranolol (95, 96) decreases vascular compliance, probably due to vasoconstriction arising from unbridled α-constriction.

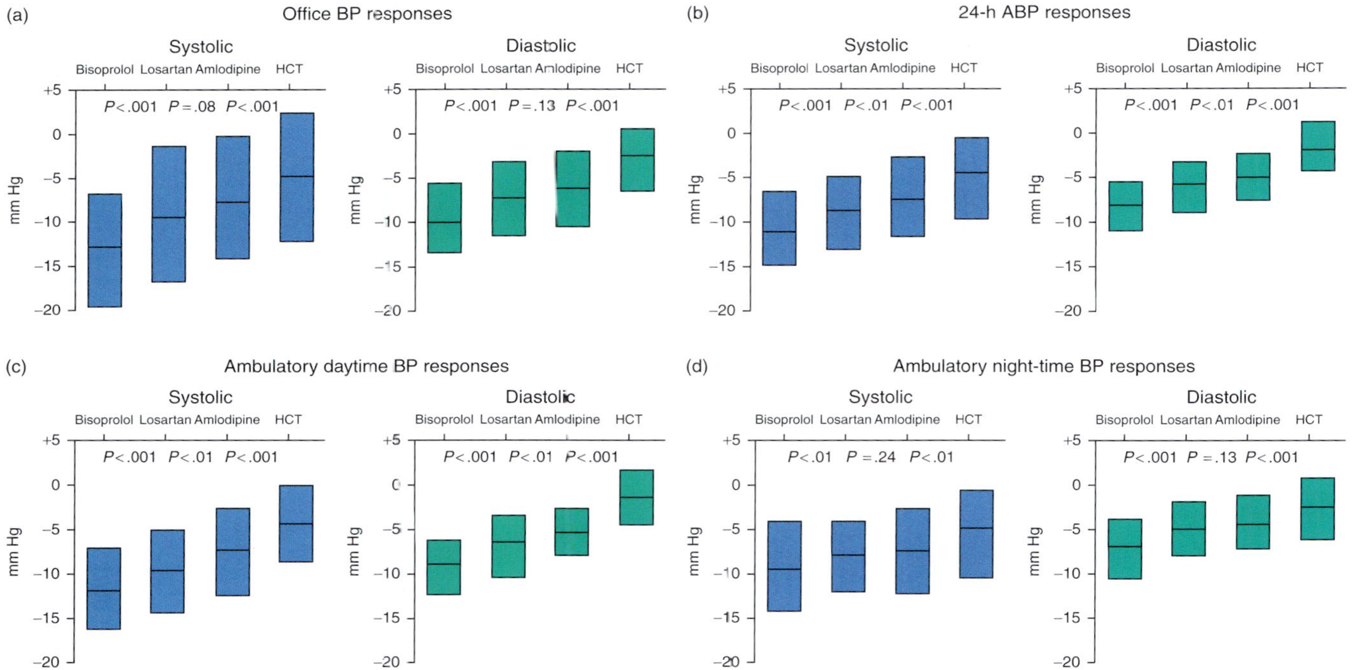

Fig. 6-28 In middle-aged hypertensive men, under randomized, double-blind, crossover conditions, bisoprolol was superior to hydrochlorthiazide, losartan, and amlodipine in reducing BP. (From Hiltunen TP, Suonsyrja T, Hannila-Handelberg T, et al. Predictors of antihypertensive responses: initial data from a placebo-controlled, randomised cross-over with four anti-hypertensive drugs (the GENRES study). *Am J Hypertens* 2007;20:311–8.)

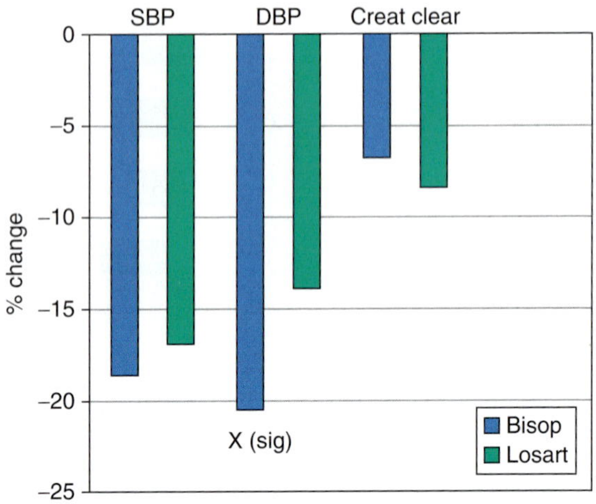

Fig. 6-29 Bisoprolol versus losartan (randomized/double-blind): effects on BP/renal function over 1 year in 72 hypertensives (mean age of 50 y). (From Parrinello G, Paterna S, Torres D, et al. One year renal and cardiac effect of bisoprolol versus losartan in recently diagnosed hypertensive patients. *Clin Drug Investig* 2009;29:591–600.)

Moderately β-1 selective atenolol does not alter vascular compliance (97), though in the elderly atenolol was as effective as an ACE inhibitor in reducing PWV in the aorta, but not in the limbs (98). Highly β-1 selective bisoprolol was highly effective in increasing arterial compliance, and reducing PWV, in middle-aged hypertensives (**Figure 6-30**) (99), being as effective as ACE inhibitors, calcium blockers, and diuretics in reducing PWV (Figure 6-23) (67). β-Blockers with high ISA (pindolol) are particularly effective in improving vascular compliance compared with propranolol (100).

ii) Central blood pressure

As a drug class, β-blockers reduce central BP less than brachial BP (**Table 6-6**) (69).

1. β-Blocker differences

In elderly patients, nebivolol (with β-3 ISA) lowered aortic P-P significantly more, and increased central AIx less, than atenolol (85). The fall in heart rate was less with nebivolol, which may be important, as fall in heart rate is linked to an increase in AIx (**Figure 6-31**). However, the link between vasodilation and the

TABLE 6-6 Studies evaluating the effects of BBs on central blood pressure (CBP) beyond peripheral blood pressure (PBP)

Author	Drug	Type of study	Duration	Assessment of CBP	Age (Y)	Number of subjects	Disease/Risk factor	Evidence of reduction of CBP beyond PBP
Asmar RG et al. Hypertension 2001 (REASON study)	Atenolol 50 mg × 1	Randomized, double-blind, active controlled	Long term (12 mo)	Noninvasive	53	64	Untreated/ wash out eHTN	NEGATIVE PP amplification (ratio): decreased significantly, $P < .05$
Deary AJ et al, Cli Sci 2002 (ADLIP Study)	Bisoprobol 5 mg × 1	Double-blind, crossover, placebo/active controlled	Midterm (6 wk)	Noninvasive	47	30 (22 M)	Untreated eHTN	NEGATIVE Change in SBP amplification: men—5 mm Hg/women—10 mm Hg§ (vs. baseline)
Morgan T et al. Am J Hypertens 2004	Atenolol 50 mg × 1	Randomized, crossover placebo/active controlled	Midterm (2 mo)	Noninvasive	77	32	Never treated eHTN	NEGATIVE Change in SBP/ PP amplification −2/−1.5 mm Hg§
Hirata K et al. J Hypertens 2005	Atenolol 100 mg	Randomized, double blind, 3 way crossover, placebo active controlled	Acute (5 h)	Noninvasive	67(±10)	30 (25 M)	High CV risk	NEGATIVE Change in SBP amplification: −3.2 mm Hg, $P < .001$

TABLE 6-6 Studies evaluating the effects of BBs on central blood pressure (CBP) beyond peripheral blood pressure (PBP) (*Continued*)

Author	Drug	Type of study	Duration	Assessment of CBP	Age (Y)	Number of subjects	Disease/Risk factor	Evidence of reduction of CBP beyond PBP
Dhakam Z et al. Am J Hypertens 2006	Atenolol 50 mg × 1	Randomized, double-blind, crossover, active/placebo controlled	Midterm (6 wk)	Noninvasive	51(>40)	21 (13 M)	Never treated eHTN	NEGATIVE PP amplification (ratio): 1.38 baseline versus 1.21, $P < .05$
Dhakam Z et al. J Hypertens 2008	Atenolol 50 mg × 1 Nebivolol 5 mg × 1	Randomized, double-blind, crossover, active/placebo controlled	Midterm (5 wk)	Noninvasive	70	16 (10M)	Low risk uncontrolled eISH	NEGATIVE PP amplification (ratio); significant reduction, $P < .001$

Abbreviations: SBP, systolic blood pressure; M, males; eHTN, essential hypertension; ISH, isolated systolic hypertension; HTN, hypertension.

From Protogerou AD, Stergiou GS, Vlachopoulos C, et al. The effect of antihypertensive drugs on central blood pressure beyond peripheral blood pressure: evidence for specific class-effects on antihypertensive drugs on pressure amplification. *Curr Pharmac Design* 2009;15:272–89.

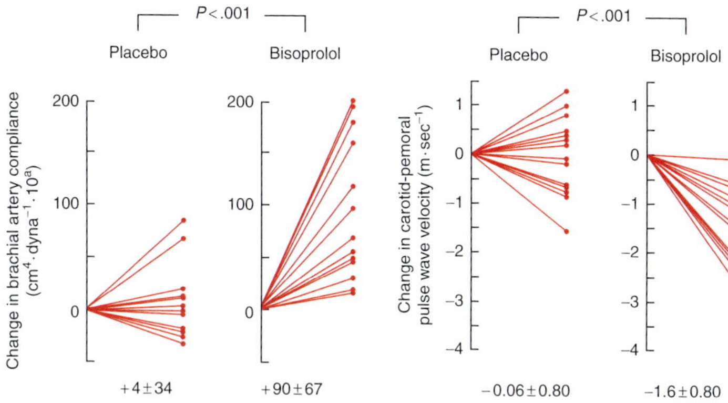

Fig. 6-30 In middle-aged hypertensives, bisoprolol reduced PWV (right) and increased brachial artery compliance (left). (From Asmar RG, Kerihuel JC, Girerd XJ, et al. Effect of bisoprolol on blood pressure and arterial haemodynamics in system hypertension. *Am J Cardiol* 1991;68:61–4.)

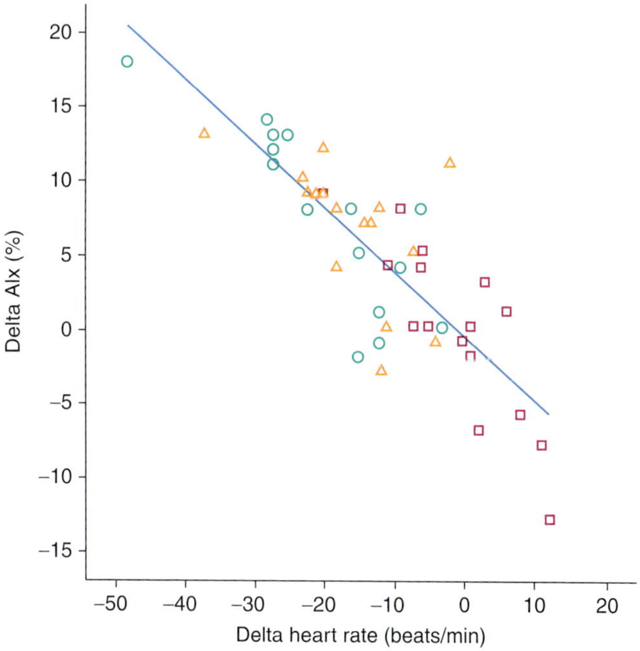

Fig. 6-31 In elderly hypertensives, there is an inverse relationship between heart rate and augmentation index (AIx). (From Dhakam Z, Yasmin, McEniery CM, et al. A comparison of atenolol and nebivolol in isolated systolic hypertension. *J Hypertens* 2008;26:351–6.)

magnitude of the reflected wave appears to be the main reason why a β-blocker with nonselective ISA, for example, dilevalol, is more effective than atenolol in reducing the magnitude of the reflected wave and central pressure in middle-aged hypertensives (101). Nonselective propranolol is particularly effective in increasing the magnitude of the reflected wave in women (102). Also, in middle-aged hypertensives, nebivolol (β-3 ISA) and metoprolol lowered brachial BP to a similar degree, but nebivolol was more effective than metoprolol in reducing central pressures and P-P (103).

2. β-Blockers versus other antihypertensive drugs

As discussed earlier (Figure 6-24) (68), in the elderly, atenolol reduced central SBP and P-P less effectively than other drug classes and tended to increase AIx. Others have confirmed that in the elderly patients with isolated systolic hypertension, atenolol, compared with an ACE inhibitor, calcium blocker, and diuretic, was ineffective in reducing central P-P, and increased central AIx (104). The ASCOT study, in the elderly, showed that the lesser effect of atenolol, versus amlodipine, on central pressures, was due to the greater magnitude of the reflected wave on atenolol (Figure 6-31a) (105). In middle-aged hypertensives, atenolol and the ACE inhibitor fosinopril lowered brachial BP equally, but the ACE inhibitor was more effective in lowering central AIx (**Figure 6-32**) (106). In a comparison of amlodipine, lisinopril, and bisoprolol, only the

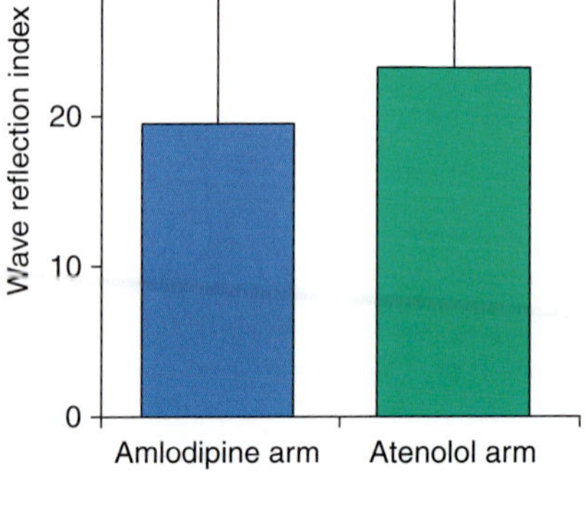

Fig. 6-31a ASCOT; the higher central SBP and P-P with atenolol (vs. amlodipine) is *not* due to low HR but through increased magnitude of reflected wave (absence of vasodilatation). (From Manisty CH, Zambanini A, Parker KH, et al. Differences in the magnitude of wave reflection account for differential effects of amlodipine versus atenolol-based regimens on central blood pressure ASCOT. *Hypertension* 2009;54:724–30.)

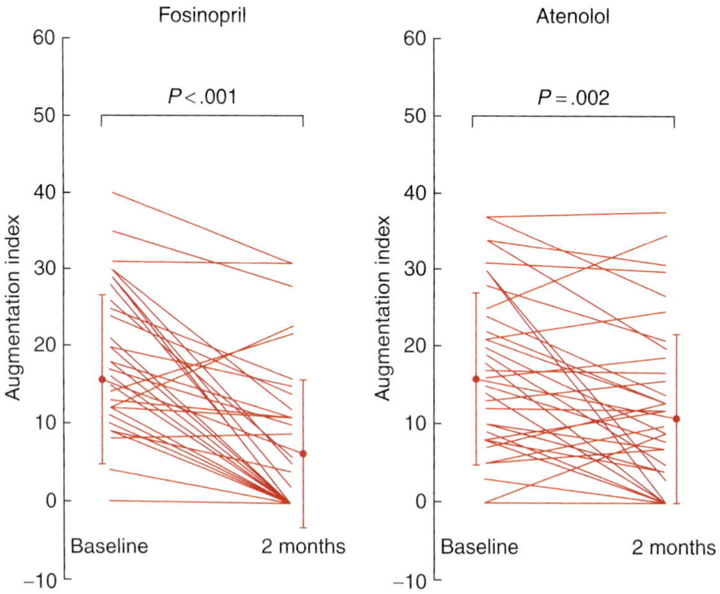

Fig. 6-32 In middle-aged hypertensives, under randomized, double-blind conditions, fosinopril reduced central AIx more than atenolol. (From Chen CH, Ting CT, Lin SJ, et al. Different aspects of fosinopril and atenolol on wave reflections in hypertensive patients. *Hypertension* 1995;25:1034–41.)

former 2 drugs lowered central AIx, whereas bisoprolol increased AIx (107). However, in young/middle-aged hypertensives, in a randomized comparison between atenolol and the ACE inhibitor perindopril, atenolol was superior in improving the PWV, whereas the ACE inhibitor was best at reducing the magnitude of the reflected wave; the result was that both drugs lowered central BP and P-P equally (108).

D) Adverse reactions

The adverse reactions responsible for patient withdrawal from the Medical Research Council (MRC) trial in those taking propranolol are shown in Table 6-4 (70). However, propranolol is not a typical BB, being nonselective and highly liphophilic (crosses blood–brain barrier with ease). Thus, propranolol scores poorly on "a quality of life" scale, opposite atenolol and enalapril (**Figure 6-33**) (109). Highly β-1 selective bisoprolol, compared to enalapril, affected quality of life to a similar degree as the ACEI (110).

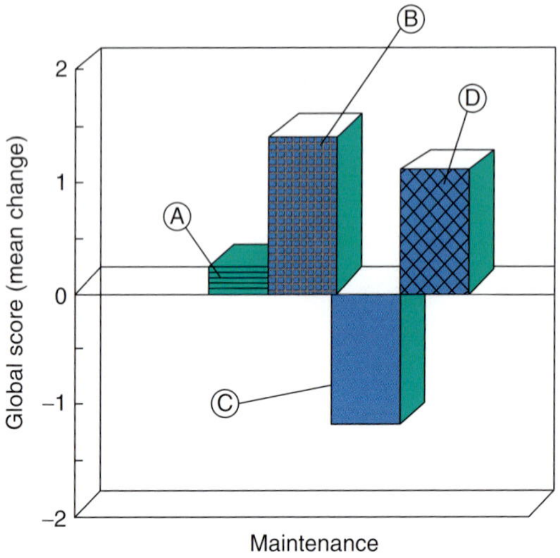

Fig. 6-33 Quality of life scores were least good with propranolol (C) compared to atenolol (D), enalapril (B), and captopril. (From Steiner SS, Friedhoff AJ, Wilson BL, et al. Antihypertensive therapy and quality of life: a comparison of atenolol, captopril, enalapril, and propranolol. *J Hum Hypertens* 1990;4:217–25.)

β-Blockers' adverse reactions have been dealt with comprehensively by Cruickshank (111). A summary of these adverse reactions are as follows:

1. β-Blockers are heterogeneous group of drugs, and adverse reactions vary markedly between the various classes.
2. β-1 blockade is shared by all BBs, and rarely causes problems; bradycardia is usually asymptomatic (unless the heart rate falls to the low 40s or less); fatigue is uncommon, and is exacerbated by the addition of β-2 blockade; cold peripheries are also uncommon; patients with peripheral arterial disease (PAD) are unaffected in terms of walking distance; all other side effects occur at placebo level. This adverse-reaction pattern would reflect side effects of a highly β-1 selective agent like bisoprolol.
3. β-2 blockade (through nonselective and only moderately β-1 selective BBs) adds a host of possible extra side effects (see Table 6-5); lethargy is increased, and effort tolerance falls; cold peripheries are more common; renal function may be impaired; bronchospasm is possible in vulnerable patients with reversible obstruction, although with "fixed" obstruction chronic obstructive pulmonary disease (COPD) all BBs are relatively

safe; metabolic disturbance is likely, involving insulin resistance, increased blood sugar/HbA1c, increased blood triglycerides, and a fall in high-density lipoprotein (HDL); sexual dysfunction can occur; weight gain of 1–2 kg occurs; the smoking/adrenaline interaction leads to marked increases in BP.

4. Additional α-blockade (e.g. carvedilol and labetalol) may induce postural hypotension, particularly at the first dose; add sexual dysfunction; on chronic dosing carvedilol tends to lose its α-blocking property, that is, tachyphylaxis.
5. High lipophilcity (e.g. propranolol, metoprolol, and nebivolol) permits easy crossing of the blood–brain barrier and may be associated with nightmares and sleep disturbances.
6. Poor metabolizer status (liver cytochrome P450 system), relevant to metoprolol and nebivolol, leads to high blood levels and loss of β-1 selectivity.
7. Intrinsic sympathomimetic activity (e.g. pindolol with β-1 and β-2 ISA, and nebivolol with β-3 ISA) can affect efficacy and adverse reactions. High levels of ISA, for example, pindolol, leads mainly to loss of efficacy as well as muscle pain (with high blood creatine phospho-kinase (CPK) levels); nebivolol has few side effects, but high blood levels in poor metabolizers will lead to loss of β-1 selectivity.

3. ACE inhibitors

A) Efficacy on lowering brachial blood pressure

Like BBs, ACE inhibitors are best at lowering BP in hypertensives with high plasma renin (112). However, an age/race subgroup (elderly and black) may be a better predictor than a renin profile (113). Interestingly, middle-aged, black African male hypertensives on a low/moderate salt intake respond better to an ACE inhibitor than to a diuretic (114).

B) Compared to other antihypertensives (white patients)

In young/middle-aged hypertensives, a double-blind, randomized, crossover study showed that the ACE inhibitor lisinopril was somewhat less effective in lowering BP than bisoprolol (Figure 6-20) (60), and was "best drug" less often than bisoprolol (10 vs. 13), but more often than amlodipine, doxazosin, and bendrofluazide (**Table 6-7**).

TABLE 6-7 In young/middle-aged hypertensives, a double-blind crossover study showed "best treatment" (*n*) was most commonly with the BB bisoprolol, followed by ACE inhibitor lisinopril

			BP on placebo		BP on repeat	
Drug	*n*	Age	Clinic	24-hour average	Clinic	24-hour average
Amlodipine	5	49.0	162 ± 6/100 ± 6	161 ± 6/104 ± 5	154 ± 14/96 ± 4	144 ± 7/95 ± 4
Doxazosin	4	46.0	161 ± 13/100 ± 7	160 ± 9/102 ± 9	155 ± 4/100 ± 6	154 ± 6/102 ± 6
Lisinopril	10	46.5	159 ± 8/99 ± 7	160 ± 12/106 ± 9	137 ± 9/86 ± 6	136 ± 7/89 ± 5
Bisoprolol	13	42.5	160 ± 99/10 ± 6	155 ± 12/107 ± 6	140 ± 17/86 ± 8	135 ± 13/86 ± 7
Bendrofluazide	2	51.5	158 ± 14/95 ± 3	150 ± 19/103 ± 16	156 ± 2/99 ± 2	148 ± 14/99 ± 11

Abbreviations: BP, blood pressure; BB, β-blockers; ACE, angiotensin-converting enzyme.

From Deary AJ, Schumann AL, Murfeet H, et al. Double-blind, placebo controlled crossover comparison of 5 classes of drugs. *J Hypertens* 2002;20:771–7.

In the HANE study (Figure 6-21) (61), in younger hypertensives, enalapril came second to atenolol in terms of response rate, and in the older patients was the least effective compared with atenolol, nifedipine, and hydrochlorthiazide.

C) ACE inhibitors and vascular compliance and central blood pressure

i) Vascular compliance

There is evidence that a local renin/angiotensin/aldosterone (RAAS) system is 1 mediator of vessel wall elasticity (115), and that ACE inhibition promotes elastogenic remodeling (116). In the elderly, both ACE inhibitors and diuretics reduce radial artery wall hypertrophy and improve carotid compliance (117). Another study showed some improvement in aortic stiffness (↓PWV), but no improvement in vascular compliance (118). On balance it appears that ACE inhibitors do improve vascular compliance (65, 100) and are effective in reducing PWV (Figure 6-23) (67).

ii) Central BP

As a drug class, ACE inhibitors lower central BP more effectively than brachial BP (**Table 6-8**) (69). The effect of ACE inhibitors upon central BP and AIx is superior to β-blockers and similar to diuretics and calcium blockers, in elderly systolic hypertensives (Figure 6-24) (68). Some have confirmed this (98, 107, 119), whereas others indicated that long-term ACE inhibition (4.5 years) did not reduce central AIx (118). In younger/middle-aged hypertensives, enalapril was superior to the diuretic indapamide in reducing central pressures (**Figure 6-34**) (120). These beneficial effects of ACE inhibitors are due to dilatation of small peripheral arteries, thereby reducing the magnitude of wave reflections, and thus lowering aortic pressure augmentation during systole, often without a corresponding reduction in brachial SBP (121, 122).

D) Adverse reactions

Although some studies indicate that quality of life is better on enalapril than on captopril (Figure 6-33) (110), others suggest the reverse to be the case (123). Captopril, containing the suphydryl group (124), has been associated with taste disturbance, or dysgeusia (125), and this may occur in up to 17% of patients (126). Skin reactions occur in about 17% of cases of ACE inhibitors (126).

Cough is not an uncommon adverse reaction with ACE inhibitors, possibly due to increased bradykinin levels, and disappears rapidly on stopping the drug (127). ACE-inhibitor-induced cough may be more common in East Asians than in Caucasians (128).

Angioedema, which can be life threatening, usually accompanying urticaria, occurs at a rate of about 1.2 in 1000, is not dose dependent, and can be either early or late onset (129). It appears to be more common in black Americans (128), women, and smokers (130). Like cough, it appears to be linked to increased bradykinin levels. Even when switched to other drugs, in particular angiotensin receptor blockers (ARBs) (131), vulnerable patients can still experience angioedema (130). It thus seems that certain patients are prone to angioedema and that 50% of those switched from ACE inhibitors will have similar problems with other drugs (130).

Unlike thiazide diuretics, and non/poorly β-1 selective β-blockers, captopril actually improves insulin resistance (132).The risk of diabetes is thus reduced (133).

TABLE 6-8 Studies evaluating the effect of ACE inhibitor treatment on central blood pressure (CBP) beyond peripheral blood pressure (PBP)

Author	Drug	Type of study	Duration[a]	Assessment of CBP	Age (Y)	Number of subjects	Disease/Risk factor	Evidence of reduction of CBP beyond PBP
London G et al. Circulation 1994	Perindopril 2/4 mg 3 times a week	Randomized, double-blind, placebo run in, 2 parallel active group	Long term (12 mo)	Noninvasive[c]	53	14 (7 M)	ESRD	POSITIVE Change in PP amplification 0–12 months: 1.00 versus 1.13 $P < .01$
London G et al. J Hypertens 1996	Quinapril 20 mg once	Placebo controlled, crossover	Acute effect (during 172 h)	Noninvasive	53.3	12 (8 M)	ESRD	POSITIVE Change in PP amplification: approximately +10 mm Hg
Mitchell GF et al. Circulation 2002 (CHOIR study)	Enalapril 40 mg × 1	Active control	Midterm (3 mo)	Noninvasive[c]	61	87	eHTN	NEUTRAL Change in PP amplification: 0 mm Hg
Deary AJ et l, Cli Sci 2002 (ADLIP Study)	Lisinopril 10 mg × 1	Double-blind, crossover, placebo/active controlled	Midterm (6 wk)	Noninvasive[b]	47	30 (22 M)	Untreated eHTN	NEUTRAL/NEGATIVE Change in PP amplification: men 0 mm Hg/ women -6 mm Hg

Stokes GS et al., Hypertension 2003	Captopril	Randomized, double-blind crossover placebo/active	Acute effect (0–8 h)	Noninvasive[b]	69.8 (59–82)	11 (5 M)	High risk eHTN	NEUTRAL No change in PP amplification
Morgan T et al. Am J Hypertens 2004	Enalapril 20/40 mg or Perindopril 4/8 mg	Randomized, crossover placebo/active controlled	Midterm (1 mo)	Noninvasive[b]	77	32	Untreated eHTN	POSITIVE Change in PP amplification: +4.7 mm Hg
Hirata K et al. J Hypertens 2005	Ramipril 10 mg	Randomized, double-blind, 3 way crossover, placebo active controlled	Acute (5 h)	Noninvasive[b]	67 (±10)	30 (25 M)	High CV risk	POSITIVE Change in SBP amplification: +1.9 mm Hg
Ahimastos A et al., Hypertension 2005	Ramipril 10 mg × 1	Randomized, double-blind, placebo controlled	Long term (6 months)	Noninvasive[c]	66	40	Peripheral arterial disease	POSITIVE Change in PP amplification: +3.2 mm Hg
Dart AM et al. Hypertension 2007 (ANBPT2, vascular)	ACEIs (enalapril suggested)	Randomized, open label design, blinded assessment of end point	Long term (4 y)	Noninvasive[c]	72 (65-84)	258 (209 M)	eHTN	POSITIVE Change in PP amplification: +1 mmHg

TABLE 6-8 Studies evaluating the effect of ACE inhibitor treatment on central blood pressure (CBP) beyond peripheral blood pressure (PBP) (*Continued*)

Author	Drug	Type of study	Duration[a]	Assessment of CBP	Age (Y)	Number of subjects	Disease/Risk factor	Evidence of reduction of CBP beyond PBP
Aznaouridis K et al. J Human Hypertens 2007	Captopril 25 mg Quinapril 20 mg	Randomized, double-blind, placebo-controlled, parallel-group	Acute effect (2 h)	Noninvasive[b]	57	25 per group (48 M)	eHTN	POSITIVE Change in PP amplification: +2.1 mm Hg (quinapril)
Jiang XG et al. J Hypertens 2007	Enalapril 10mg × 1	Randomized, double blind, active controlled	Midterm (2 mo)	Noninvasive	53	101 (55 M)	Uncomplicated eHTN	POSITIVE Change in PP amplification: +3 mm Hg

Abbreviations: SBP, systolic blood pressure; M, males; eHTN, essential hypertension; ESRD, end-stage renal disease; CV, cardiovascular.

[a]Of the observation period after the administration of the active drug.

[b]Sphygmocor apparatus (radial artery tonometry and application of generalized transfer functions for the assessment of aortic blood pressure).

[c]Direct carotid tonometry (Fitchet–Kelly method).

Note: Post-hoc calculation of the change of SBP amplification—the level of statistical significance was not assessed.

From Protogerou AD, Stergiou GS, Vlachopoulos C, et al. The effect of antihypertensive drugs on central blood pressure beyond peripheral blood pressure: evidence for specific class-effects on antihypertensive drugs on pressure amplification. *Curr Pharmac Design* 2009;15:272–89.

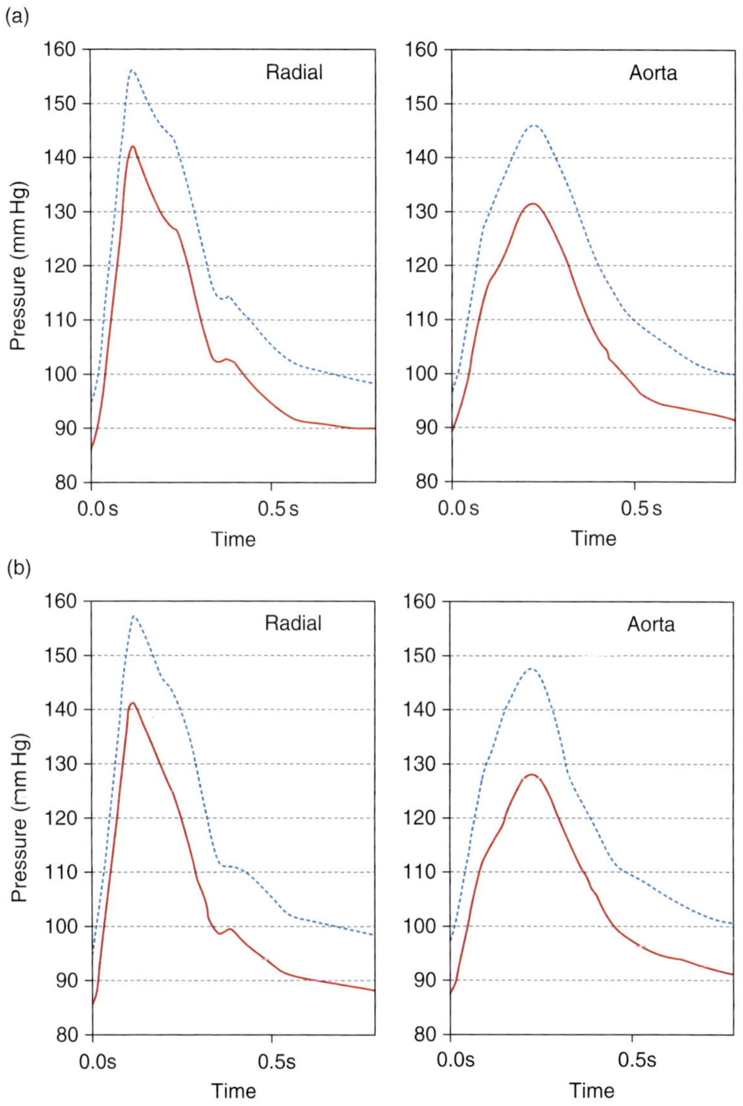

Fig. 6-34 In middle-aged hypertensives, enalapril (B) was more effective than indapamide (A) in reducing aortic BP. (From Jiang X-J, O'Rourke MF, Zhang Y-Q, et al. Superior effect of an angiotensin-converting enzyme inhibitor over a diuretic for reducing aortic systolic pressure. *J Hypertens* 2007;25:1095–9.)

ACE inhibitors reduce renal elimination of potassium, and cases of hyperkalemia can occur, which may be serious and life threatening when spironolactone is co-prescribed (134). This ACE inhibitor problem poses a greater risk in the presence of diabetes or renal failure (135).

Angiotensin II can induce increased sympathetic nerve activity (136), and this can be reversed by ACE inhibition (136, 137), particularly in renal failure (138).

4. Angiotensin receptor blockers

A) Efficacy in lowering brachial blood pressure

In young (18–36 years) subjects with hypertensive parents, candesartan lowered mean 24-hour BP by 4/3 mm Hg over a 2-year period (139). In middle-aged prehypertensives, randomized to placebo or candesartan, over 4 years formal hypertension was 63% less common in the ARB group (140).

An ARB lowers BP to the same degree as an ACE inhibitor (141), but less than the highly β-1 selective BB bisoprolol (Figures 6-28, and 6-29) (90, 91)—in middle-aged hypertensives. Candesartan was likewise less effective than metoprolol in lowering BP in young/middle-aged hypertensives (142).

B) Efficacy in improving vascular compliance and lowering central blood pressure

Angiotensin receptor blockers are as effective as ACE inhibitors and calcium blockers in improving vascular compliance (143). Like ACE inhibitors, ARBs appear to lower central pressures more than peripheral (**Table 6-9**) (69). Central P-P is also reduced because of the vasodilatory action of the ARB (141).

In the middle-age hypertensives, valsartan was more effective than placebo and hydrochlorthiazide in reducing central AIx (144).

C) Adverse reactions

Angiotensin receptor blockers are generally very well tolerated and, unlike ACE, they do not cause a dry cough (145). Although angioedema is essentially an ACE-inhibitor problem, when such cases are switched to an ARB, or other drugs, they may continue to experience this potentially death-threatening condition (130); such subjects are clearly predisposed to angioedema.

Losartan improves insulin sensitivity (146), possibly through a direct action on the pancreas (133). ARBs are, compared to diuretics and non/poorly β-1 selective β-blockers, associated with less type 2 diabetes (**Figure 6-35**) (147). Losartan, unlike other ARBs, does not precipitate gout (148).

TABLE 6-9 Studies evaluating the effect of ARBs on central blood pressure (CBP) beyond peripheral blood pressure (PBP)

Author	Drug	Type of study	Duration[a]	Assessment of CBP	Age (Y)	Number of subjects	Disease/ Risk factor	Evidence of reduction of CBP beyond PBP
Mahmud A, Feely J. J Human Hypertens 2000	Valsartan 80 mg × 1	Age-matched control group	Short term (2 wk)	Noninvasive	56.9 (41–69)	18 (6 M)	Uncontolled eHTN	POSITIVE Change in PP amplification: 6.5, mm Hg $P < .001$
Stokes GS et al., Hypertension 2003 (a)	Eprosartan 600 mg × 1	Randomized, double-blind crossover placebo/ active	Acute effect (0–8 h)	Noninvasive	69.8 (59–82)	11 (5 M)	High risk eHTN	NEUTRAL Change in SBP amplification: 0 mm Hg

TABLE 6-9 Studies evaluating the effect of ARBs on central blood pressure (CBP) beyond peripheral blood pressure (PBP) (*Continued*)

Author	Drug	Type of study	Duration[a]	Assessment of CBP	Age (Y)	Number of subjects	Disease/ Risk factor	Evidence of reduction of CBP beyond PBP
Dhakam Z et al. Am J Hypertens 2006	Eprosartan 400 mg × 1	Randomized, double-blind, crossover	Midterm (6 wk)	Noninvasive	51 (>40)	21 (13 M)	Never treated eHTN	POSITIVE PP amplification (ratio) 1.38 baseline versus 1.42 $P < .05$
Aznaouridis K et al. J Human Hypertens 2007	Telmisartan 80 mg	Randomized, double-blind, placebo controlled, parallel group	Acute effect (2 h)	Noninvasive	57	25	HTN	NEUTRAL Change in SBP amplification: -0.5 mm Hg

From Protogerou AD, Stergiou GS, Vlachopoulos C, et al. The effect of antihypertensive drugs on central blood pressure beyond peripheral blood pressure: evidence for specific class-effects on antihypertensive drugs on pressure amplification. *Curr Pharmac Design* 2009;15:272–89.

[a] eHTN, essential hypertension.

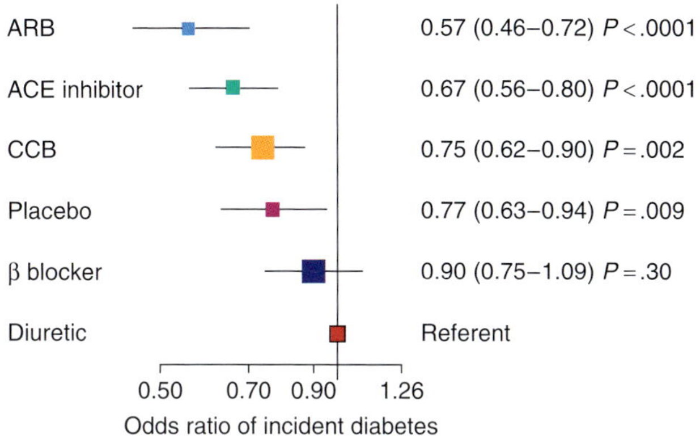

Fig. 6-35 Trials including 143 153 patients indicate that compared to a diuretic (reference) diabetes is less likely with ARBs, ACE inhibitors, and calcium blockers. (From Elliot WJ, Meyer PM. Incident diabetes in clinical trials of antihypertensive drugs: a network analysis. *Lancet* 2007;369:201–7.)

Angiotensin receptor blockers, like ACE, can induce hyperkalemia in up to 10%–38% of hospital patients, and patients with diabetes or renal impairment are particularly at risk (135). The hyperkalemia can be severe in the presence of spironolactone and induce muscle paralysis, bradyarrythmia, and marked hypotension, requiring hemodialysis (**Figure 6-36**) (134).

A meta-analysis suggested that ARBs are associated with an increased risk of cancer (149). However, this has been refuted by others (150, 151), and some even suggest a reduced cancer risk (152). ACE inhibitors, β-blockers, calcium blockers, and diuretics are also not associated with cancer (153).

Angiotensin II increases sympathetic nerve activity (154, 155). Angiotensin II levels increase in the presence of ARBs, but in older patients (156) or those with renal failure (138), there is a decrease in sympathetic nerve activity. Others have not confirmed the fall in sympathetic nerve activity (157). However, in younger hypertensives, ARBs have been shown to increase sympathetic nerve activity (**Figure 6-37**) (142, 158). The significance of increased sympathetic nerve activity in younger/middle-aged hypertensives is discussed in Chapter 8.

5. Calcium blockers

A) Efficacy in lowering brachial blood pressure and its variability

As mentioned earlier (77), β-blockers are more effective in younger, high-renin hypertensives and less effective in older, low-renin cases

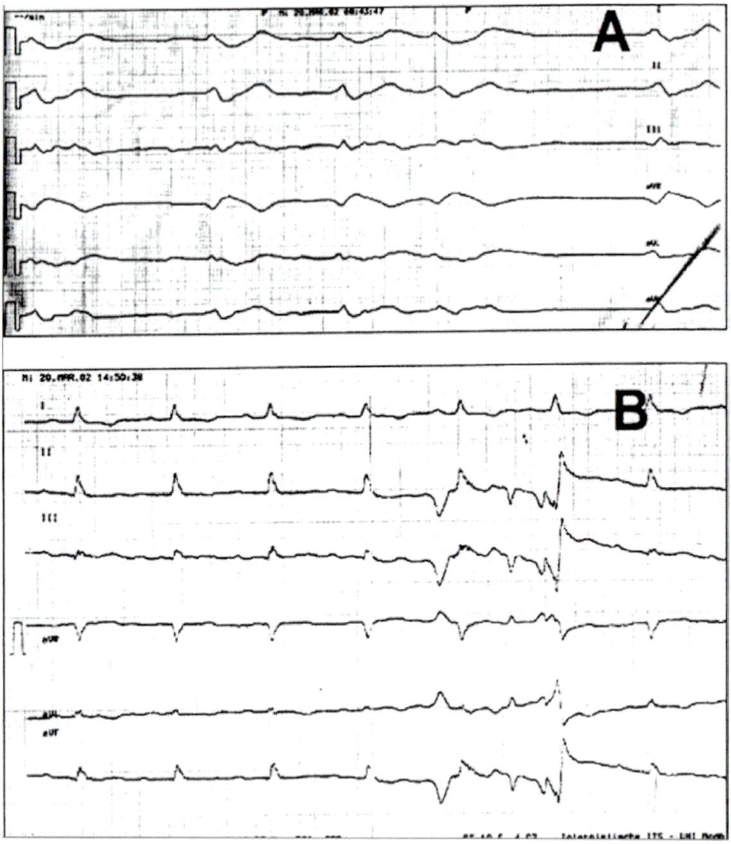

Fig. 6-36 ECGs of patients on ARB + spironolactone with muscle paralysis, bradyarrhythmia (A) and serum K = 9.65 mmol/L; after dialysis, no paralysis or bradyarrhythmia (B), serum K = 4.65 mmol/L. (From Wrenger E, Muller R, Moesenthin M, et al. Interaction of spironolactone with ACE-inhibitors or angiotensin receptor blockers; analysis of 44 cases. *BMJ* 2003;327:147–9.)

that are sodium/volume-mediated; it is opposite to with calcium antagonists (**Figure 6-38**) (159).

In younger/middle-aged hypertensives, calcium blockers are less effective than highly β-1 selective bisoprolol (Figures 6-20 and 6-28) and (Table 6-7) (60, 90, 91).

Variability of SBP appears to be a good predictor of stroke, and calcium blockers are the best class of drugs to reduce the variability (160, 161).

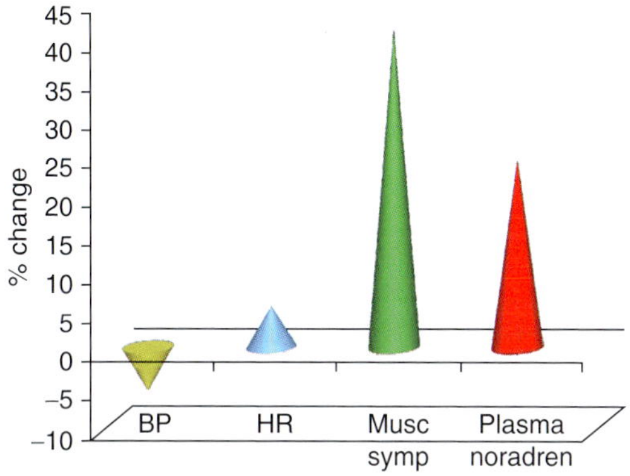

Fig. 6-37 ARBs and sympathetic nerve activity; double-blind, randomized, crossover, placebo-controlled study in young, hypertensive men. (From Heusser K, Vitkovsky J, Raasch W, et al. Elevation of sympathetic nerve activity by eprosartan in young male subjects. *Am J Hypertens* 2003;16:658–64.)

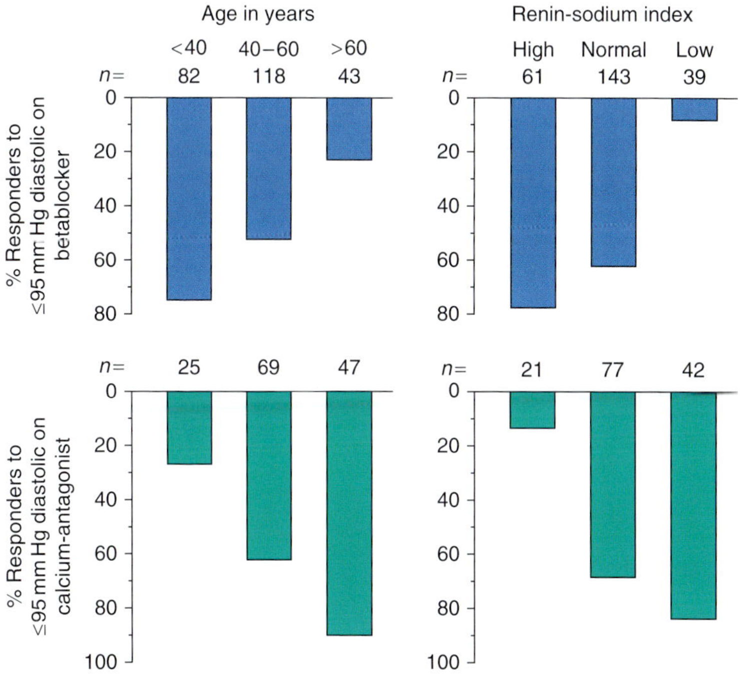

Fig. 6-38 In younger, high-renin hypertensives, the response rate to β-blockers is excellent (upper graphs) and poor to calcium blockers (lower graphs); the reverse is true in elderly, low-renin hypertensives. (From Buhler FH. Age and pathophysiology- orientated antihypertensive response to calcium antagonists. *J Cardiovasc Pharmacol* 1988;12(supp B):156–62.)

B) Efficacy in improving vascular compliance and reducing central BP

Calcium blockers improve vascular compliance (97, 143), as shown by a decrease in PWV (67) (Figure 6-23).

Like ACE inhibitors and ARBs, calcium blockers reduce central BP to a greater extent than brachial BP (**Table 6-10**) (69). Others have shown the efficacy of calcium blockers in reducing central BP and AIx (Figure 6-24) (68, 104, 107). This benefit of calcium blockers in reducing central BP is due to their ability, unlike atenolol, to reduce the magnitude of the peripheral reflected wave through vasodilatation (105).

C) Adverse Reactions

Because of their negative inotropic effect, calcium blockers should not be given to the subjects with poor systolic function (162). Nondihdropindine calcium blockers (e.g. verapamil and diltiazem), due to their negative chronotropic action, can induce bradycardia, and therefore should not be co-prescribed with BBs, as heart block can occur (163). Verapamil can also cause constipation (163).

Calcium blockers, due to their vasodilatory action, can induce peripheral edema, headaches, flushing, and tachycardia (163); eye pain (possibly due to ocular vasodilation) can occur (125).

Metabolic disturbance does not occur with calcium blockers, and the risk of diabetes, compared to diuretics, is reduced (Figure 6-35) (147).

In middle-aged hypertensives, four different dihydropyridine calcium blockers lowered BP to a similar extent, but increased plasma noradrenaline and heart rate to varying degrees (**Figure 6-39**) (164). Verapamil appears not to increase sympathetic nerve activity (165).

6. Other drugs

A) α-1 blockers

In younger/middle-aged hypertensives, doxazosin was less effective in lowering BP than β-1 selective bisoprolol (Table 6-7, Figure 6-20) (60), and atenolol (166). In the elderly, doxazosin was as effective as a diuretic, calcium blocker, or ACE inhibitor in lowering BP (167). In terms of adverse reactions, there is no metabolic disturbance (168), but symptoms include dizziness, postural hypotension, syncope, headache, asthenia (168, 169).

TABLE 6-10 Studies evaluating the effect of dihydropyridine calcium blockers on central blood pressure (CBP) beyond peripheral blood pressure (PBP)

Author	Drug	Type of Study	Duration[a]	Assessment of CBP	Age (Y)	Number of subjects	Disease/ Risk factor	Evidence of reduction of CBP beyond PBP
London G et al. Circulation 1994	Nitredipine 20/40 mg × 1	Randomized, double-blind, placebo run in, 2 parallel active group	Long term (12 mo)	Noninvasive[c]	53	10 (7 M)	End-stage renal disease	POSITIVE Change in PP amplification 0–12 months: 1.02 versus 1.10, $P < .01$
Deary AJ et al. Cli Sci 2002 (ADLIP Study)	Amlodipine 5 mg ×1	Double-blind, crossover, placebo/active controlled	Midterm (6 wk)	Noninvasive[b]	47	30 (22 M)	Untreated eHTN	NEUTRAL Change in SBP amplification versus placebo: men +1/women-3, mm Hg[d]
Morgan T et al. Am J Hypertens 2004	Amlodipine or Felodipine 5/10 mg × 1	Randomized, cross-over, placebo/active controlled	Mid-term (1 months)	Noninvasive[b]	77	32	Never treated eHTN	POSITIVE Change in SBP amplification versus placebo: +2.7 mm Hg[d]

Abbreviations: SBP, systolic blood pressure; M, males; eHTN, essential hypertension; BB, β-blocker; ACEI, angiotensin-1-converting enzyme inhibitor.

[a]Of the observation period after the administration of the active drug.

[b]Sphygmocor apparatus (radial artery tonometry and application of generalized transfer functions for the assessment of aortic blood pressure).

[c]Direct carotid tonometry (Fitchet–Kelly method).

[d]Post-hoc calculation of the change of SBP amplification-the level of statistical significance was not assessed.

From Protogerou AD, Stergiou GS, Vlachopoulos C, et al. The effect of antihypertensive drugs on central blood pressure beyond peripheral blood pressure: evidence for specific class-effects on antihypertensive drugs on pressure amplification. *Curr Pharmac Design* 2009;15:272–89.

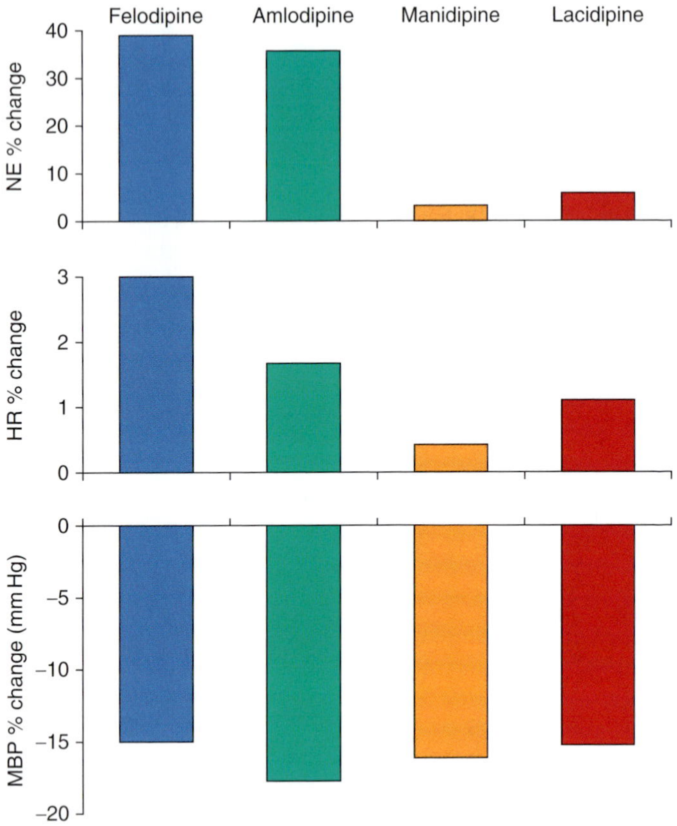

Fig. 6-39 Effect of various dihydropyridine calcium blockers on plasma noradrenaline (NE), heart rate, and BP in middle-aged hypertensives. (From Fogari R, Zoppi A, Corradi L, et al. Effects of different dihydropyridine calcium antagonists on plasma norepinephrine in essential hypertension. *J Hypertens* 2000;18:1871–5.)

B) α-2 blockers (centrally acting agents)

α-2 receptors are found in the brain and are blocked by antihypertensive drugs, such as methyldopa and clonidine, resulting in reduced sympathetic nerve activity. Methyldopa and transdermal clonidine have a similar antiyhypertensive efficacy to atenolol (170). α-2 blockers have the major problem of drowsiness and sedation (171).

C) Nitrates

Nitrates are NO donors that dilate small, peripheral arteries, and reduce the magnitude of the reflected wave from the periphery, thus reducing central pressures (69, 121). In elderly/systolic hypertensives, extended-release nitrate was superior to randomized placebo in reducing brachial SBP and P-P, with no significant effect on the DBP, and also reduced AIx by 25% (172). There was no loss of efficacy (tolerance) over 9 years. It is thus suitable for adding onto conventional therapy in cases of refractory hypertension in the elderly (172). Adverse reactions include headache, flushing, and palpitations, and there is an increase in plasma renin activity and sympathetic nerve activity (173).

D) Renin inhibitors and vaccination against angiotensin II

i) Aliskiren

It is an oral renin inhibitor that, unlike ACE inhibitors and ARBs (which increase plasma renin levels), decreases plasma renin concentration (174). In middle-aged hypertensives, it lowers BP more effectively than hydrochlorthiazide does, and has a similar adverse reaction profile to the diuretic, but is not prone to hypokalemia (175). It lowers BP to a similar degree to ACE inhibitors and ARBs (**Figure 6-40**) (176).

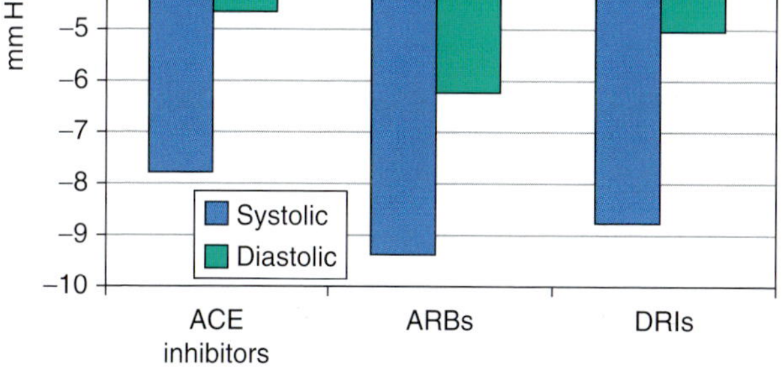

Fig. 6-40 The renin inhibitor aliskiren (DRI) lowers BP to a similar degree as ACE inhibitors and ARBs. (From Messerli FH, Bangalore S. Antihypertensive efficacy of aliskiren. *Circulation* 2009;119:371–3.)

ii) Vaccination

Active immunization to induce antibodies against angiotensin is a novel concept whose long-term safety is unknown, for example, could an autoimmune disease be induced? (177). Given intravenously, versus randomized placebo, it lowered morning BP by 23/15 mm Hg, with occasional flu-like symptoms (178). One big advantage of this approach is that only three injections a year would be necessary.

E) Endothelin-receptor antagonism

Endothelin-1 is a powerful vasoconstrictor. Under double-blind, randomized, placebo-controlled conditions, the endothelin-receptor antagonist lowered BP by 8/5 mm Hg (179). However, the future does not look bright for this class of drug, due to the adverse reaction profile (179, 180) that includes nasal stuffiness, facial edema, heart failure, and myocardial infarction.

F) Aspirin

Aspirin is an inhibitor of cyclooxygenases (COX) responsible for arachidonic acid metabolism and prostaglandin production, and also induces NO release from the vascular endothelium. In middle-aged mild hypertensives, the potential antihypertensive effect of 100 mg of aspirin, taken either on awakening or at bedtime, was studied (181). It is clear that the timing of aspirin intake is important, with only aspirin taken at bedtime having a significant antihypertensive action in both "dippers" and "nondippers" (**Figure 6-41**). The fall in nocturnal BP is particularly notable in nondippers who took aspirin at bedtime. Others were unable to differentiate between aspirin taken in the morning or night, in terms of fall in BP (182).

G) Melatonin, phosphodiesterase-5 inhibition, statins

i) Melatonin

Patients with hypertension and ischemic heart disease show a blunted day/night rhythm in vasodilatation, and suppressed nighttime melatonin levels (melatonin is secreted by the pineal gland). In a randomized, placebo-controlled, double-blind trial, melatonin taken 1 hour before bedtime for 3 months was shown to lower nocturnal BP by 6/4 mm Hg (183).

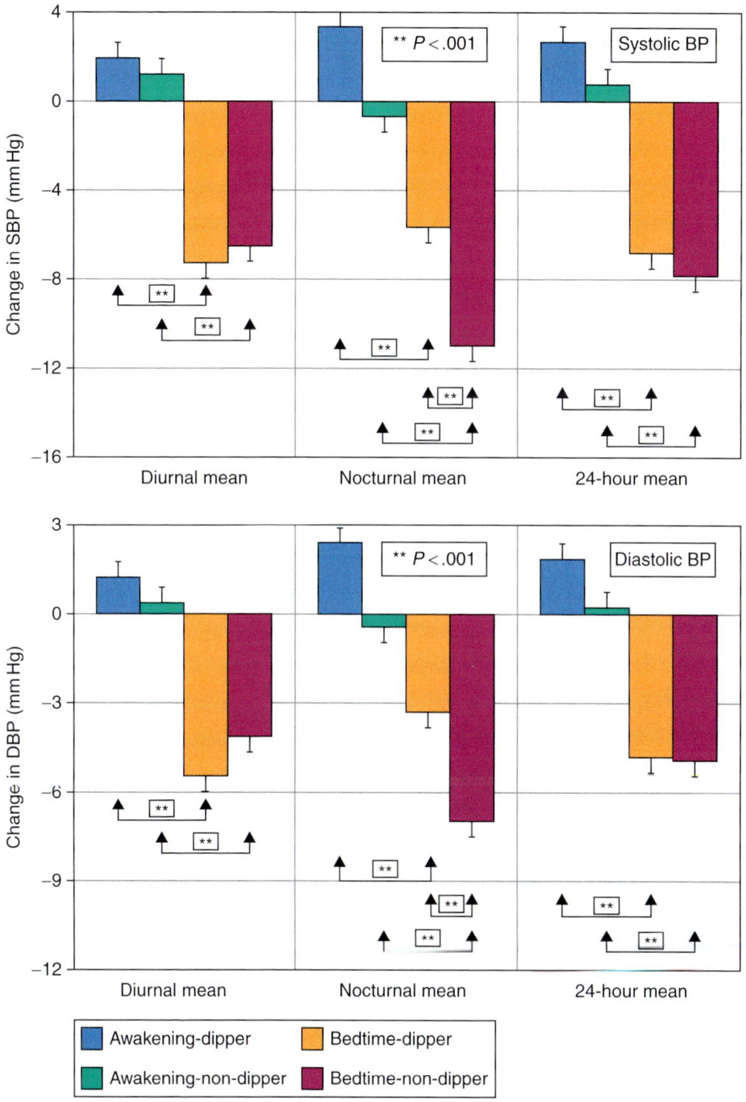

Fig. 6-41 In middle-aged hypertensives, aspirin 100 mg given at bedtime effectively lowers BP, particularly in nondippers. (From Hermida RD, Ayala DE, Calvo C, et al. Differing administration time-dependent effects of aspirin on blood pressure in dipper and nondipper hypertensives. *Hypertension* 2005;46:1060–8.)

ii) Statins

Statins appear not to lower BP (184).

iii) Phosphodiesterase-5 inhibition

These drugs (of which Viagra is a member) have promise in lowering BP without sympathetic activation and an increase in heart rate; their efficacy being similar to other commonly used antihypertensive drugs (185).

7. Ways to optimize blood pressure control

A) Improved "out-of-hospital" systems

Educational packages to general practitioners in developing countries have been shown to improve adherence to antihypertensive drug therapy (186). Home BP values could be uploaded to computers and integrated into a central care system (187). Those who are uncomfortable with computers could be referred to a local pharmacist (187, 188).

B) Noninvasive hemodynamics to achieve better drug selection and blood pressure control

Impedance cardiography has emerged as a reliable noninvasive method to measure hemodynamics in physician clinics (189). Important information on cardiac output, systemic resistance, and intravascular volume can be gathered. A randomized study, comparing standard care with care employing impedance cardiography in middle-aged hypertensives, showed better control of BP in the latter (**Figure 6-42**) (190). Thus, a high cardiac output would result in prescribing a β-blocker or centrally acting agent, and a high systemic resistance would encourage ACE inhibitors, ARBs, or calcium blockers.

C) Pharmacogenomics and response to therapy

There are candidate genes that characterize individuals and their response to certain antihypertensive drug therapy (191). However, this approach does not consistently predict BP response (192); but recent information indicates otherwise (193), where in a large study (n = 51,512) those with the G-allele of the *NEDD4L* gene (controls tubular sodium excretion) responded best to β-blockers and diuretics compared to calcium blockade, in terms of BP control and cardiovascular events.

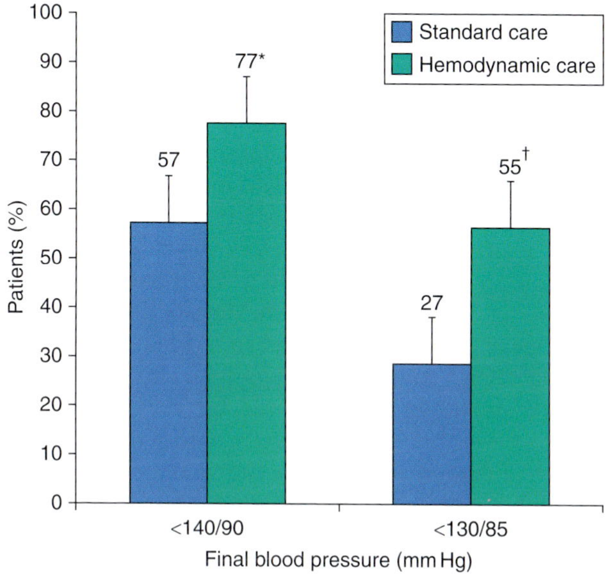

Fig. 6-42 Noninvasive hemodynamic profiling improved the percentage of middle-aged, obese hypertensives who achieved the goal BP. (From Smith RD, Levy P, Ferrario CM, et al. Value of noninvasive hemodynamics to achieve blood pressure control in hypertensive subjects. *Hypertension* 2006;47:771–7.)

8. Resistant hypertension

It has been estimated that in the United States of America, about two-thirds of hypertension is either untreated or undertreated (194), and that 20%–30% is supposedly resistant hypertension (195). However, if ambulatory BP monitoring is employed, removing the so-called white-coat hypertension cases, about 12%–15% of hypertension is genuinely resistant (196, 197). Often, apparently resistant cases are either undertreated or not treated at all (198). The factors that are associated with genuine resistant hypertension are wrong choice of drugs (199), patients taking other drugs that may increase BP (200), male sex, type 2 diabetes, LVH, central obesity, high alcohol intake, the elderly, non-Hispanic black subjects, kidney dysfunction, smokers, and sleep apnea (195–204, 205). Such cases should be taking at least 3 drugs, 1 of which should be a diuretic, and have tried sodium restriction (201). Good results with spironolactone have been obtained in resistant cases (206).

Many cases of resistant hypertension do not respond to variations of combinations of antihypertensive drugs, and renal sympathetic denervation, or carotid baroreflex activation, could be an option—see later.

9. Combination therapy, free and fixed dose

A) Free combination

It has been estimated that 75% of patients will require combination therapy to achieve BP targets (207). By combining drugs with complementary modes of action, there is an increased chance of achieving BP targets (208). Such an approach is superior to up-titrating a single drug. A meta-analysis of 42 trials showed that combining 2 drugs with different modes of action gives about a 5 times greater additional fall in BP than doubling the dose of a single drug (209).

The European Society of Hypertension (ESH)/European Society of Cardiology (ESC) guidelines on combination therapy conclude that (i) the drugs should have different, but complementary modes of action; (ii) the antihypertensive effect of the combination should be greater than that of either of the individual drugs; and (iii) the combination has a favorable tolerability profile (208).

Suitable drug combinations are shown in **Figure 6-43** (210) and (**Table 6-11**) (211), with the recommendation that such combinations should be the initial treatment if the patient's BP is greater than 20/10 mm Hg above the target level, unless cardiovascular status is brittle (211). The author of this book would disagree with (Table 6-11) on 2 counts—(1) A β-blocker/diuretic or calcium blocker combination

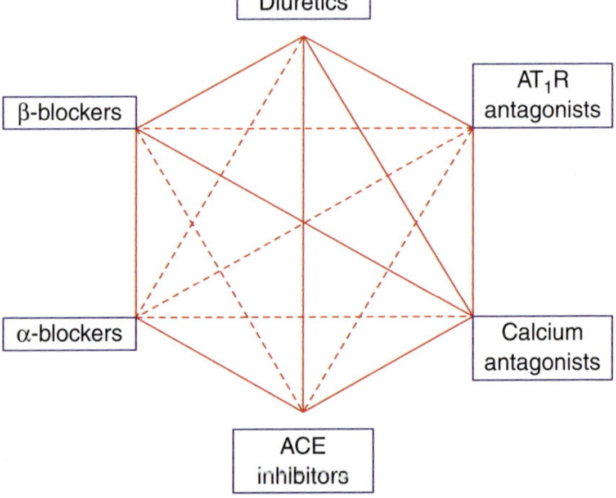

Fig. 6-43 Schematic representation showing the most rational (thick lines) antihypertensive drug combinations. (From Unger T, Paulis L, Sica DA. Therapeutic perspectives in hypertension. *Eur Heart J* 2011;32:2739–47.)

TABLE 6-11 Drug combinations in hypertension

Preferred
ACE inhibitor/diuretic
ARB/diuretic
ACE inhibitor/CCB
ARB/CCB
Acceptable
β-blocker/diuretic
CCB (dihydropyridine)/β-blocker
CCB/diuretic
Renin inhibitor/diuretic
Renin inhibitor/CCB
Dihydropyridine CCB/nondihydropyridine CCB
Unacceptable
ACE inhibitor/ARB
Renin inhibitor/ARB
Renin inhibitor/ACE inhibitor
RAS inhibitor/β-blocker
CCB (nondihydropyridine)/β-blocker
Centrally acting agent/β-blocker

Abbreviations: ACE, angiotensin-converting enzyme; ARB, angiotensin receptor blockers; CCB, calcium channel blockers.

From Sever PS, Messerli FH. Hypertension management 2011: optimal combination therapy. *Eur Heart J* 2011;32:2499–506.

should be a preferred choice, provided the β-blocker was highly β-1 selective, for example, bisoprolol, which causes no metabolic disturbance and avoids the β-blocker/smoking interaction (see Chapter 8). It is a β-blocker/calcium blocker combination that compared so favorably with ACE inhibition/calcium blocker combination in the classic UKPDS Study in middle-aged, obese hypertensives with diabetes (see Chapter 8). (3) ARB/diuretic combinations have a major query hanging over them because both the diuretic and the ARB are linked to a significant increase in sympathetic nerve activity in younger subjects (212), thus increasing the risk of myocardial infarction in young/middle-aged diastolic hypertensives (see Chapters 5 and 8).

B) Fixed-dose combination

i) Two drugs

The advantages of single-pill regimens are (1) more simple administration, (3) more rapid achievement of BP goal, and (4) better patient adherence to therapy (208, 210).

Fixed-dose combinations improve patient compliance to treatment compared to free combinations of the same drugs (213), which leads to improved BP control and reduced adverse events and morbidity, that is, it is more cost effective (214).

ii) Three drugs

Such fixed-dose combinations exist, for example, RAAs inhibitor plus amplodipine plus a thiazide diuretic (210). These combinations provide a more profound fall in BP without (generally) increasing adverse reactions or safety. However, there can be dose-independent adverse reactions, loss of dose flexibility, and possible inappropriate dosing. Hence, individually tailored therapy is traded for reduced costs and simplification (210).

iii) Five drugs

The so-called Polycap polypill contains a thiazide 12.5 mg, atenolol 50 mg, ramapril 5 mg, simvastatin 20 mg, and aspirin 100 mg, and is effective in reducing BP, low-density lipoprotein (LDL) cholesterol, thromboxane, and heart rates, with excellent tolerability (215). Such drugs could potentially be widely used in secondary prevention and selected high-risk individuals without cardio vascular disease, with the prospect of a 50%–75% reduction in risk (216). In contrast, low-risk individuals would require a large trial to quantify benefits (216).

10. Renal sympathetic denervation and baroceptor activation in patients with resistant hypertension

A) Renal sympathetic denervation

Both renal afferent and efferent sympathetic nerves contribute toward the development and progression of hypertension (**Figure 6-44**) (217). The denervation procedure involves femoral artery catheterization, the tip of the catheter being placed in the distal renal artery. Radiofrequency energy is then applied to the endothelial lining, the catheter is then pulled back 1–2 cm, rotated, and further energy is applied. The procedure is repeated 4–5 times in the same artery before moving to the other renal artery. The hope is that the holy grail of "a once and forever treatment of hypertension" will be available.

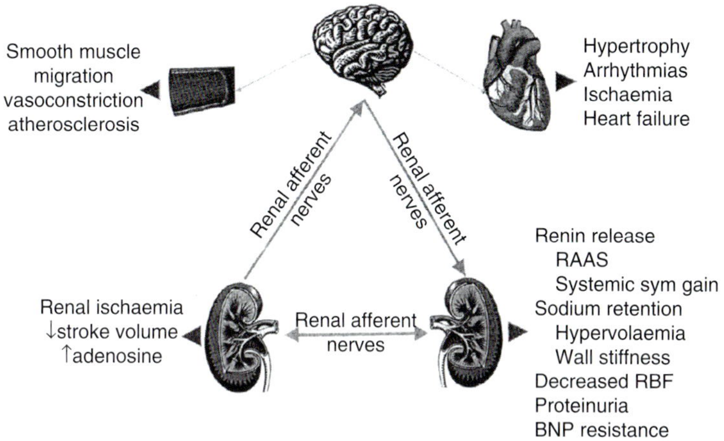

Fig. 6-44 Renal sympathetic afferent and efferent nerve activity contributes to the development and maintenance of hypertension. (From Krum H, Schlaich M, Sobotka P, et al. Novel procedure- and device-based strategies in the management of systemic hypertension. *Eur Heart J* 2011;32:537–44.)

A randomized, controlled study in 106 middle-aged (mean age of 58 years), resistant hypertensives, the so-called SYMPLICITY HTN-1 trial, resulted in a 32/12 mm Hg fall in BP, with 84% experiencing a fall in SBP of 10 mm Hg, over 6 months (218). In this study, at 6 months, 71% of patients were classified responders, increasing to 100% at 3-year follow-up (219). There were no serious procedure-related, or device-related, adverse events. Noradrenaline spillover is reduced by 47%, there is improvement of renal function (220), and the fall in BP is evident for at least 2 years (Figure 6-45) (221). A study in middle-aged (mean age of 49 years) resistant hypertensives showed that not only was BP lowered for 6 months, but also sleep apnea was markedly reduced, as was blood sugar and HbA1-c (222). Post-apneic rises in BP and atrial fibrillation are preventedd by renal sympathetic denervation (225). Albuminuria is also markedly reduced (226). However, it should be emphasized that only 39% of resistant cases achieve optimal control of BP by this method.

There is a concern that renal nerve fibers may regenerate; it is thus reassuring that good BP control continues 2 years after the procedure (**Figure 6-45**) (221).

Renal sympathetic denervation has been shown to reduce left ventricular hypertrophy and improve cardiac function—see Chapter 7 (223).

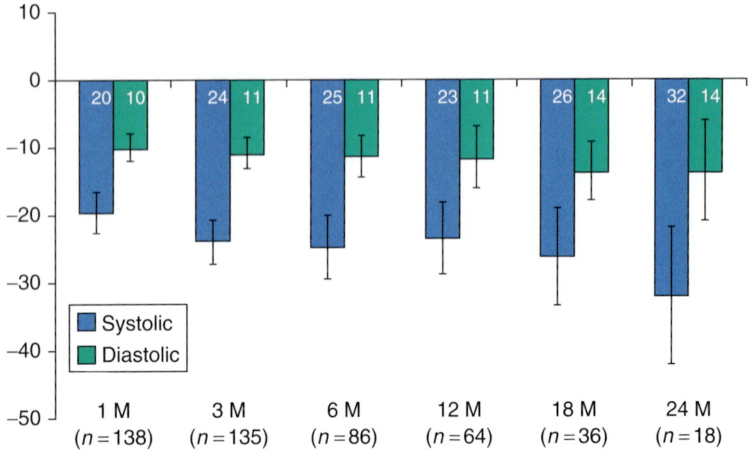

Fig. 6-45 Effect of catheter-based renal sympathetic denervation on BP over 2 years in middle-aged resistant hypertensives. (From Symplicity HTN-1 Investigators. Catheter-based renal sympathetic denervation for resistant hypertension. *Hypertension* 2011;57:911–17.)

Not all patients are suitable for renal denervation (224); contraindications being (i) previous renal artery intervention, (ii) evidence of renal artery atherosclerosis, (iii) multiple renal arteries, (iv) GFR < 45 ml/min, (v) unstable angina or a myocardial infarction/stroke within the past 3–6 months.

B) Baroceptor Activation

This procedure involves active surgical intervention (217). The Rheos device implantation involves both carotid sinuses being surgically exposed; an experienced surgeon can perform the operation within 2.5–3.0 hours, followed by a few days post-operative care. Blood pressure control is still present 3 years post-op (**Figure 6-46**) (217). Clearly, this procedure is a long way from routine practice (210), but for some patients the opportunity to reduce the intensity of polypharmacy may prove attractive (227). Recent information indicates that baroceptor activation is equivalent to renal sympathetic denervation in lowering BP (in obesity-related hypertension), but superior in that it also suppresses systematic sympathetic activity (lowers plasma noradrenaline levels) and lowers heart rate (**Figure 6-47**) (228).

11. Hypertension in children

As in young/middle-aged adults, hypertension in children/adolescents is linked to obesity and lack of exercise—see Chapter 4. It is

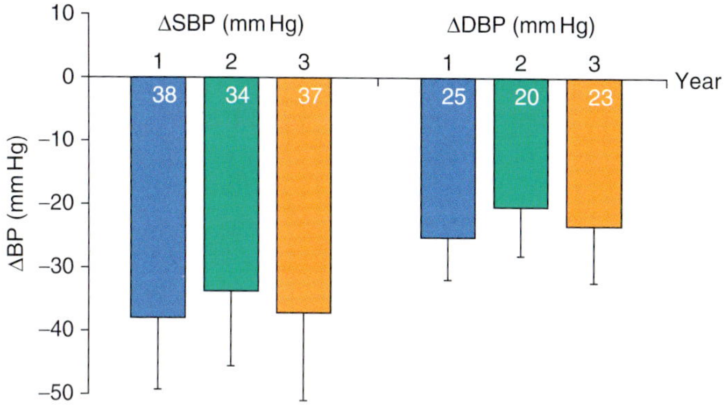

Fig. 6-46 Rheos baroreflex stimulation lowers BP over 3 years in the cases of resistant hypertension. Krum H et al. 2011 (217).

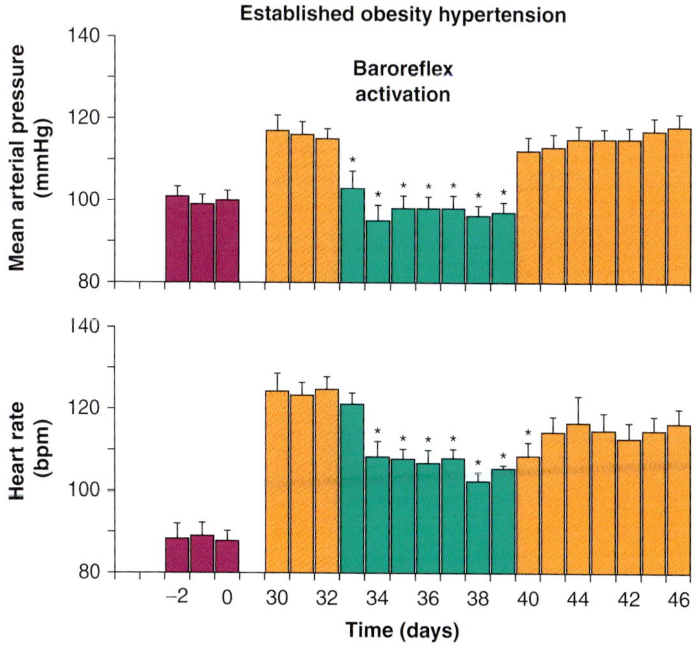

Fig. 6-47 Prolonged baroreflex activation lowers both blood pressure and heart rate. Lohmeier T et al. 2012 (228).

thus not surprising that randomized, controlled studies have shown that losing weight plus aerobic exercise are effective in lowering BP (229–231), and that volume of exercise might be more important than intensity (232).

Drug therapy for childhood hypertension is still a difficult area, with no outcome data available. The first randomized trial in hypertensive children aged less than 6 years showed that the ARB valsartan was superior to placebo in lowering BP, with few adverse reactions (233). The antihypertensive effect of valsartan in children is similar to that of the ACEI enalapril (234). The recommendations of the European Society of Hypertension 2009 (235) are shown in Table 6-11. The concern that the author of this book has with these recommendations relates to increased sympathetic nerve activity and its possible harm. As indicated in Chapter 4, childhood hypertension is linked to increased sympathetic activity, and certain drug groups—diuretics, dihydropyridine calcium blockers, and ARBs, increase sympathetic activity; in young/middle-aged hypertensives these three drug groups increase the risk of myocardial infarction (see Chapter 8). Thus, the author's preference would be for β-1 selective, β-blockade, or ACE-inhibition.

12. Hypertension and pregnancy

This is a contentious area. The prevalence of chronic hypertension in pregnancy in the United States is about 3% (236). Chronic hypertension increases the risk of preeclampsia and the risk of low fetal weights and premature birth (236). Antihypertensive drugs that may be considered for treatment are shown in **Table 6-12** (236).

ACE inhibitors and ARBs should not be used in the first trimester due to an increased risk of oligohydramnios, neonatal anuria, growth abnormalities, skull hypoplasia, fetal death, and teratogenic effects (236). Concerning fetal malformations, there are data to suggest that these are just as likely with commonly used antihypertensive agents, other than ACE inhibitors, used in the first trimester (237).

There seems to be a general consensus that the first-line drugs to be considered for the treatment of hypertension in pregnancy are methyldopa, labetalol, and nifedipine (238–240). Interestingly, low-dose aspirin, given at bedtime, has been found to be protective against preeclampsia, gestational hypertension, intrauterine growth retardation, and preterm delivery in high-risk pregnant women (241).

TABLE 6-12 Recommended initial doses for selected antihypertensive drugs for the management of hypertension in children and adolescents

Class	Drug	Dose	Interval
Diuretics	Amiloride	0.4–0.6 mg/kg per day	q.d.
	Chlorthalidone	0.3 mg/kg per day	q.d.
	Furosemide	0.5–2.0 mg/kg per dose	q.d.–b.i.d.
	Hydrochlorothiazide	0.5–1 mg/kg per day	q.d.
	Spironolactone	1 mg/kg per day	q.d.–b.i.d.
β-Adrenergic blockers	Atenolol	0.5–1 mg/kg per day	q.d.–b.i.d.
	Metoprolol	0.5–1.0 mg/kg per day	q.d. (ER)
	Propanolol	1 mg/kg per day	b.i.d.–t.i.d.
Calcium channel blockers	Amlodipine	0.06–0.3 mg/kg per day	q.d.
	Felodipine	2.5 mg per day	q.d.
	Nifedipine	0.25–0.5 mg/kg per day	q.d.–b.i.d. (ER)
Angiotensin-converting enzyme inhibitors	Captopril	0.3–0.5 mg/kg per dose	b.i.d.–t.i.d.
	Enalapril	0.08–0.6 mg/kg per day	q.d.
	Fosinopril	0.1–0.6 mg/kg per day	q.d.
	Lisinopril	0.08–0.6 mg/kg per day	q.d.
	Ramipril	2.5–6 mg per day	q.d.
Angiotensin-receptor blockers	Candesartan	0.16–0.5 mg/kg per day	q.d.
	Irbesartana	75–150 mg per day	q.d.

TABLE 6-12 Recommended initial doses for selected antihypertensive drugs for the management of hypertension in children and adolescents (*Continued*)

Class	Drug	Dose	Interval
	Losartan	0.75–1.44 mg/kg per day	q.d
	Valsartan	2 mg/kg per day	q.d.

From Lurbe E, Cifkova R, Cruickshank JK, et al. Management of high blood pressure in children and adolescents; recommendations of the European Society of Hypertension. *J Hypertens* 2009;27:1719–42.

TABLE 6-13 Common drugs used in chronic hypertension in pregnancy

Drug	Class or mechanism of action	Usual range of dose	Comments
Methyldopa	Centrally acting alpha agonist	250 mg–1.5 g orally twice daily	Often used as first-line therapy Long-term data suggest safety in offspring
Labetalol	Combined α- and β-blocker	100–1200 mg orally twice daily	Often used as first-line therapy May exacerbate asthma Intravenous formulation is available to treat hypertensive emergencies
Metoprolol	β-blocker	25–200 mg orally twice daily	May exacerbate asthma Possible association with fetal growth restriction
			Other β-blockers (e.g., pindolol and propranolol) have been safely used Some experts recommend avoiding atenolol

TABLE 6-13 Common drugs used in chronic hypertension in pregnancy (*Continued*)

Drug	Class or mechanism of action	Usual range of dose	Comments
Nifedipine (long-acting)	Calcium-channel blocker	30–120 mg orally once daily	Use of short-acting nifedipine is typically not recommended, given risk of hypotension Other calcium-channel blockers have been safely used
Hydralazine	Peripheral vasodilator	50–300 mg orally in 2 or 4 divided doses	Intravenous formulation is available to treat hypertensive emergencies
Hydrochlorothiazide	Diuretic	12.5–50 mg orally once daily	Previous concerns about increased risk of an adverse outcome are not supported by recent data

From Seely EW, Ecker J. Chronic hypertension in pregnancy. *N Engl J Med* 2011;365:439 46.

SUMMARY AND CONCLUSIONS

1. Changes in lifestyle can be effective in lowering raised BP; these include (a) loss of excess weight, (b) aerobic (and to a lesser extent anaerobic) exercise that not only affects BP, but also improves blood chemistry and lowers plasma noradrenaline levels, (c) dietary adjustment, for example, the DASH diet that is rich in fruit and vegetables and low in saturated fat, can lower BP as much as drug monotherapy; the DASH diet, plus low sodium content, is particularly effective in lowering BP. (d) avoiding alcohol abuse, (e) reducing dietary salt content can, in some subjects, lower BP as much as drug monotherapy, and is particularly relevant in countries with high salt intake, for example, Japan and China, (though there is some concern regarding the stimulation

of the renin-angiotensin system associated with low-salt diets). (f) antistress and yoga techniques, and (g) governmental health plans and input from the food industry can have major beneficial effects.

2. Thiazide-type diuretics and spironolactone—are effective in lowering BP in low-plasma renin/salt sensitive subjects, that is, the elderly and black hypertensives; chlorthalidone and spironolactone appear to be more effective in lowering BP than hydrochlorthiazide; diuretics can improve vascular compliance, but possibly less so than calcium blockers or ACE inhibitors; diuretics lower central BP effectively, but not more so than brachial BP; adverse reactions of thiazide-like agents include impaired glucose tolerance, gout, impotence, and increased sympathetic nerve activity; spironolactone avoids or prevents these problems, but can induce gynecomastia, sexual dysfunction, and hyperkalemia; unlike thiazide diuretics, spironolactone does not increase sympathetic nerve activity.
3. β-Blockers—the active antihypertensive ingredient is β-1 blockade, and high β-1 selectivity, for example, bisoprolol, is the most effective way to lower brachial BP in white young/middle-aged hypertensives (high sympathetic nerve activity); β-1 blockade improves vascular compliance, but lowers central BP less than brachial BP in the elderly (additional vasodilatory properties, e.g. nebivolol with ISA, induce a further fall in central BP); adverse reactions with (a) nonselective, for example, propranolol, or only moderately β-1 selective β-blockers, for example, atenolol and metoprolol, include metabolic disturbance (involving increased insulin resistance, blood sugar, and blood lipids), increase in weight, sexual dysfunction, cigarette smoking/adrenaline/hypertensive interaction, bronchoconstriction in reversible airways disease, renal dysfunction; (b) with additional α-blocking properties, for example, carvedilol, there can be postural hypotension/dizziness, and added sexual dysfunction; (c) high lipophilicity, for example, metoprolol and nebivolol, results in high brain concentrations and possible sleep disturbance; (d) poor metabolizer status involving cytochrome P 450 system, for example, metoprolol and nebivolol, leads to high blood levels and loss of β-1 selectivity; (e) most of these potential problems can be avoided by high β-1 selectivity, for example bisoprolol, where occasional fatigue and cold peripheries are the prime adverse reactions, and renoprotection is similar to an ACEI/ARB.

4. ACE inhibitors—like BBs, they act best in high-renin hypertension, for example, young/middle-aged, but lower brachial BP less effectively than highly β-1 selective bisoprolol; they improve vascular compliance and lower central BP more effectively than brachial BP; adverse reactions include: (a) captopril, with a sulfhydril grouping, can cause dysgeusia (taste disturbance); (b) other ACE inhibitors can cause skin reactions, but more commonly cough (possibly due to high bradykinin levels); rarely the life-threatening angioedema, and urticaria can occur in susceptible patients; hyperkalemia can occur, particularly if spironolactone is co-prescribed.
5. ARBs—in young/middle-aged hypertensives, ARBs lower BP less effectively than highly β-1 selective bisoprolol, but in the elderly, lower central BP more effectively than brachial BP; adverse reactions include (a) ARBs are generally well tolerated, but like ACE inhibitors can, induce hyperkalemia, particularly where there is renal dysfunction, or spironolactone is co-presented; (b) in younger hypertensives, ARBs increase sympathetic nerve activity.
6. Calcium blockers—in younger/high-renin hypertensives, calcium blockers are less effective in lowering BP than highly β-1 selective bisoprolol; in the elderly, they improve vascular compliance and lower central BP more effectively than brachial BP, and they reduce variability of SBP; nondihydropyridine calcium blockers can induce constipation (verapamil), and can induce bradycardia and heart block (particularly if BBs are co-prescribed), and, where cardiac function is impaired, induce heart failure; dihydropyridine calcium blockers should be avoided if poor cardiac systolic function is present, and being vasodilators, they can induce palpitations, flushing, peripheral edema and headaches; they increase sympathetic nerve activity.
7. Other drugs—(a) α-1 blockers, for example, doxazosin, are less effective in lowering BP than bisoprolol in younger patients, but in the elderly, they lower brachial BP to a similar degree as diuretics, calcium blockers, and ACE inhibitors; adverse reactions include postural hypotension, dizziness, and syncope. (b) α-2 blockers (centrally acting), for example, methyldopa and clonidine, lower BP effectively, but have the major adverse reaction problem of drowsiness and sedation. (c) Nitrates—highly effective in lowering central BPs, but adverse reactions include headaches, flushing, and palpitations, and they increase sympathetic nerve activity. (d) Renin inhibitors (including vaccination

against angiotensin II)—lower BP to a similar degree as ACE inhibitors and ARBs; vaccination (to angiotensin) need be given only three times a year, but can induce flu-like symptoms, and long-term safety is unknown. (e) Endothelin receptor antagonists—lower BP moderately, but adverse reactions include nasal stuffiness, facial edema, and heart failure/myocardial infarction. (f) Aspirin—low dose (100 mg), given at bedtime, induces a significant fall in BP over 24 hours, particularly in "nondippers"; the adverse reactions to aspirin are well known.

8. Optimizing BP control—(a) involve home BP measurement and pharmacists in an integrated central care system; (b) impedance cardiography can assess hemodynamics noninvasively, and aids selection of appropriate drug; (c) pharmacogenomics can help choose the correct antihypertensive drugs for a particular patient.
9. Drug combination therapy—75% of hypertensives require 2 or more antihypertensive agents to achieve adequate BP control; combining drugs with complimentary antihypertensive actions is more effective than dose titration of a single drug; suitable combinations are β-blocker (BB)/dihydropyridine calcium blocker, BB/thiazide diuretic (but metabolic disturbance with nonselective BB), diuretic/ACE inhibitor, diuretic/ARB, diuretic/ calcium blocker, ACE/ calcium blocker; the BB should preferably be highly β-1 selective.
10. Fixed-dose combination therapy—could be initial therapy if BP is at least 20/10 mm Hg above target levels; this once-daily approach improves patient compliance to therapy, BP control is achieved more quickly, thus morbidity/mortality is reduced, and the approach is cost effective.
11. Resistant hypertension—about 12%–15% of primary hypertension is genuinely resistant to lifestyle/drug therapy; such cases are candidates for procedures such as renal sympathetic denervation and baroceptor activation, the so-called once and forever treatment; the jury is still out on these procedures, though good control of BP continues for at least 2–3 years postintervention.
12. Childhood/adolescent primary hypertension is closely linked to obesity and high sympathetic nerve activity; antihypertensive drugs that further increase sympathetic activity, that is, diuretics, dihydropyridine calcium blockers, and ARBs, should therefore be avoided; the author's preference would be β-1 selective blockade.
13. Primary hypertension of pregnancy increases maternal and fetal risk; the first-line drugs for this condition are methyldopa, labetalol, and nifedipine.

REFERENCES

1. Woolf KJ, Bisognano JD. Nondrug interventions for treatment of hypertension. *J Clin Hypertens* 2011;13:829–35.
2. Weinster RL, James LD, Darnell BE, et al. Obesity-related hypertension: evaluation of the separate effects of energy restriction and weight reduction on heamodynamic and neuroendocrine status. *Am J Med* 1991;90:460–8.
3. Harsha DW, Bray GA. Weight loss and blood pressure control (Pro). *Hypertension* 2008;51:1420–5.
4. Wildman RP, Farhat GN, Patel AS, et al. Weight change is associated with change in arterial stiffness among healthy young adults. *Hypertension* 2005;45:187–92.
5. Niebauer J, Cooke JP. Cardiovascular effects of exercise: role of endothelial shear stress. *J Am Coll Cardiol* 1996;28:1652–60.
6. Cornelissen VA, Fagard RH. Exercise intensity and post exercise hypotension. *J Hypertens* 2004;22:1859–61.
7. Erol MK, Yilmaz M, Oztasyonar Y, et al. Aortic distensiblity is increasing in elite athletes. *Am J Cardiol* 2002;89:1002–4.
8. Ferrier KE, Waddell TK, Gatzka CD, et al. Aerobic exercise training does not modify large artery compliance in isolated systolic hypertension. *Hypertension* 2001;38:222–6.
9. Cornelissen VA, Fagard RH. Effects of endurance training on blood pressure, blood pressure-regulating mechanisms, and cardiovascular risk factors. *Hypertension* 2005;46:667–75.
10. Totsikas C, Rohm J, Kantartzis K, et al. Cardiorespiratory fitness determines the reduction in blood pressure and insulin resistance during lifestyle intervention. *J Hypertens* 2011;29:1220–7.
11. Franks PW, Bhattacharyya S, Luan J, et al. Association between physical activity and blood pressure is modified by variants in the G-protein coupled receptor 10. *Hypertension* 2004;43:224–8.
12. Fagard RH. Physical activity, physical fitness and the incidence of hypertension. *J Hypertens* 2005;23:265–7.
13. Hu G, Barengo NC, Tuomilehto J, et al. Relationship of physical activity and body mass index to the risk of hypertension: a Prospective Study in Finland. *Hypertension* 2004;43:25–30.
14. Cornelissen VA, Fagard RH. Effect of resistance training on resting blood pressure: a meta-analysis of randomised controlled trials. *J Hypertens* 2005;23:251–9.
15. Appel LJ, Moore TJ, Obarzanek E, et al. A clinical trial of the effects of dietary patterns on blood pressure. *N Engl J Med* 1997;336:1117–24.
16. Moore TJ, Conlin PR, Ard J, et al. DASH diet is effective treatment of stage 1 isolated systolic hypertension. *Hypertension* 2001;38:155–8.
17. Lopez HF, Martin KL, Nashar K, et al. DASH diet lowers blood pressure and lipid-induced oxidative stress in obesity. *Hypertension* 2003;41:422–30.
18. Akita S, Sacks FM, Svetkey LP, et al. Effects of the DASH diet on the pressure-naturesis relationship. *Hypertension* 2003;42:8–13.

19. Nori US, Agarwal AK, Von Visger JR. Dietary therapy in hypertension. *N Engl J Med* 2010;363:1580–1.
20. Duffy SJ, Gokce N, Holbrook M, et al. Treatment of hypertension with ascorbic acid. *Lancet* 1999;354:2048–9.
21. Fotherby MD, Williams J, Forster LA, et al. Effect of vitamin C on ambulatory blood pressure and plasma lipids in older persons. *J Hypertens* 2000;18:411–5.
22. Chen L, Caballero B, Mitchell DC, et al. Reducing consumption of sugar-sweetened beverages is associated with reduced blood pressure. *Circulation* 2010;121:2398–406.
23. Appel LJ, Sacks FM, Carey VJ, et al. Effects of protein, monosaturated fat, and carbohydrate intake on blood pressure and serum lipids. *JAMA* 2005;294:2455–64.
24. Tambert D, Roesen R, Lehmann C, et al. Effects of low habitual cocoa intake on blood pressure and bioactive nitric oxide. *JAMA* 2007;298:49–60.
25. Baer HJ, Glynn RJ, Hu FB et al. Risk factors for mortality in the Nurses' Health Study. *Am J Epidemiol* 2010;173:319–29.
26. West SG, Gebauer SK, Kay CD et al. Diets containing pistachios reduce systolic blood pressure and peripheral vascular responses to stress in adults with hyperlipidemia. *Hypertension* 2012;60:58–63.
27. Corti R, Binggeli C, Sudano I, et al. Coffee acutely increases sympathetic nerve activity and blood pressure independently of caffeine content. *Circulation* 2002;106:2935–40.
28. Papamichael CM, Karatzi KN, Papaioannou TG, et al. Acute combined effects of olive oil and wine on pressure wave reflections: another beneficial influence of the Mediterranean diet antioxicants. *J Hypertens* 2008;26:223–9.
29. Rakic V, Puddey IB, Burke V, et al. Influence of pattern of alcohol intake on blood pressure in regular drinkers: a controlled trial. *J Hypertens* 1998;16:165–74.
30. Moreira LB, Fuchs FD, Moraes RS, et al. Alcohol intake and blood pressure: the importance of time since the last drink. *J Hypertens* 1998;16:175–80.
31. Hougaku H, Fleg JL, Lakatta EG, et al. Effect of light-to-moderate alcohol consumption on age-associated arterial stiffening. *Am J Cardiol* 205;95:1006–10.
32. Sacks FM, Svetkey LP, Vollmer WM, et al. Effects on blood pressure of reduced dietary sodium and the dietary approaches to stop hypertension (DASH) diet. *N Engl J Med* 2001;344:3–10.
33. Obarzanek E, Proschan MA, Vollmer WM, et al. Individual blood pressure responses to changes on salt diet: results from the DASH-sodium trial. *Hypertension* 2003;42:459–67.
34. Brag GA, Vollmer WM, Sacks FM, et al. A further subgroup analysis of the effects of the DASH diet and three dietary sodium levels on blood pressure. *Am J Cardiol* 2004;94:222–7.

35. Sacks FM, Campos H. Dietary therapy in hypertension. *N Engl J Med* 2010;362:2102–12.
36. Chen J, Gu D, Huang J, et al. Metabolic syndrome and salt-sensitivity of blood pressure in non-diabetic people in China. *Lancet* 2009;373:829–35.
37. Matyas E, Jeitler K, Horvath K, et al. Benefit assessment of salt reduction in patients with hypertension: systematic overview. *J Hypertens* 2011;29:821–8.
38. He FJ, Marciniak M, Visagie E, et al. Effect of modest salt reduction on blood pressure, urinary albumin and pulse wave velocity in White, Black and Asian mild hypertensives. *Hypertension* 2009;54:482–8.
39. Gates PE, Tanaka H, Hiatt WR, et al. Dietary sodium restriction rapidly improves large elastic artery compliance in older adults with systolic hypertension. *Hypertension* 2004;44:35–41.
40. Gaudal NA, Galloe AM, Garred P. Effects of sodium restriction on blood pressure, renin, aldosterone, catecholamines, cholesterols and triglyceride: a meta-analysis. *JAMA* 1998;279:1383–91.
41. Tikellis C, Pichering RJ, Tsorotes D et al. Activation of the renin-angiotensin system mediates the effects of dietary salt intake on atherogenesis in the apolipoptotein E knockout mouse. *Hypertension* 2012;60:98–105.
42. Miller 3rd ER, Erlinger TP, Young DR, et al. Results of Diet, Exercise and Weight Loss Intervention Trial (DEW-IT). *Hypertension* 2002;40:612–8.
43. Writing Group of the PREMIER Collaborative Research Group. Effects of comprehensive lifestyle modification on blood pressure control. Main results of the PREMIER Clinical Trial. *JAMA* 2003;289: 2083–93.
44. Esposito K, Pontillo A, Di Palo C, et al. Effect of weight loss and lifestyle changes on vascular inflammatory markers in obese women. *JAMA* 2003;289:1799–1804.
45. Mori TA, Burke V, Puddey IB, et al. Effect of fish diets and weight loss on serum leptin concentration in overweight, treated hypertensive subjects. *J Hypertens* 2004;22:1983–90.
46. Jones DW. Dietary sodium and blood pressure. *Hypertension* 2004;43:932–5.
47. Whelton PK, He J, Appel LJ. Primary prevention of hypertension: clinical and public health advisory from the National High Blood Pressure Education Program. *JAMA* 2002;288:1882–8.
48. Bibbins-Domingo K, Chertow GM, Coxson PG, et al. Projected effect of dietary salt reductions on future cardiovascular disease. *N Engl J Med* 2010;362:590–9.
49. Yang G. Salt intake in individuals with metabolic syndrome. *Lancet* 2009;373:792–4.
50. Webster JL, Dunford EK, Hawkes C, et al. Salt reduction initiatives around the world. *J Hypertens* 2011;29:1043–50.

51. MacMahon S, Yan L. Responding to China's hypertensive crisis. *Lancet* 2009;374:1728–9.
52. Sharp D. Labelling salt in food: if yes, how? *Lancet* 2004;364:2079–81.
53. Appel LJ, Brands MW, Daniels SR, et al. Dietary approaches to prevent and treat hypertension: a scientific statement from the American Heart Association. *Hypertension* 2006;47:296–308.
54. Niarchos AP. Pathophysiology, diagnosis and treatment of hypertension in the elderly. *Cardiovasc Rev Rep* 1980;1:621–7.
55. Richardson DW, Freund J, Gear AS, et al. Effect of propranolol on elevated arterial blood pressure. *Circulation* 1968;37:534–42.
56. Dorsch MP, Gilespie BW, Erickson SR, et al. Chorthalidone reduces cardiovascular events compared with hydrochlorthiazide. *Hypertension* 2011;57:689–94.
57. Ernst ME, Carter BL, Goerdt CJ, et al. Comparative antihypertensive effects of hydrochlorthiazide and chlorthalidone on ambulatory and office blood pressure. *Hypertension* 2006;47:352–8.
58. Kaplan NM. The choice of thiazide diuretics. *Hypertension* 2009;54:951–3.
59. Rosendorff C. Spironolactone for all hypertensive patients? *J Hypertens* 2010;28:13–4.
60. Deary AJ, Schumann AL, Murfeet H, et al. Double-blind, placebo controlled crossover comparison of 5 classes of drugs. *J Hypertens* 2002;20:771–7.
61. Philipp T, Anlauf M, Distler A, et al. Randomised,double-blind, multicentre comparison of hydrochlorthiazide, atenolol, nitrendipine and enalapril in antihypertensive treatment: results of the HANE study. *BMJ* 1997;315:154–9.
62. Giannattasio C, Mancia G. Arterial distensibility in humans. Modulating mechanisms, alterations in diseases and effects of treatment. *J Hypertens* 2002;20:1889–99.
63. Levenson J, Gariepy J, Megnien JL, et al. Diuretics and arteriolar resistance and arterial compliance in human hypertension. *Eur Heart J* 1992;13:48–52.
64. Winer N, Weber MA Sowers JR. The effect of antihypertensive drugs on vascular compliance. *Curr Hypertens Rep* 2001;3:297–304.
65. Benetos A, Lafleche A, Asmar R, et al. Arterial stiffness, hydrochlorthiazide and converting enzyme inhibition in essential hypertension. *J Hum Hypertens* 1996:10:77–82.
66. Asmar RG, Benetos A, Chaouche-Teyara K, et al. Comparison of effects of felodipine versus hydrochorhiazide on arterial diameter and PWV in essential hypertension. *Am J Cardiol* 1993;72:794–8.
67. Ong K-T, Delerme S, Pannier B, et al. Aortic stiffness is reduced beyond blood pressure lowering by short-term and long-term antihypertensive treatment. *J Hypertens* 2011;29:1034–42.
68. Morgan T, Lauri J, Bertram D, et al. Effect of different antihypertensive drug classes on central aortic pressure. *Am J Hypertens* 2004;17:118–23.

69. Protogerou AD, Stergiou GS, Vlachopoulos C, et al. The effect of antihypertensive drugs on central blood pressure beyond peripheral blood pressure: evidence for specific class-effects on antihypertensive drugs on pressure amplification. *Curr Pharmac Design* 2009;15:272–89.
70. Miall WE, Greenberg G. *Mild Hypertension – Is There Pressure to Treat?* Cambridge: Cambridge University Press; 1987, pp 70.
71. Eriksson JW, Jansson P-A, Carlberg B, et al. Hydrochorthiazide, but not candesartan, aggravates insulin resistance and causes visceral and hepatic fat accumulation. *Hypertension* 2008;52:1030–7.
72. Kurtz TW. Chlorthalidone: don't call it "thiazide-like" anymore. *Hypertension* 2010;56:335–7.
73. Carter BL, Einhorn PT, Brands M, et al. Thiazide-induced dysglycemea. *Hypertension* 2008,52:30–6.
74. Menon DV, Arbique D, Wang Z, et al. Differential effects of chorthalidone versus spironolactone on muscle sympathetic nerve activity in hypertensive patients. *J Clin Endocrinol Metab* 2009;94:1361–6.
75. Wray DW, Supiano MA. Impact of aldosterone receptor blockade compared with thiazide therapy on sympathetic nervous system function in geriatric hypertension. *Hypertension* 2010;55:1217–23.
76. Raheja P, Price A, Wang Z, et al. Spironolactone prevents chlorthalidone-induced sympathetic activation and insulin resistance in hypertensive patients. *Hypertension* 2012;60:319–25.
77. Buhler FR. Age and cardiovascular response adaptation. *Hypertension* 1983;5:94–100.
78. Channaraya V, Marya RK, Somasundaram M et al. Efficacy and tolerability of a beta-1 selective beta-blocker, bisoprolol, as a first-line antihypertensive in Indian patients diagnosed with essential hypertension (BRIGHT): an open-label, multicentric observational study. *BMJ Open* 2012;2. doi: 10.1136/bmjopen-2011-000683.
79. Robb OJ, Petrie JC, Webster J, et al. ICI 118,551 does not reduce blood pressure in hypertensive patients responsive to atenolol and propranolol. *Br J Clin Pharmacol* 1985;19:541–2.
80. Zacharias FJ, Cowen KJ. Comparison of propranolol and atenolol in hypertension. *Postgrad Med J* 1977;53:111–3.
81. Neutel JM, Smith DH, Ram CV, et al. Application of ambulatory blood pressure monitoring in differentiating between antihypertensive agents. *Am J Med* 1993;94:181–7.
82. Buhler FR, Berglund G, Anderson OK, et al. Double-blind comparison of the cardioselective beta-blockers bisoprolol and atenolol in hypertension. *J Cardiovasc Pharmacol* 1986:8:122–7.
83. Cruickshank JM, Prichard BN. *Beta-blockers in clinical practice*. 2nd ed., Edinburgh: Churchill Livingstone, 1994, p 353–498.
84. Veterans Administration Cooperative Study Group. Oxprenolol vs propranolol: a randomised, double-blind multicentre trial in hypertensive patients taking hydrochlorthiazide. *Hypertension* 1981;3:250–6.

85. Dhakam Z, Yasmin, McEniery CM, et al. A comparison of atenolol and nebivolol in isolated systolic hypertension. *J Hypertens* 2008;26:351–6.
86. Broeders MA, Doevendans PA, Bekkers BC, et al. Nebivolol a third generation beta-blocker that augments vascular nitric oxide release. *Circulation* 2000;102:677–84.
87. Puri R, Liew YH, Nicholls SJ, et al. Coronary beta-2 adrenoceptors mediate endothelium-dependent vasoreactivity in humans. *Eur Heart J* 2012;33:495–504.
88. Ignaro LJ. Experimental evidences of nitric oxide-dependent vasodilatory activity of nebivolol, a third generation beta-blocker. *Blood Press* 2004;13:2–16.
89. Lehtonen A, Allonen H, Kleimola T. Antihypertensive effect and plasma levels of labetalol. A comparison with propranolol and dihydrallazine. *Int J Pharmacol Biopharm* 1979;17:71–5.
90. Hiltunen TP, Suonsyrja T, Hannila-Handelberg T, et al. Predictors of antihypertensive responses: initial data from a placebo-controlled, randomised cross-over with four anti-hypertensive drugs (the GENRES study). *Am J Hypertens* 2007;20:311–8.
91. Parrinello G, Paterna S, Torres D, et al. One year renal and cardiac effect of bisoprolol versus losartan in recently diagnosed hypertensive patients. *Clin Drug Investig* 2009;29:591–600.
92. Olivan MJ, Garcia MJ, Rodriguez BA, et al. Bisoprolol and nifedipine SR in the treatment of hypertension in the elderly. *J Cardiovasc Pharmacol* 1990;16:95–9.
93. Kuusela TA, Jartu TT, Tahvanainen KV, et al. Effects of terbutaline on peripheral vascular resistance and arterial compliance. *J Cardiovasc Pharmacol* 2004;44:74–81.
94. Benetos A, Huguet F, Alvaladejo P, et al. Role of adrenergic tone in mechanical and functional properties of carotic artery during aging. *Am J Physiol* 1993;265:1132–8.
95. Laurant S, Boutouyrie P. Recent advances in arterial stiffness and wave reflection in human hypertension. *Hypertension* 2007;49:1202–6.
96. Ting CT, Chen CH, Chang MS, et al. Short and long-term effects of antihypertensive drugs on arterial reflections, compliance and impendence. *Hypertension* 1995;26:524–30.
97. De Cesaris R, Ranieri G, Filetti V, et al. Large artery compliance in essential hypertension. Effects of calcium antagonism and beta-blocking. *Am J Hypertens* 1992;5:624–8.
98. Hirata K, Vlachopoulos C, Adji A, et al. Benefits for angiotensin-converting enzyme inhibitor "beyond blood pressure lowering": beyond blood pressure or beyond the brachial artery? *J Hypertens* 2005;23:551–6.
99. Asmar RG, Kerihuel JC, Girerd XJ, et al. Effect of bisoprolol on blood pressure and arterial haemodynamics in system hypertension. *Am J Cardiol* 1991;68:61–4.

100. Simon AC, Levenson J, Pithois-Merli I. Large arteries in hypertension: heterogeneous haemodynamic response to beta-adrenoceptor antagonists with and without intrinsic sympathometic activity. *Br J Clin Pharmacol* 1987;24:45–9.
101. Kelly R, Daley J, Avolio A, et al. Arterial dilation and reduced wave reflection. *Hypertension* 1989;14:14–21.
102. Casey DP, Curry TB, Joyner MJ, et al. Acute beta-adrenergic blockade increases aortic wave reflection in young men and women. *Hypertension* 2012;59:145–50.
103. Kampus P, Serg M, Kals J, et al. Differential effects of nebivolol and metoprolol on central aortic pressure and left ventricular wall thickness. *Hypertension* 2011;57:1122–8.
104. Mackenzie IS, McEniery CM, Dhakam Z, et al. Comparison of effects of antihypertensive agents on central blood pressure and arterial stiffness in isolated systolic hypertension. *Hypertension* 2009;54:409–13.
105. Manisty CH, Zambanini A, Parker KH, et al. Differences in the magnitude of wave reflection account for differential effects of amlodipine-versus atenolol-based regimens on central blood pressure ASCOT. *Hypertension* 2009;54:724–30.
106. Chen CH, Ting CT, Lin SJ, et al. Different aspects of fosinopril and atenolol on wave reflections in hypertensive patients. *Hypertension* 1995;25:1034–41.
107. Neal DA, Brown MJ, Wilkinson IB, et al. Haemodynamic effects of amlodipine, bisoprolol and lisinopril in hypertensive patients after liver transplantation. *Transplantation* 2004;77:748–66.
108. Pannier BM, Guerin AP, Marchais SJ, et al. Different aortic reflection wave responses following long-term angiotensin-converting enzyme inhibition and beta-blocker in essential hypertension. *Clin Exper Pharmac Physiol* 2001;28:1074–7.
109. Steiner SS, Friedhoff AJ, Wilson BL, et al. Antihypertensive therapy and quality of life: a comparison of atenolol, captopril, enalapril and propranolol. *J Hum Hypertens* 1990;4:217–25.
110. Breed JG, Ciampricotti S, Byington R, et al. Quality of life perception during antihypertensive treatment: a comparative study of bisoprolol and enalapril. *J Cardiovasc Pharmacol* 1992;20:750–5.
111. Cruickshank JM. *The Modern Role of Beta-Blockers in Cardiovascular Medicine*. Shelton, Connecticut: People's Medical Publishing House-USA; 2011.
112. Leotta G, Rabbia F, Testa E, et al. Efficacy of antihypertensive treatment based on plasma renin activity. *Blood Press* 2010;19: 218–24.
113. Preston RA, Materson BJ, Reda DJ, et al. Age-race subgroup compared with renin profile as predictors of blood pressure response to antihypertensive therapy. *JAMA* 1998;280:1168–72.
114. Falconnet C, Bochud M, Bovet P, et al. Gender differences in the response to an ACE-inhibitor and a diuretic in hypertensive patients of African descent. *J Hypertens* 2004;22:1213–20.

115. Safar ME, Temmar M, Kakou A, et al. Sodium intake and vascular stiffness in hypertension. *Hypertension* 2009;54:203–9.
116. Ahimastos AA, Natoli AR, Lawler A, et al. Ramipril reduces large-artery stiffness in peripheral arterial disease and promotes elastogenic remodeling in cell culture. *Hypertension* 2005;45:1194–9.
117. Girerd X, Giannattasio C, Moulin C, et al. Regression of radial artery wall hypertrophy and improvement of carotid artery compliance after long-term antihypertensive treatment in elderly hypertensives. *J Am Coll Cardiol* 1998;31:1064–73.
118. Mitchell GF, Dunlap ME, Warnica W, et al. Long-term trandolopril treatment is associated with reduced aortic stiffness. *Hypertension* 2007;49:1271–7.
119. Mackenzie IS, McEniery CM, Dhakam Z, et al. Comparison of the effects of antihypertensive agents on central blood pressure and arterial stiffness in isolated systolic hypertension. *Hypertension* 2009;54:409–13.
120. Jiang X-J, O'Rourke MF, Zhang Y-Q, et al. Superior effect of an angiotensin-converting enzyme inhibitor over a diuretic for reducing aortic systolic pressure. *J Hypertens* 2007;25:1095–9.
121. O'Rourke M. Arterial stiffening and vascular/ventricular interaction. *J Hum Hypertens* 1994;8:9–15.
122. Avolio AP, Van Bortel LM, Boutouyrie P, et al. Role of pulse-pressure amplification in arterial hypertension. *Hypertension* 2009;54: 375–83.
123. Testa MA, Anderson RB, Nackley JF, et al. Quality of life and antihypertensive therapy in men. A comparison of captopril with enalapril. *N Engl J Med* 1993;328:907–13.
124. Girard M. The safety of ACE-inhibitors in moderate hypertension. *Adverse Drug React Toxicol Rev* 1991;10:169–85.
125. Coulter DM. Eye pain with nifedipine and disturbance of taste with captopril: a mutually controlled study showing a method of postmarketing surveillance. *BMJ* 1988;296:1086–8.
126. Mangrella M, Motola G, Russo F, et al. Hospital intensive monitoring of adverse reactions of ACE inhibitors. *Minerva Med* 1998;89:91–7.
127. Coulter DM, Edwards LR. Cough associated with captopril and enalapril. *BMJ* 1987;294:1521–3.
128. Mc Dowell SE, Coleman JJ, Ferner RE. Systematic review and meta-analysis of ethnic differences in risks of adverse reactions to drugs used in cardiovascular medicine. *BMJ* 2006;332:1177–80.
129. Pillans PL, Coulter DM, Black P. Angioedema and urticaria with angiotensin converting enzyme inhibitors. *Eur J Clin Pharmacol* 1996;51:123–6.
130. Beltrami L, Zanichelli A, Zingale L, et al. Long-term follow-up of 111 patients with angiotensin-converting enzyme inhibitor-related angioedema. *J Hypertens* 2011;29:2273–7.

131. Howes LG, Tran D. Can angiotensin receptor antagonists be used safely in patients with previous ACE-inhibitor-induced angioedema? *Drug Saf* 2002;25:73–6.
132. Lind L, Pollare T, Berne C, et al. Long-term metabolic effects of antihypertensive drugs. *Am Heart J* 1994;128:1177–83.
133. Jandeleit KA, Tikellis C, Ried CM, et al. Why blockade of the renin-angiotensin system reduces the incidence of new-onset diabetes. *J Hypertens* 2005;23:463–73.
134. Wrenger E, Muller R, Moesenthin M, et al. Interaction of spironolactone with ACE-inhibitors or angiotensin receptor blockers; analysis of 44 cases. *BMJ* 2003;327:147–9.
135. Palmer BF. Managing hyperkalaemia caused by inhibitors of renin-angiotensin-aldosterone system. *N Engl J Med* 2004;351:585–92.
136. Grassi G. Renin-angiotensin-sympathetic crosstalks in hypertension: reappraising the relevance of peripheral interactions. *J Hypertens* 2001;19:1713–6.
137. Miyajima E, Shigemasa T, Yamada Y, et al. Angiotensin II blunts, while angiotensin-converting enzyme inhibitor augments, reflex sympathetic inhibition in humans. *Clin Exp Pharmacol Physiol* 1999;26:797–802.
138. Ligtenberg G, Blankestijn PJ, Oey PL, et al. Reduction of sympathetic hyperactivity by enalapril in patients with chronic renal failure. *N Engl J Med* 1999;340:1321–8.
139. Skov K, Eiskjaer H, Hansen HE, et al. Treatment of young subjects at high familial risk of future hypertension with an angiotensin-receptor blocker. *Hypertension* 2007;50:89–95.
140. Julius S, Nesbitt SD, Egan BM, et al. Feasibility of treating prehypertension with an angiotensin-receptor blocker. *N Engl J Med* 2006;354:1685–97.
141. Safar ME, Protogerou A, Blacker J. Central blood pressure under angiotensin and calcium channel blockade. *Hypertension* 2009;54:704–6.
142. Moltzer E, Raso FU, Karamermer Y, et al. Comparison of candesartan versus metoprolol for treatment of system hypertension after repaired aortic coarctation. *Am J Cardiol* 2010;105: 217–22.
143. Resnick LM, Lester MH. Differential effects of antihypertensive drug therapy on arterial compliance. *Am J Hypertens* 2002;15: 1096–100.
144. Klingbeil AV John S, Schneider MP, et al. AT1-receptor blockade improves augmentation index: a double-blind, randomised, controlled study. *J Hypertens* 2002;20:2423–8.
145. Matchar DB, McCrory DC, Orlando LA, et al. Systematic review: comparative effectiveness of ACE-inhibitors and angiotensin 11 receptor blockers for treating essential hypertension. *Ann Intern Med* 2008;148:16–29.

146. Olsen MH, Fossum F, Hoieggen A, et al. Long-term treatment with losartan versus atenolol improves insulin sensitivity in hypertension (LIFE). *J Hypertens* 2005;23:891–8.
147. Elliot WJ, Meyer PM. Incident diabetes in clinical trials of antihypertensive drugs: a network analysis. *Lancet* 2007;369:201–7.
148. Choi HK, Soriano LC, Zhang Y, et al. Antihypertensive drugs and risk of gout among patients with hypertension: population based case-control study. *BMJ* 2012;344:d8190. doi:10.1133336/bmj.d8190.
149. Sipahi I, Debanne SM, Rowland DY, et al. Angiotensin-receptor blockade and risk of cancer: a meta-analysis of randomised controlled trials. *Lancet Oncol* 2010;11:627–36.
150. The ARB Trialists Collaboration. Effects of telmisartan, irbesartan, valsartan, candesartan and losartan on cancers in 15 trials enrolling 138,769 individuals. *J Hypertens* 2011;29:623–35.
151. Bhaskaran K, Douglas I, Evans S, et al. Angiotensin receptor blockers and risk of cancer: cohort study among people receiving antihypertensive drugs in UK General Practice Research Database. *BMJ* 2012;344:19.
152. Huang C-C, Chan W-L, Chen Y-C, et al. Angiotensin II receptors blockers and risk of cancer in patients with systemic hypertension. *Am J Cardiol* 2011;107:1028–33.
153. Coleman CI, Baker WL, Kluger J, et al. Antihypertensive medication and their impact on cancer incidence. *J Hypertens* 2008;26:622–9.
154. Goodfriend TL, Elliot ME, Catt KJ. Angiotensin receptors and their antagonists. *N Engl J Med* 1996;334:1649–54.
155. Lohmeier TE. Angiotensin II infusion model of hypertension. Is there an important sympathetic component? *Hypertension* 2012;59:539–41.
156. Bechir M, Enseleit F, Chenevard R, et al. Effect of Losartan on muscle sympathetic activity and baroceptor function in systemic hypertension. *Am J Cardiol* 2005;95:129–31.
157. Krum H, Lambert E, Windebank E, et al. Effect of angiotensin II receptor blockade on autonomic nervous system function in patients with essential hypertension. *Am J Physiol Heart Care Physiol* 2006;290:1706–12.
158. Heusser K, Vitkovsky J, Raasch W, et al. Elevation of sympathetic nerve activity by eprosartan in young male subjects. *Am J Hypertens* 2003;16:658–64.
159. Buhler FH. Age and pathophysiology-orientated antihypertensive response to calcium antagonists. *J Cardiovasc Pharmacol* 1988;12(supp B):156–62.
160. Webb AJ, Fischer U, Mehta Z, et al. Effects of antihypertensive-drugs class on interindividual variation in blood pressure and risk of stroke: a systematic review and meta-analysis. *Lancet* 2010;375: 906–15.
161. Schillaci G, Pucci G, Parati G. Blood pressure variability: an additional target for antihypertensive treatment? *Hypertension* 2011;58:133–5.

162. Nathan S, Pepine CJ, Bakris GL. Calcium antagonists. *Hypertension* 2005;46:637–42.
163. Elliot J, Ram CV. Calcium channel blockers. *J Clin Hypertens* 2011;13:687–9.
164. Fogari R, Zoppi A, Corradi L, et al. Effects of different dihydropyridine calcium antagonists on plasma norepinephrine in essential hypertension. *J Hypertens* 2000;18:1871–5.
165. Binggeli C, Corti R, Sudano I, et al. Effects of chronic calcium channel blockade on sympathetic nerve activity on hypertension. *Hypertension* 2002;39:892–6.
166. Lijnen P, Fagard R, Staessen J, et al. Short-term double-blind comparison of doxazosin and atenolol in patients with mild to moderate hypertension. *J Cardiovasc Pharmacol* 1988;12:461–6.
167. Furberg CD, Psaty BM, Pahor M, et al. Clinical implications of recent findings for the ALLHAT and other studies of hypertension. *Am Intern Med* 2001;135:1074–8.
168. Pessina AC, Ciccariello L, Perrone F, et al. Clinical efficacy and tolerability of alpha-blocker doxazosin as add-on therapy in patients with hypertension and impaired glucose metabolism. *Nutr Metab Cardiovasc Dis* 2006;16:137–47.
169. Chapple CR. A comparison of varying alpha-blockers and other pharmotherapy options for lower urinary tract symptoms. *Rev Urol* 2005;7:22–30.
170. Cruickshank JM, Prichard BN. *Beta-blockers in clinical practice.* Edinburgh: Churchill Livingstone; 1994. p 437–8.
171. Reid JL. Alpha-adrenergic receptors and blood pressure control. *Am J Cardiol* 1986;57:6E–12E.
172. Stokes GS, Bune AJ, Huon N, et al. Long-term effectiveness of extended-release nitrate for the treatment of systolic hypertension. *Hypertension* 2005;45:380–4.
173. Noll G, Wenzel RR, de Marchi S, et al. Differential effects of captopril and nitrates on muscle sympathetic nerve activity in volunteers. *Circulation* 1997;95:2286–92.
174. Ingelfinger JR. Aliskeren and dual therapy in type-2 diabetes mellitus. *N Engl J Med* 2008;23:2503–5.
175. Schmieder RE, Philipp T, Guerediaga J, et al. Long-term antihypertensive efficacy and safety of the oral direct renin inhibitor aliskiren. *Circulation* 2009;119:417–25.
176. Messerli FH, Bangalore S. Antihypertensive efficacy of aliskiren. *Circulation* 2009;119:371–3.
177. Samuelsson O, Herlitz H. Vaccination against high blood pressure: a new strategy. *Lancet* 2008;371:788–9.
178. Tissot AC, Maurer P, Nussberger J, et al. Effect of immunisation against angiotensin II with CYT006-AngQb on ambulatory blood pressure: a double blind, randomised, placebo controlled phase 11a study. *Lancet* 2008;371:821–7.

179. Weber MA, Black H, Bakris G, et al. A selective endothelin-receptor antagonist to reduce blood pressure in patients with treatment resistant hypertension. *Lancet* 2009;374:1423–31.
180. Sica DA. Endothelin receptor antagonism: what does the future hold? *Hypertension* 2008;52:460–1.
181. Hermida RD, Ayala DE, Calvo C, et al. Differing administration time-dependent effects of aspirin on blood pressure in dipper and non-dipper hypertensives. *Hypertension* 2005;46:1060–8.
182. Dimitrov Y, Baguet JP, Hottelart C, et al. Is there a BP benefit of changing the time of aspirin administration in treated hypertensive patients? *Eur J Prev Cardiol* 2012;19:706–11.
183. Scheer FA, Van Montifrans GA, Someren EJ, et al. Daily nighttime melatonin reduces blood pressure in male patients with essential hypertension. *Hypertension* 2004;43:192–7.
184. Mancia G, Parati G, Revera M, et al. Statins, antihypertensive treatment, and blood pressure control in clinic and over 24 hours: evidence from PHYLLIS randomised double-blind trial. *BMJ* 2010;340:846.
185. Taddei S, Ghiadoni L. Phosphodiesterase 5 inhibition to treat essential hypertension: is this the beginning of the story? *Hypertension* 2006;48:546–8.
186. Qureshi NN, Hatcher J, Chaturvedi N, et al. Effect of general practitioner education on adherence to antihypertensive drugs: cluster randomised controlled trial. *BMJ* 2007;335:1030–3.
187. Jones DW, Peterson ED. Improving hypertension control rates: technology, people or systems? *JAMA* 2008;299:2896–8.
188. Heisler M, Hofer TP, Schmittdiel JA, et al. Improving blood pressure control through a clinical pharmacist outreach program in patients with diabetes mellitus in 2 high-performing health systems. *Circulation* 2012;125:2863–72.
189. Flack JM. Non-invasive hemodynamic measurements: an important advance in individualising drug therapies for hypertensive patients. *Hypertension* 2006;47:646–7.
190. Smith RD, Levy P, Ferrario CM, et al. Value of noninvasive hemodynamics to achieve blood pressure control in hypertensive subjects. *Hypertension* 2006;47:771–7.
191. Turner ST, Schwartz GL, Chapman AB, et al. Antihypertensive pharmacogenetics: getting the right drug into the right patient. *J Hypertens* 2001;19:1–11.
192. Mellen PB, Herrington DM. Pharmacogenomics of blood pressure response to antihypertensive treatment. *J Hypertens* 2005;23:1311–25.
193. Svensson-Farbom P, Wahlstrand B, Almgren P, et al. A functional variant of the NEDD4L gene is associated with beneficial treatment response with beta-blockers and diuretics in hypertensive patients. *J Hypertens* 2011;29:388–95.
194. Wang TJ, Vasan RS. Epidemiology of uncontrolled hypertension in the United States. *Circulation* 2005;112:1651–62.

195. Calhoun DA, Jones D, Textor S, et al. Resistant hypertension: diagnosis, evaluation and treatment. *Hypertension* 2008;51:1403–19.
196. de la Sierra A, Segura J, Banegas JR, et al. Clinical features of 8295 patients with resistant hypertension classified on the basis of ambulatory BP monitoring. *Hypertension* 2011;57:898–902.
197. Pimenta E, Calhoun DA. Resistant hypertension: Incidence, prevalence, and prognosis. *Circulation* 2012;125:1594–6.
198. Egan BM, Zhao Y, Axon N, et al. Uncontrolled and apparent treatment resistant hypertension in the United States, 1988 to 2008. *Circulation* 2011;124:1046–58.
199. Hanselin MR, Saseen JJ, Allen RR, et al. Description of antihypertensive use in patients with resistant hypertension prescribed four or more agents. *Hypertension* 2011;58:1008–13.
200. Rossi GP, Seccia TM, Maniero C, et al. Drug-related hypertension and resistance to antihypertensive treatment: a call for action. *J Hypertens* 2011;29:2295–309.
201. Jordan J, Grassi G. Belly fat and resistant hypertension. *J Hypertens* 2010;28:1131–3.
202. Gupta AK, Nasothimiou EG, Chang CL, et al. Baseline predictors of resistant hypertension in the ASCOT trial: a risk score to identify those at risk. *J Hypertens* 2011;29:2004–13.
203. Persell SD. Prevalence of resistant hypertension in the United States, 2003–8. *Hypertension* 2011;57:1076–80.
204. Goncalves SC, Martinez D, Gus M, et al. Obstructive sleep apnea and resistant hypertension: a case-control study. *Chest* 2007;132:1858–70.
205. Abdel-Kader K, Dohar S, Shah N, et al. Resistant hypertension and obstructive sleep apnea in the setting of kidney disease. *J Hypertens* 2012;30:960–6.
206. Nishizaka MK, Zaman MA, Calhoun DA. Efficacy of low-dose spironolactone in subjects with resistant hypertension. *Am J Hypertens* 2003;16:925–30.
207. Gradman A, Basile J, Carter B, et al. Combination therapy in hypertension. *J Am Soc Hypertens* 2010;4:42–50.
208. Mancia G, de Backer G, Dominiczak A, et al. Guidelines for the management of arterial hypertension. *J Hypertens* 2007;25:1105–87.
209. Wald D, Law M, Morris J, et al. Combination therapy versus monotherapy in reducing blood pressure: meta-analysis in 11,000 participants for 42 trials. *Am J Med* 2009;122:290–300.
210. Unger T, Paulis L, Sica DA. Therapeutic perspectives in hypertension. *Eur Heart J* 2011;32:2739–47.
211. Sever PS, Messerli FH. Hypertension management 2011: optimal combination therapy. *Eur Heart J* 2011;32:2499–506.
212. Fu Q, Zhang R, Witkowski S, et al. Persistent sympathetic activation during chronic antihypertensive therapy. A potential mechanism for long term morbidity? *Hypertension* 2005;45:513–21.

213. Hess G. Medication utilization patterns and hypertension related expenditure among patients who were switched from fixed-dose to free-combinations antihypertensive therapy. *Pharm Ther* 2008;33:2121–58.
214. Gupta A, Arshad S, Poulter N. Compliance, safety and effectiveness of fixed-dose combinations of antihypertensive drugs: a meta-analysis. *Hypertension* 2010;55:399–407.
215. The Indian Polycap Study. Effects of a plypill (Polycap) on risk factors in middle-aged individuals with cardiovascular disease (TIPS) in a phase 11 double-blind, randomised trial. *Lancet* 2009;373:1341–51.
216. Lonn E, Bosch J, Teo KK, et al. The Polypill in the prevention of cardiovascular diseases. *Circulation* 2010;122:2078–88.
217. Krum H, Schlaich M, Sobotka P, et al. Novel procedure- and device-based strategies in the management of systemic hypertension. *Eur Heart J* 2011;32:537–44.
218. SYMPICITY HTN-2 investigators. Renal sympathetic denervation in patients with treatment-resistant hypertension: a randomised controlled trial. *Lancet* 2010;376:1903–9.
219. SYMPLICITY HTN-2. *Cardiovascular News*, Issue 25, May 2012, p 1–4.
220. Krum H, Sclaich M, Whitbown R, et al. Catheter-based renal sympathetic denervation for resistant hypertension. *Lancet* 2009;373: 1375–81.
221. Symplicity HTN-1 Investigators. Catheter-based renal sympathetic denervation for resistant hypertension. *Hypertension* 2011;57: 911–17.
222. Witkowsky A, Prejbisz A, Florczak E, et al. Effects of renal sympathetic denervation on blood pressure, sleep apnoea course and glycemic control in patients with resistant hypertension and sleep apnoea. *Hypertension* 2011;58:559–650.
223. Brandt MC, Mahfoud F, Reda S, et al. Renal sympathetic denervation reduces left ventricular hypertrophy and improves cardiac function in patients with resistant hypertension. *J Am Coll Cardiol* 2012;59:901–9. doi:10.1016/jack.2011.11.034
224. Schmieder RE, Redon J, Grassi G, et al. ESH Position Paper: renal denervation – an interventional therapy of resistant hypertension. *J Hypertens* 2012;30:837–41.
225. Linz D, Mahfoud F, Schotten U, et al. Renal sympathetic denervation suppresses postapneic blood pressure rises and atrial fibrillationin a model for sleep apnea. *Hypertension* 2012;60:172–8.
226. Mahfoud F, Cremers B, Janker J et al. Renal hemodynamics and renal function after catheter-based renal sympathetic denervation in patients with resistant hypertension. *Hypertension* 2012;60: 419–24.
227. Krum H, Sobotka P, Mahfoud F, et al. Device-based antihypertensive therapy. *Circulation* 2011;123:209–15.

228. Lohmeier TE, Iliescu R, Liu B, et al. Systemic and renal-specific sympathoinhibition in obesity hypertension. *Hypertension* 2012;59:331–8.
229. Rocchini AF, Katch V, Anderson J, et al. Blood pressure in obese adolescents: effect of weight loss. *Pediatrics* 1988;82:16–23.
230. Burke V, Thompson C, Taggart AC, et al. Differences in response to nutrition and fitness education programmes in relation to baseline levels of cardiovascular risk in 10 to 12 year-old children. *J Hum Hypertens* 1996;10:99–106.
231. Ewart CK, Young DR, Hagberg JM. Effects of school-based aerobic exercise on blood pressure in adolescent girls at risk of hypertension. *Am J Pub Health* 1988;88:949–51.
232. Leary DS, Ness AR, Davey Smith G, et al. Physical activity and blood pressure in children. *Hypertension* 2008;51:92–8.
233. Flynn JT, Meyers KE, Neto JP, et al. Efficacy and safety of the angiotensin receptor blocker valsartan in children with hypertension aged 1 to 5 years. *Hypertension* 2008;52:222–8.
234. Schaefer F, Litwin M, Zachwieja J, et al. Efficacy and safety of valsartan compared to enalapril in hypertensive children: a 12-week, randomised, double-blind, parallel-group study. *J Hypertens* 2011;29:2484–90.
235. Lurbe E, Cifkova R, Cruickshank JK, et al. Management of high blood pressure in children and adolescents; recommendations of the European Society of Hypertension. *J Hypertens* 2009;27:1719–42.
236. Seely EW, Ecker J. Chronic hypertension in pregnancy. *N Engl J Med* 2011;365:439–46.
237. Li D-K, Yang C, Andrade S, et al. Maternal exposure to angiotensin converting enzyme inhibitors in the first trimester and risk of malformations in offspring: a retrospective cohort study. *BMJ* 2011;343:887.
238. Podymow T, August P. Update on the use of antihypertensive drugs in pregnancy. *Hypertension* 2008;51:960–9.
239. Caton AR, Bell EM, Druschel CM, et al. Antihypertensive medication use during pregnancy and the risk of cardiovascular malformations. *Hypertension* 2009;54:63–70.
240. Redman CW. Hypertension in pregnancy. *Heart* 2011;97:1967–9.
241. Hermida RC, Ayala DE, Iglesias M. Administration-time dependent influence of aspirin on blood pressure in pregnant women. *Hypertension* 2003;41:651–6.

End-Organ Damage in Essential Hypertension

CHAPTER 7

In essential hypertension, the mode of death relates primarily to the heart, and includes myocardial infarction, sudden death, and heart failure. Death from cardiac causes is followed (in frequency) by stroke and kidney disease (1) (**Table 7-1**).

Before a major event or death, there are usually signs, and possibly symptoms, of major end-organ damage. Such end-organ damage can be modified, or reversed, by appropriate antihypertensive therapy.

RENAL DYSFUNCTION

1. General

The two most relevant measures used to evaluate renal function are an estimated glomerular filtration rate (eGFR), estimated via a formula, and the presence of albumin in the urine (2). Formulae to assess eGFR rely on the accuracy of serum creatinine measurement (2). **Table 7-2** shows the five different stages of renal dysfunction (3). The various classifications of abnormal levels of urinary albumin excretion are summarized in **Table 7-3**. Albuminuria is expressed as milligrams of albumin excreted per gram of creatinine (4).

TABLE 7-1 Causes of death in essential hypertension

Mode of death	%
Heart (MI, CCF, arrhythmia)	35–50
Stroke	15
Kidney	10
Other	30

Abbreviations: congestive heart failure (CCF), myocardial infarction (MI).
From Pickering GW. *High Blood Pressure*. 2nd ed. London: JA Churchill Ltd; 1968.

TABLE 7-2 Patients at risk and the 5 stages of chronic kidney disease

Stage	Description	GFR
At increased risk	Risk factors for kidney disease (diabetes, high BP familial history, older age, ethnic group)	>90
Stage 1	Kidney damage (albuminuria) and normal renal function	>90
Stage 2	Kidney damage and mild decrease in GFR	60–89
Stage 3	Moderate decrease in GFR	30–59
Stage 4	Severe decrease in GFR	15–29
Stage 5	Kidney failure (dialysis needed soon)	<15

Abbreviations: BP, blood pressure; GFR, glomerular filtration rate.
From National Kidney Foundation. K/DOQI clinical practice guidelines for chronic kidney disease: evaluation, classification and stratification: part 5. Evaluation of laboratory measurement for clinical assessment of kidney disease. *Am J Kidney Dis* 2002;39(suppl 2):S1–S266.

Not only high blood pressure (BP) compromises the kidney and other key organs, but also increased sympathetic nerve activity (SNA) can be harmful (**Figure 7-1**) (5). A wide pulse-pressure (P-P) is a poor prognostic sign for renal dysfunction (6). A low eGFR is also a poor prognostic sign for premature cardiovascular events and death (**Figure 7-2**) (7).

TABLE 7-3 Classification of abnormal UA excretion

	24 h UA (mg/24 h)	Overnight UA (μg/min)	Spot urine UA (mg/L)	Albumin/creatinine ratio		
				Gender	mg/mmol	mg/g
Normal	<15	<10	<10	M	<1.25	<10
				F	<1.75	<15
High normal	15 to <30	10 to <20	10 to <20	M	1.25 to <2.5	10 to <20
				F	1.75 to <3.5	15 to <30
Microalbuminuria	30 to <300	20 to <200	20 to <200	M	2.5 to <25	20 to <200
				F	3.5 to <35	30 to <300
Macroalbuminuria	>3	>200	>200	M	>25	>200
				F	>35	>300

Abbreviations: UA, urinary albumin.
From De Jong P, Curhan GC. Screening, monitoring and treatment of albuminuria: public health perspectives. *J Am Soc Nephrol* 2006;17:2120–6.

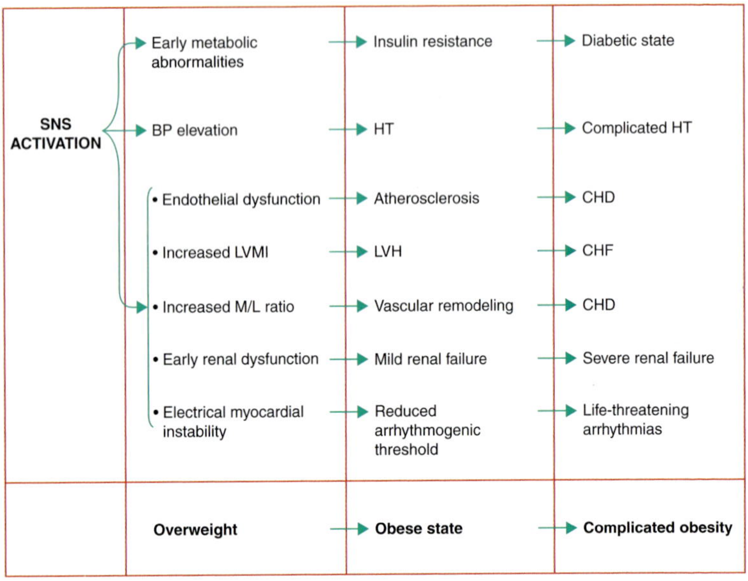

Fig. 7-1 Role of the sympathetic nervous system in the progression of metabolic disturbance and end-organ damage in relation to weight. (From Grassi G, Seravalle G, Dell'Oro R. Sympathetic activation in obesity. A non-innocent bystander. *Hypertension* 2010;56:338–40.)

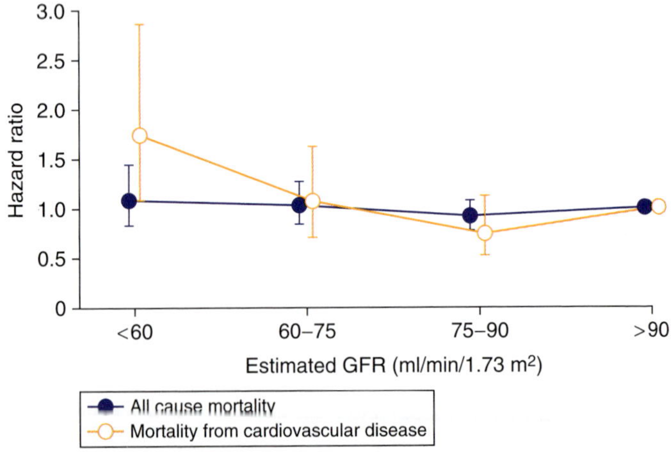

Fig. 7-2 A low eGFR (< 60 ml/min/1.73 m^2) is linked to increased cardiovascular (CV) mortality in women. (From Weiner DE, Rifkin DE. Kidney function and the risk of cardiovascular disease. *BMJ* 2009:339:2–3.)

2. Antihypertensive therapy and renal function

A) Angiotensin receptor blockers and angiotensin-converting enzyme inhibitors

The African American Study of Kidney Disease and Hypertension (AASK) trial (8), in 1094 black Americans with hypertensive renal disease, compared 2 levels of antihypertensive control drugs and 3 drugs (metoprolol, amlodipine, and ramipril) under randomized conditions over 2–6 years. The calcium blocker was inferior to both the β-blocker (BB) and the angiotensin-converting enzyme inhibitor (ACEI) in preventing death and end-stage renal failure, whereas the ACEI was superior to the BB only in slowing the rate of GFR decline.

Based on the fact that only 24-hour ambulatory blood pressure monitoring (ABPM) can detect true differences in BP control (9), claims that ACE/angiotensin receptor blockers (ARBs) have renoprotective properties beyond BP control have been doubted. A meta-analysis of trials involving antihypertensive drugs and renal outcomes partly confirmed this view (10). Although ACE/ARB treatment appeared superior to other antihypertensive drugs in (a) reducing the risk of end-stage renal disease and a doubling of the serum creatinine in both persons with and without diabetes (**Figure 7-3**) and (b) reducing the risk of an increase in serum creatinine, albuminuria, but not a change in GFR (in persons with and without diabetes) (**Figure 7-4**), these advantages largely disappeared when differences in BP were taken into account (**Figure 7-5**). Since the 2005 meta-analysis (10), the ONTARGET study (Ongoing Telmisartan Alone and in combination with Ramipril Global Endpoint Trial) in high-risk subjects (11) showed that the ARB telmisartan and ACEI ramipril had similar renoprotective properties, but the combination of the 2 drugs worsened the major renal outcomes. Although ACEIs and ARBs appeared superior to calcium antagonists in slowing the progression of renal dysfunction in Japanese hypertensive (13, 29), a follow-up of the Antihypertensive and Lipid-Lowering Treatment to Prevent Heart Attack Trial (ALLHAT) study in 33,357 elderly hypertensives showed that the ACEI was not different from the calcium blocker amlodipine, or the diuretic chlorthalidone, in reducing renal outcomes (137), irrespective of the baseline renal function or diabetic status (15).

In spite of continued good BP control (12), a study in children aged 3–18 years indicated that the initial ACEI-induced fall in urinary protein-to-creatinine ratio was reversed over a 5-year period (**Figure 7-6**).

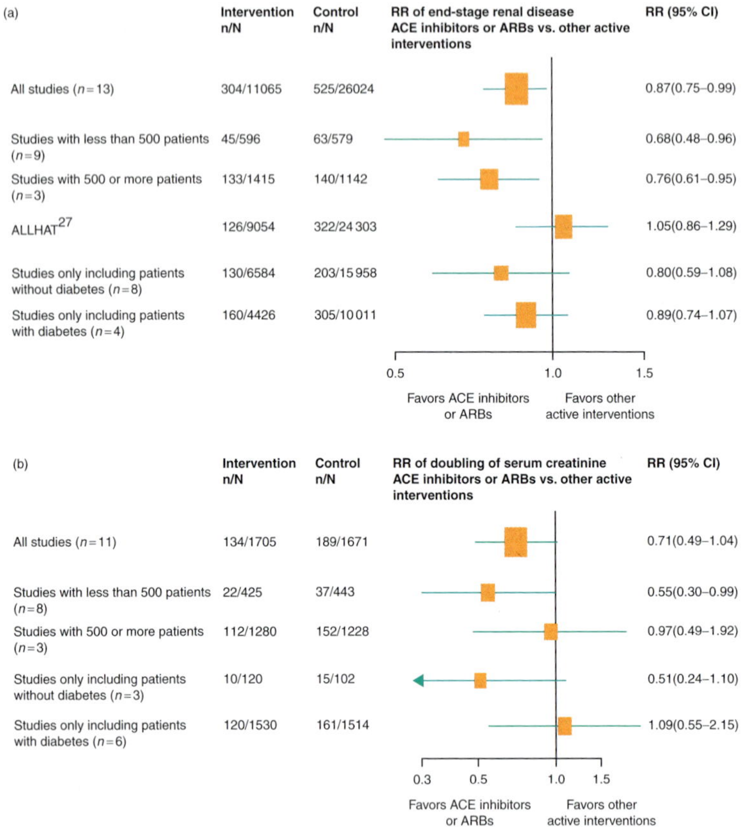

Fig. 7-3 Effect of ACEIs and ARBs versus other drugs on the relative risk of (A) end-stage renal disease and (B) doubling of serum creatinine. (From Casas JP, Chua W, Loukogeorgakis S, et al. Effect of inhibitors of the renin-angiotensin system and other anti-hypertensive drugs on renal outcomes: systematic review and meta-analysis. *Lancet* 2005;366:2026–33.)

Also of concern are the results of two studies in persons with diabetes involving the ARB olmesartan (16, 17). Although the ARB slowed the progression of renal dysfunction, there was an excess of cardiovascular deaths in the ARB group (see Chapter 8). The FDA is suitably concerned.

B) Beta-blockers (BBs)

Beta-2 stimulation is renoprotective in the sense that it improves renal blood flow and GFR, and these renal actions are inhibited by the specific β-2 blocker ICI 118,551 (18). Accordingly, BBs decrease effective renal plasma flow and GFR, mainly via β-2 blockade (19).

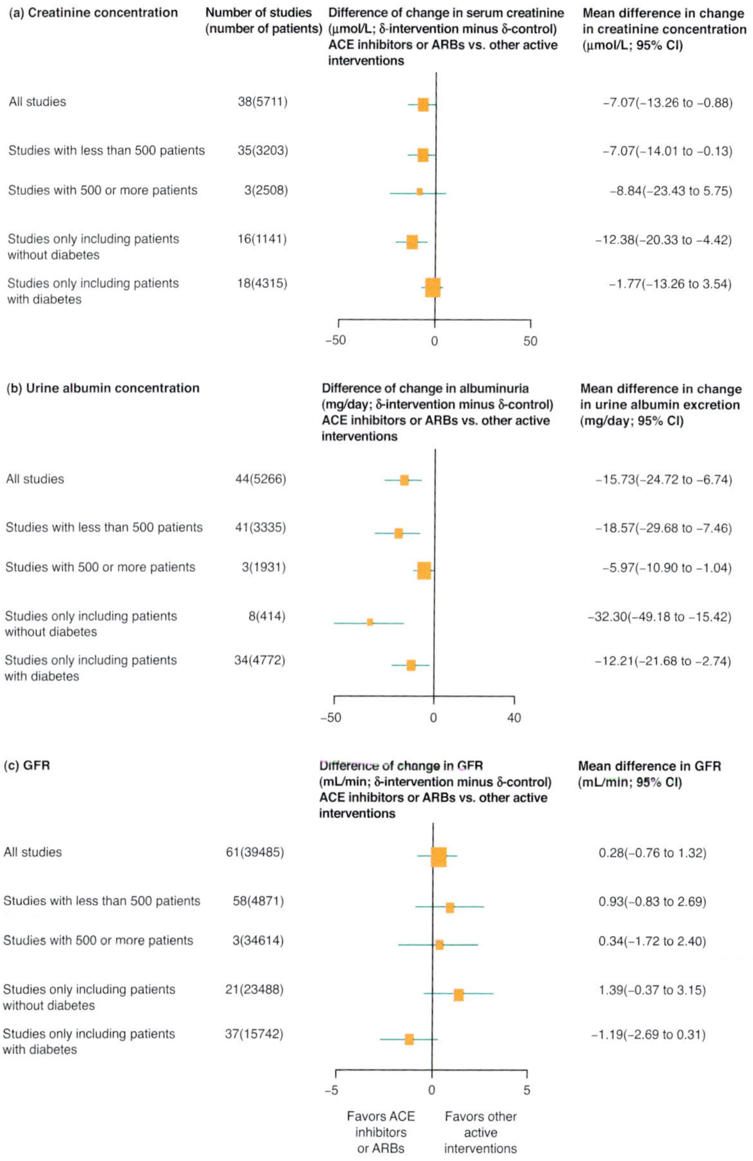

Fig. 7-4 Effect of ACEIs and ARBs versus other drugs on relative risk of (A) creatinine concentration, (B) urine albumin excretion, and (C) eGFR. (From Casas JP, Chua W, Loukogeorgakis S, et al. Effect of inhibitors of the renin-angiotensin system and other anti-hypertensive drugs on renal outcomes: systematic review and meta-analysis. *Lancet* 2005;366:2026–33.)

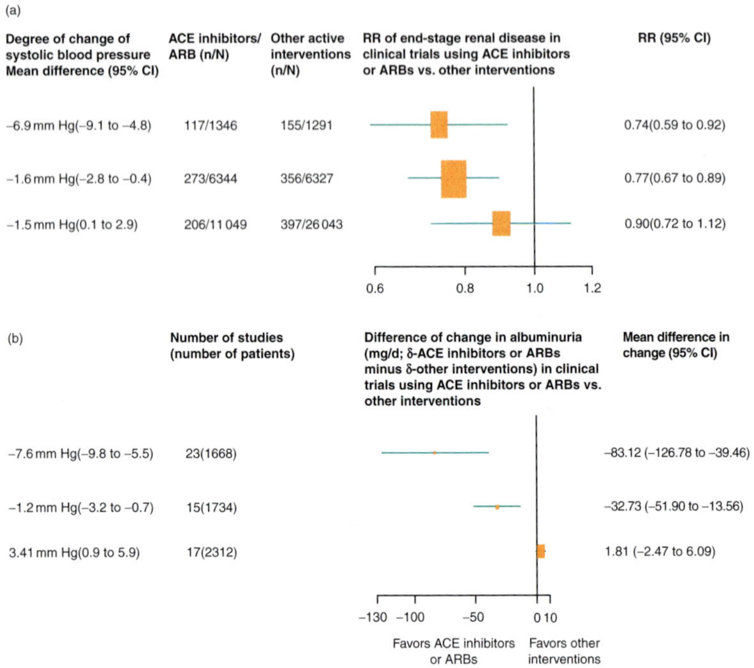

Fig. 7-5 Effect of ACEIs and ARBs on relative risk of (A) endstage renal disease and (B) urine albumin excretion, according to difference achieved in SBP between randomized groups. (From Casas JP, Chua W, Loukogeorgakis S, et al. Effect of inhibitors of the renin-angiotensin system and other anti-hypertensive drugs on renal outcomes: systematic review and meta-analysis. *Lancet* 2005;366:2026–33.)

Moderately β-1 selective atenolol, when given to a patient with malignant hypertension and renal failure, was able to reduce blood urea from 340 mg% to 114 mg%, maintained for 3 years (**Figure 7-7**) (20). It has already been noted in the AASK trial (8) that moderately β-1 selective metoprolol was similar to the ACEI ramipril in preventing end-stage renal failure and death, but inferior in slowing the fall in GFR. In the UK Prospective Diabetes Study (UKPDS) (21) involving obese, hypertensive, type 2 diabetes, over 9 years follow-up, atenolol did not differ from the ACEI captopril in its effect on albuminuria (**Figure 7-8**), proteinuria, plasma creatinine concentration, or in the proportion of patients who had a two-fold increase in plasma creatinine concentration. In a comparison of highly β-1 selective bisoprolol and the ARB losartan, the BB was at least as renoprotective (assessed by fall in creatinine clearance) as the ARB over 1 year (see Figure 6-29 in Chapter 6) (22).

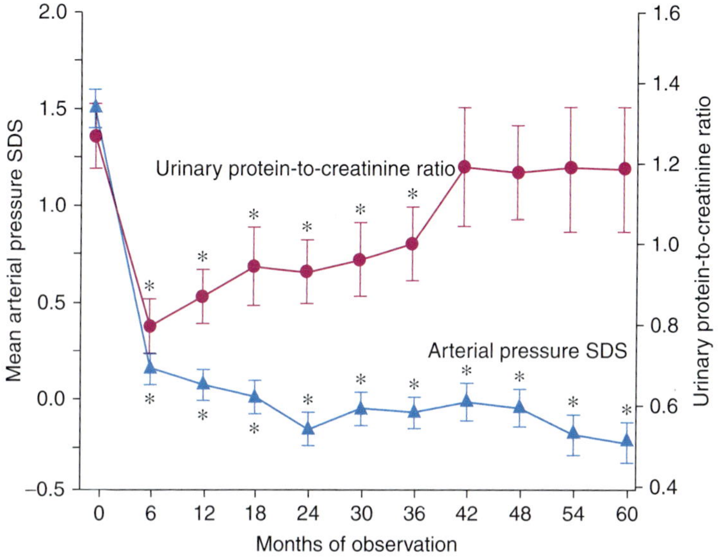

Fig. 7-6 In children, in spite of good BP control the reno-protective effects of ACEIs begin to wear off after 6 mo and have gone after 3 years. (From The ESCAPE Trial Group. Strict blood pressure control and progression of renal failure in children. *N Engl J Med* 2009;361:1639–50.)

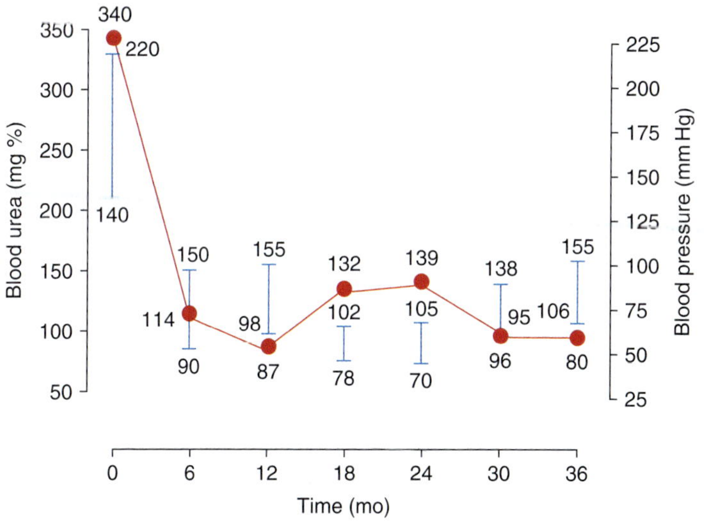

Fig. 7-7 Patient with malignant hypertension on atenolol-based therapy; based good BP-control led to fall in blood urea, but excessive fall in BP led to blood urea increase. (From Zacharias FJ. Long-term clinical experience with atenolol. *Royal Society of Medicine, International Congress and Symposium Series No 19*. 1979;19:75–91.)

% of patients with albuminuria (50 mg/l)	Captopril	Atenolol
Baseline	16%	20%
After 9 years follow-up	31%	26%

Fig. 7-8 Renoprotection in hypertensive type 2 diabetes; atenolol at least as good as g captopril in controlling albuminuria. (From UK Prospective Diabetes Study Group. Efficacy of atenolol and captopril in reducing risk of macrovascular and microvascular complications in type-2 diabetes: UKPDS39. *BMJ* 1998;317:713–20.)

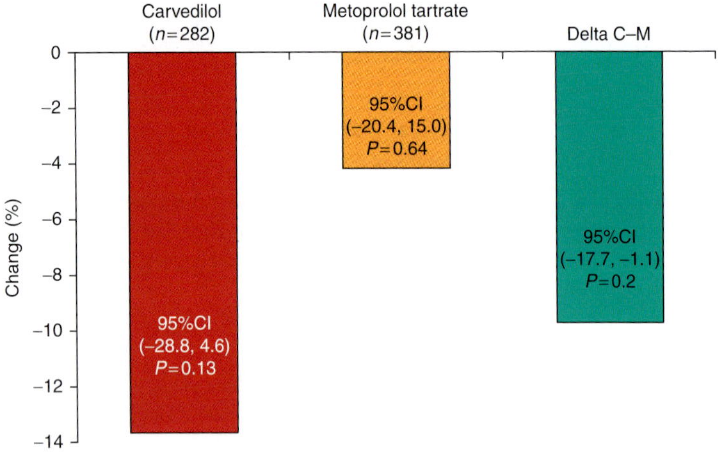

Fig. 7-9 In type-2 diabetics, at same BP-control carvedilol was superior p to metoprolol in reducing urinary albumin:creatinine ratio. (From Bakris GL, Fonseca V, Katholi RE, et al. Differential effects of beta-blockers on albuminuria in patients with type 2 diabetes. *Hypertension* 2005;46:1309–15.)

In a between-BB comparison in hypertensives with diabetes over 5 months, modestly β-1 selective metoprolol tartrate and nonselective carvedilol (with additional α-blocking properties) were similar in decreasing BP, but carvedilol was superior in reducing microalbuminuria (**Figure 7-9**) (23). Clearly, the α-blocking property of carvedilol reduces renal vascular resistance and prevents reductions in renal blood flow and GFR (24).

C) Calcium antagonists

In a study of 1715 hypertensive patients with type-2 diabetes and nephropathy, placebo, amlodipine, and the ARB irbesartan were

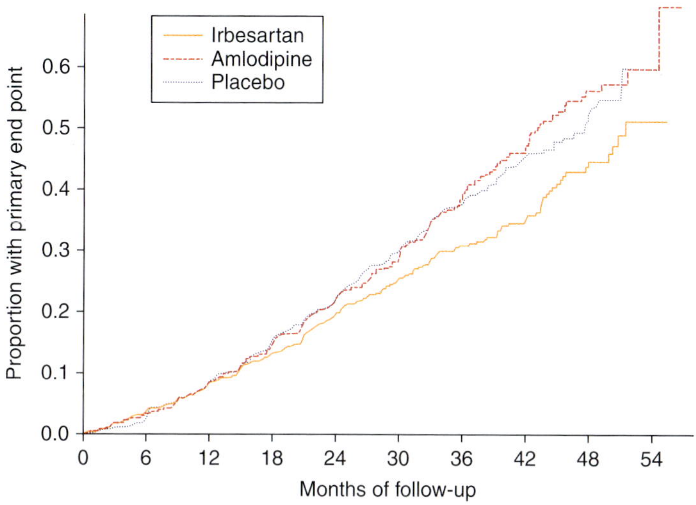

Fig. 7-10 In a randomized placebo-controlled trial of patients with type-2 diabetic nephropathy irbesartan was superior to amlodipine in preventing the primary endpoint (end-stage renal failure + all-cause death). (From Lewis EJ, Hunsicker LG, Clarke WR, et al. Renoprotective effect of the angiotensin receptor antagonist irbesartan in patients with nephropathy due to type-2 diabetes. *N. Engl J Med* 2001;345:851–60.)

compared under randomized conditions over 2.6 years (25); the primary end point (doubling of serum creatinine, development of end-stage renal disease, and death from any cause) was significantly 20% less on the ARB than placebo, and 23% less than on amlodipine, independent of BP (**Figure 7-10**). Further disappointing news for the calcium blockers (felodipine) came from the REIN = Renal Epidemiology and Information Network (REIN-2) study of hypertensive patients without diabetes nephropathy, where intensified control of BP with felodipine was associated with a nonsignificant increase in the appearance of end-stage renal disease over a 3-year period (26).

It has already been noted that, in the AASK trial (8), the calcium blocker amlodipine was inferior to both ACEI and BB in preventing death and end-stage renal failure. For this reason, the calcium blocker was withdrawn from the study (27). Also, nondihydropyridine verapamil did not reduce microalbuminuria in hypertensive patients with type 2 diabetes (28). In a recent study (29) of 1021 Japanese hypertensives randomized to valsartan or amlodipine, over 3.4 years, only the ARB reduced urinary albumin.

Why are calcium antagonists placebo possibly less renoprotective than other antihypertensive agents? Maybe it is because calcium blockers alter renal autoregulation so that, via vasodilatation, high BP is transmitted to the microcirculation (30). However, all these surmisings are somewhat irrelevant when the follow-up results of the ALLHAT study in 33,357 elderly hypertensives are considered (29, 14). Compared with the ACEI lisinopril and the diuretic chlorthalidone, the rate of GFR decline was slowest in persons with and without diabetes, with the calcium blocker amlodipine, although there was no difference between the 3 drugs in terms of renal outcomes. These results are in keeping with the results of a study in persons with type-2 diabetes, where the calcium blocker nisoldipine was similar to the ACEI enalapril in terms of renoprotection (31).

D) Diuretics

In young/middle-aged hypertensives (Medical Research Council [MRC] mild hypertension study), the diuretic bendrofluazide increased blood urea significantly more than placebo over 5 years (32). In the Heart Attack Primary Prevention in Hypertension Study (HAPPHY) in middle-aged hypertensives (33), there was a small increase in serum creatinine in both the diuretic and BB (metoprolol) groups over an 8-year follow-up period.

In the elderly patients with isolated systolic hypertension, the Systolic Hypertension in the Elderly Program (SHEP) study (n = 4736) revealed that, compared with placebo over 5 years, chlorthalidone-based therapy reduced the risk of the end point relating to renal dysfunction by 9 versus 13 (34). In the even larger ALLHAT study in the elderly (n = 33,357) (29, 14), chlorthalidone-based therapy was equal to ACEI and calcium blocker therapy in preventing end-stage renal disease, independent of initial renal function or diabetic status.

LEFT VENTRICULAR HYPERTROPHY

1. How do we recognize left ventricular hypertrophy?

A) Electrocardiogram

An electrocardiogram of a patient with left ventricular hypertrophy (LVH) is shown in **Figure 7-11** (35). LVH is present when the R-wave in the limb lead AVL is greater than 13 mm and in the precordial leads when the S-wave in lead V1, plus the R-wave in leads V5 or V6, exceeds 35 mm (a mm = 1 small square on electrocardiogram). The depressed S-T segments and inversed T-waves

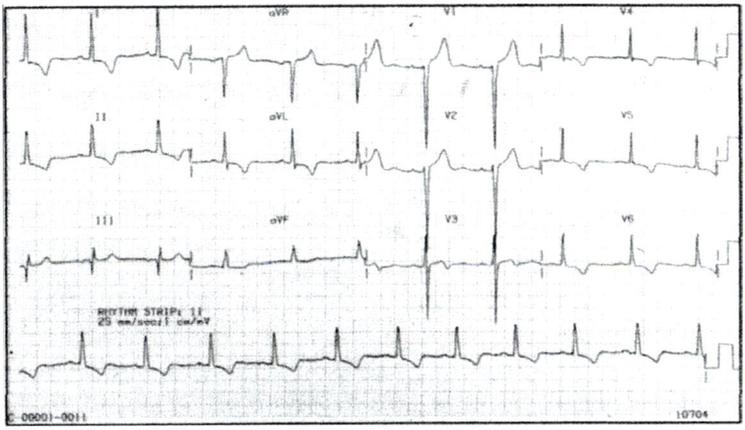

Fig. 7-11 ECG LVH and strain; tall R-waves in leads 1 and aVL and deep S waves S-V5-6, SV1 + RV5 = 47 mm, inverted T-waves aVL and V5-6. (From Goldman MJ. *Principles of Clinical Electrocardiography*. Canada: Lange Medical Publication; 1970, p. 100.)

indicate the "strain pattern." This "strain pattern" is very rare in the young, but in the elderly, it occurs in 3.5% of men and 1.6% of women (36).

Electrocardiogram remains the first tool to detect LVH because of its low cost and wide accessibility. It is good at predicting echocardiographic LVH in the elderly, but compared with echocardiography, electrocardiographic (ECG) LVH has good specificity but poor sensitivity (37).

B) Echocardiography

This technique is able to assess left ventricular mass (LVM) from either wall thickening or chamber dilatation (**Figure 7-12**) (38). Wall thickening occurs more commonly in response to pressure overload, and chamber dilatation occurs more commonly in response to volume overload and neurohumoral factors. The ratio of LV wall thickness to diastolic diameter is termed as relative wall thickness, and when increased it is termed as concentric LVH, and when not increased, it is termed as eccentric LVH (Figure 7-12).

Generally, concentric LVH is more common in black subjects and older hypertensives (particularly women), and eccentric LVH is more common in the young and obese people (38). LVM increases with increasing age (**Figure 7-13**) (37, 39) and is linked to increasing

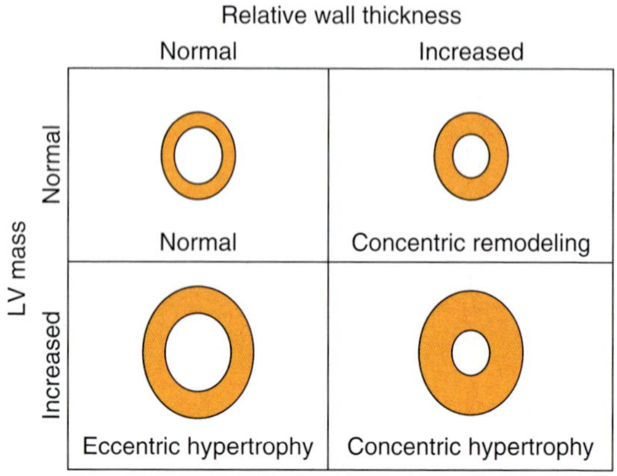

Fig. 7-12 Illustration of eccentric hypertrophy (increased LVM + normal relative wall thickness) and concentric hypertrophy (increased LVM + increased relative wall thickness). (From Drazner MH. The progression of hypertensive heart disease. *Circulation* 2011;123:327–34.)

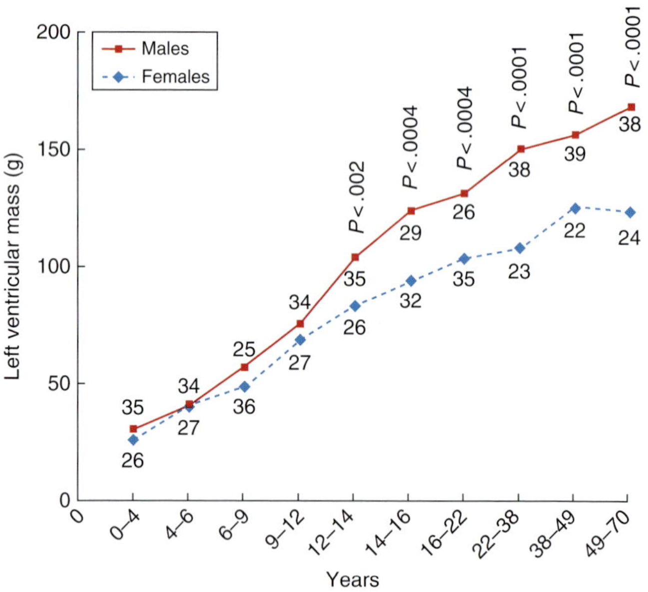

Fig. 7-13 LVM increases with age in both males and females. (From de Simone G, Izzo R, Trimarco B. Left ventricular hypertrophy: old marker, new problems and new possibilities. *J Hypertens* 2011;29:480–2.)

weight, type-2 diabetes, and smoking (39). There is a genetic component to the development of LVH (40).

2. Pathological and nonpathological LVH

These two types of LVH are shown in **Figure 7-14** (41). The nonpathological, or physiological, hypertrophy was usually linked to athletes and has different gene cluster expression involved in cardiomyocyte cell growth (**Figure 7-15**) (42). So called "Athlete's Heart" has only modest increases in LV wall and septal thickness and diastolic LV size (43), and is linked to both strength and endurance sports (44) and has normal LV function (45).

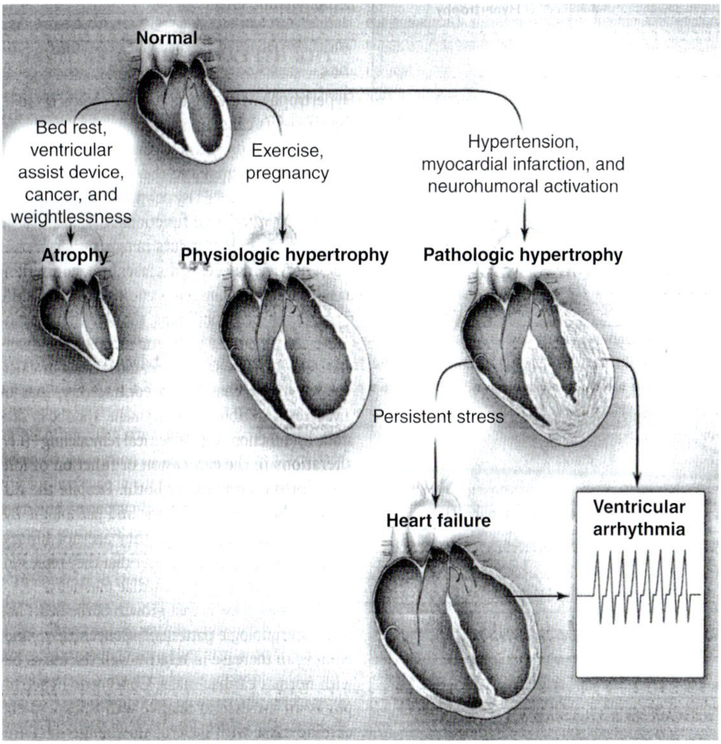

Fig. 7-14 LVH: pathological LVH arising from high BP or chronic beta-1 stimulation can give rise to heart failure or lethal arrhythmias. (From Hill JA, Olson EN. Cardiac plasticity. *New Engl J Med* 2008;358:1370–80.)

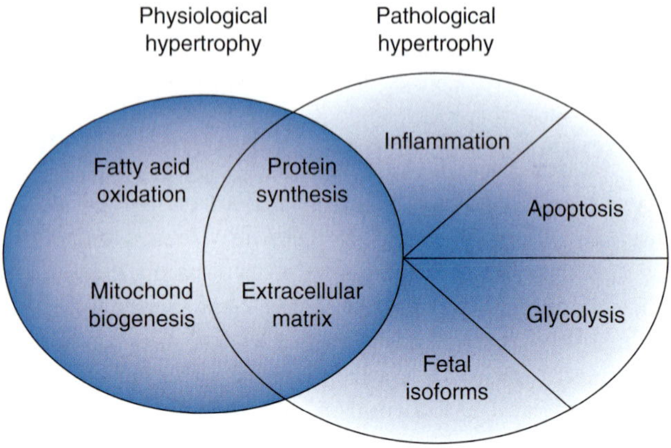

Fig. 7-15 Diagram depicting shared and distinct gene cluster expression g p profiles of physiological and pathological LV hypertrophy. (From Dorn II GW. The fuzzy logic of physiological cardiac hypertrophy. *Hypertension* 2007;49:962–70.)

3. LV wall stress and inappropriate LVM

Hypertensive hearts fall into the following three main categories in terms of LV wall stress (force on the myocardial cell): those with low wall stress (inappropriate hypertrophy), those with normal wall stress (appropriate hypertrophy), and those with high wall stress (inadequate hypertrophy) (46). High wall stress (inadequate hypertrophy) is linked to a high myocardial oxygen requirement and the reverse for inappropriate hypertrophy with low wall stress (46). Inappropriate hypertrophy is probably linked to neurohumoral factors and relates to myocardial β-receptors (47) where the response is increased, in contrast to LVH with normal wall stress, where β-receptor response is normal or decreased (48). Indeed inappropriate LVM appears independent of BP, which can be normal, and may be a phenotypic expression of nonobstructive cardiomyopathy (49). Patients with inappropriate LVM are particularly prone to poor systolic and diastolic function (50), and in younger/middle age, hypertension is present to a greater or lesser extent in about 50% of cases (**Figure 7-16**) (51).

4. LVH and myocardial blood flow

In the normal myocardium, coronary flow has the potential to increase 5–8 fold, whereas in LVH coronary flow, reserve is

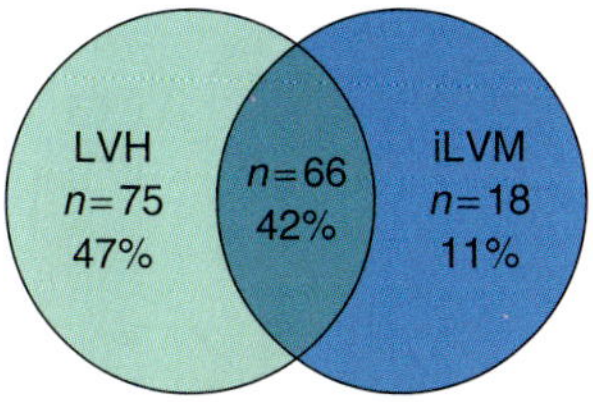

Fig. 7-16 Number and percentage of hypertensive patients that have appropriate LVH or inappropriate LVH (iLVH); 42% have both types. (From Jennings LR, McMullen JR. Left-ventricular hypertrophy: beyond the image and defining human cardiac phenotype in hypertension. *J Hypertens* 2007;25:941–7.)

diminished, possibly leading to angina (52). Compared with controls, eccentric LVH is associated with an approximate 25% fall in flow reserve, compared with a 50% fall with concentric hypertrophy (53).

5. LVH and B-type natriuretic peptide and C-reactive protein

LVH has been associated with an underlying inflammatory process and is also a precursor of heart failure; thus, a normal C-reactive protein concentration and a normal B-type natriuretic peptide level can rule out the presence of LVH, making an echocardiogram unnecessary (54).

6. Underlying causes of LVH

A) Blood pressure

In 2545 untreated hypertensives who had an echocardiogram and 24 hour BP measurement, in age groups from less than 40 years to age 60 years plus, there was a clear relationship between increasing mean 24-hour diastolic, systolic, and P-P and the degree of LVM (**Figure 7-17**) (55). Home BP is as good as 24 hour BP measurements as a predictor of LVM (56).

In young/middle-aged subjects (mean age about 40 years), both brachial and central BPs were similarly related to LVM, posterior wall thickness, and interventricular wall thickness (57, 58). The relationship between central SBP and LVM is shown in **Figure 7-18** (57). Central pressures correlate more strongly with concentric LVH (more common in older patients) (57) and LV diastolic dysfunction (58).

In older hypertensives, there is a strong relationship between LVM and magnitude of the reflected wave from the periphery

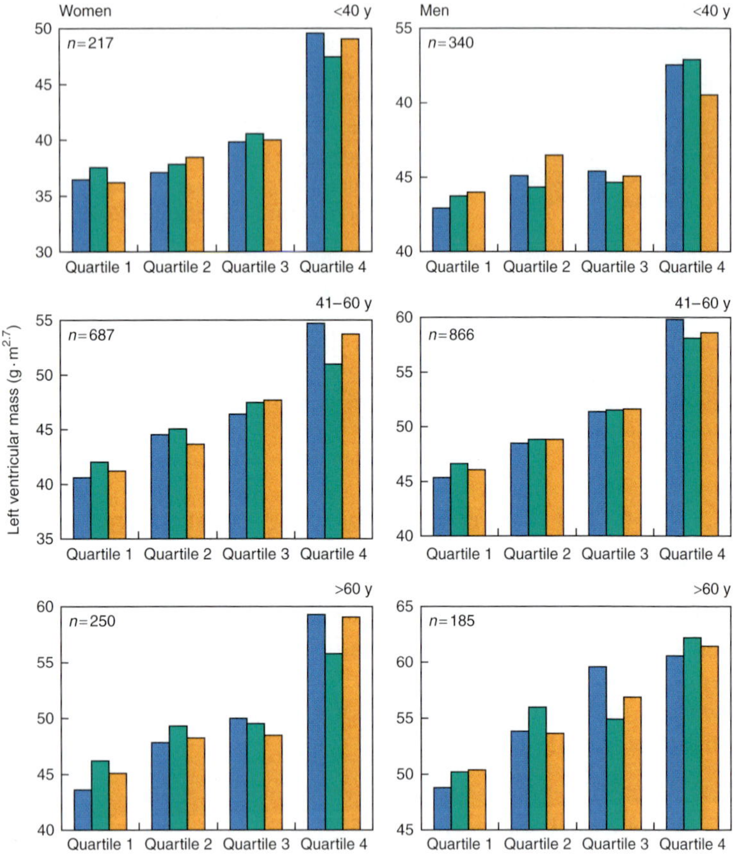

Fig. 7-17 Increase in LVM with increasing quartiles of BP according to age, in men (right) and women; column – white = 24 hr SBP, hatched = 24 hr diastolic blood pressure (DBP), black = 24 hr P-P. (From Verdecchia P, Schillaci G, Borgioni C, et al. Prevalent influence of systolic over pulse pressure on left-ventricular mass in essential hypertension. *Europ Heart J* 2002;23;658–65.)

(**Figure 7-19**) (59). Vasodilators such as ACE, ARB, or calcium blockers are able to reduce the magnitude of the reflected wave (59).

B) Obesity and sympathetic nerve activity (SNA)

In young men, LVH is closely linked to insulin resistance, whereas in young women, it is obesity that is linked to LVH (60). The obesity in women is associated not only to LVH but also to hypertrophy

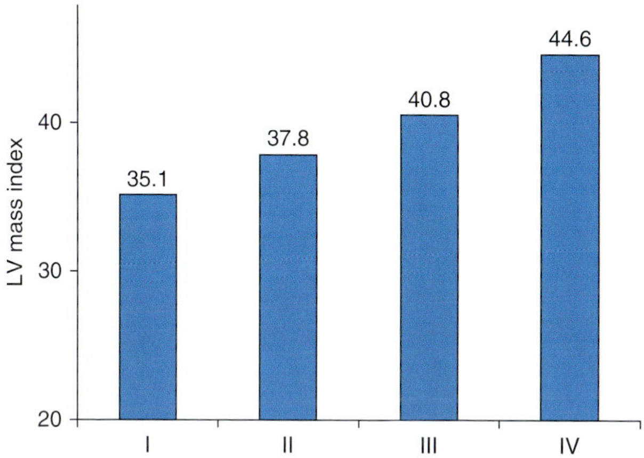

Fig. 7-18 In middle-aged hypertensives, LVM index increased with increasing quartiles of central SBP. (From Roman MJ, Okin PM, Kizer JR, et al. Relations of central and brachial blood pressure to left-ventricular hypertrophy and geometry: the Strong Hear Study. *J Hypertens* 2010;28:384–8.)

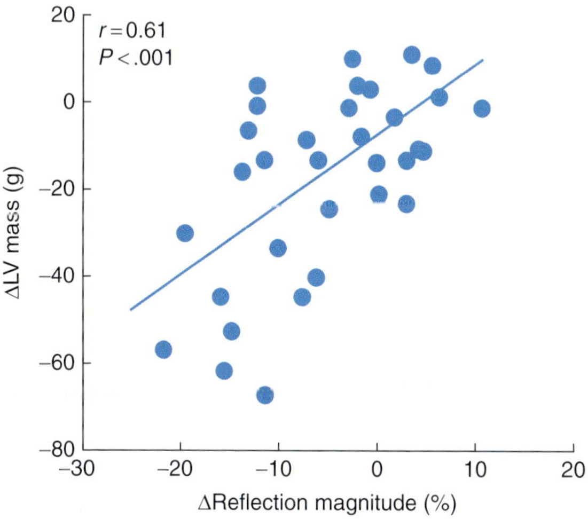

Fig. 7-19 LVM correlates highly with the magnitude of the reflected wave from the periphery to the aorta. (From Hashimoto J, Westerhof BE, Westerhof N, et al. Different role of wave reflection magnitude and timing on left-ventricular mass reduction during antihypertensive treatment. *J Hypertens* 2008;26:1017–24.)

of the right ventricle (**Figure 7-20**) (61). This same study showed a relationship between LVH and insulin and leptin levels (61). Others have noted that in obese middle-aged subjects, LVH was linked to insulin levels (62), as well as a raised cardiac output (63).

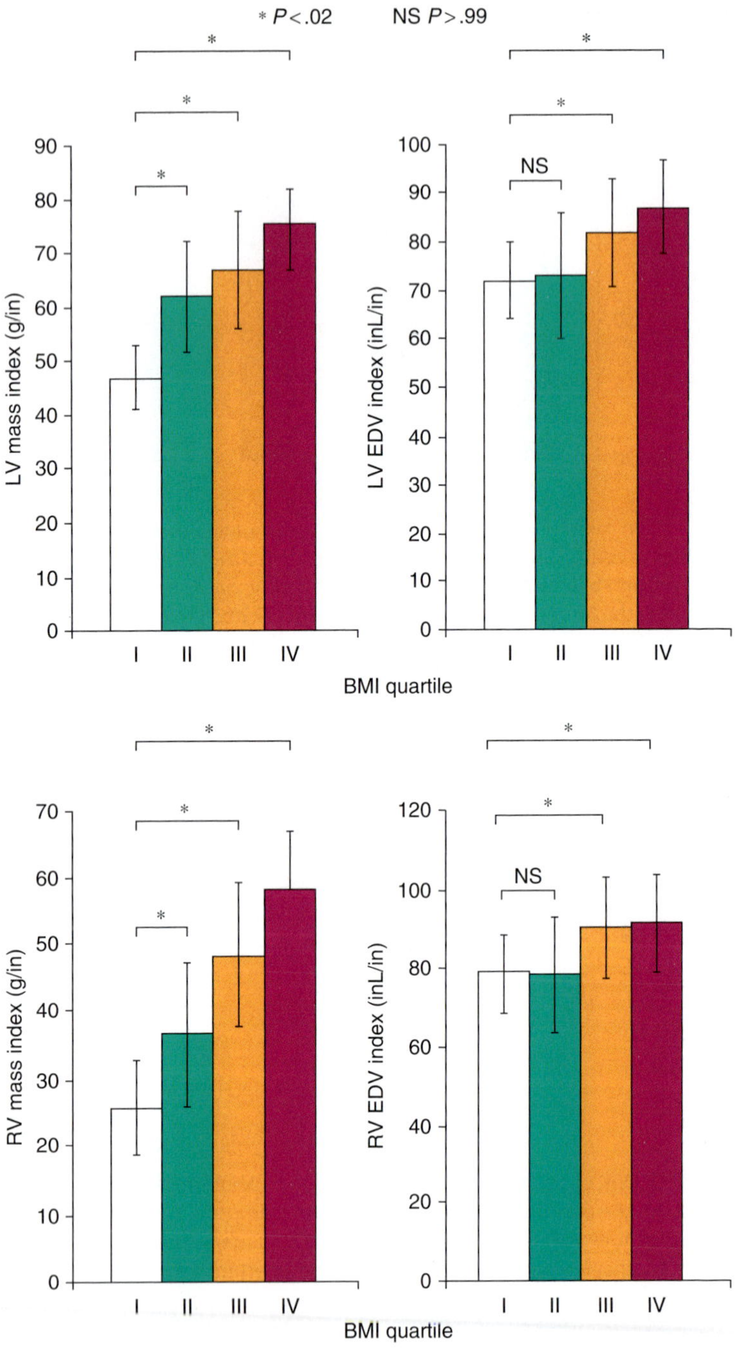

Fig. 7-20 Both LVM/EDV and RVM/EDV increase with increasing body mass index. (From Rider OJ, Petersen SE, Francis JM, et al. Ventricular hypertrophy and cavity dilatation in relation to body mass index in women with uncomplicated obesity. *Heart* 2011;97:203–8.)

In rats, LVH often precedes hypertension and is linked to a high cardiac output and increased SNA (64). Sympathectomy results in a reversal of LVH and a diminution of a cardiac fibrosis (65).

In overweight university students, increased SNA was closely linked to increased LVM and LV wall-thickness (66) and the same applied to middle-aged hypertensives (**Figure 7-21**) (67). Others have confirmed this using plasma noradrenaline levels as a measure of SNA (68). Importantly, cardiac noradrenaline levels were shown to increase progressively from normal subjects, hypertensives with normal LVM, hypertensives with raised LVM, and patients with hypertrophic obstructive cardiomyopathy (**Figure 7-22**) (69). Plasma noradrenaline is also linked to concentric LVH in patients with end-stage renal failure (70). Interestingly, in middle-aged hypertensives with LVH, the levels of β-adrenergic receptor kinase-1 (β ARK1) in lymphocytes were positively related to the presence of LVH (**Figure 7-23**) (71). Beta-ARK1 concentrations are likely to reflect robust, sustained sympathetic stimulation.

Although sympathetic nervous stimulation is linked to increased cardiac muscle mass, angiotensin II appears to be linked to cardiac fibrosis (72).

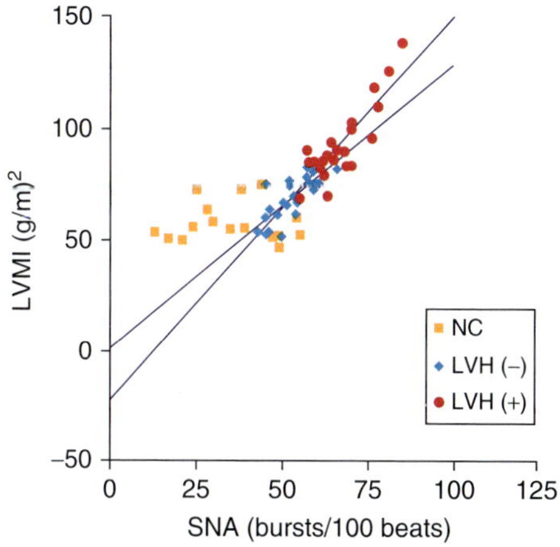

Fig. 7-21 In 52 subjects (mean age: 52 y). SNA closely related to the degree of LVM. (From Burns J, Sivananthan MV, Balls S, et al. Relationship between central sympathetic drive and magnetic resonance imaging-determined left-ventricular mass in essential hypertension. *Circulation* 2007;115:1999–2005.)

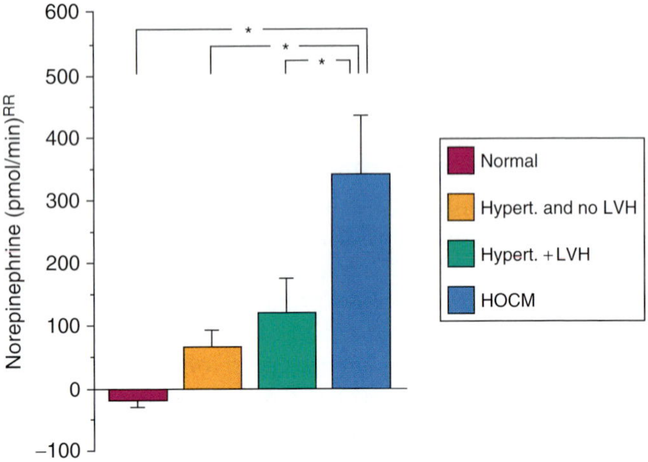

Fig. 7-22 Relationship between cardiac release of noradrenaline and LVH. (From Kelm M, Schafer S, Mingers S, et al. Left ventricular mass is linked to cardiac noradrenaline in normotensive and hypertensive patients. *J Hypertens* 1996;14:1357–64.)

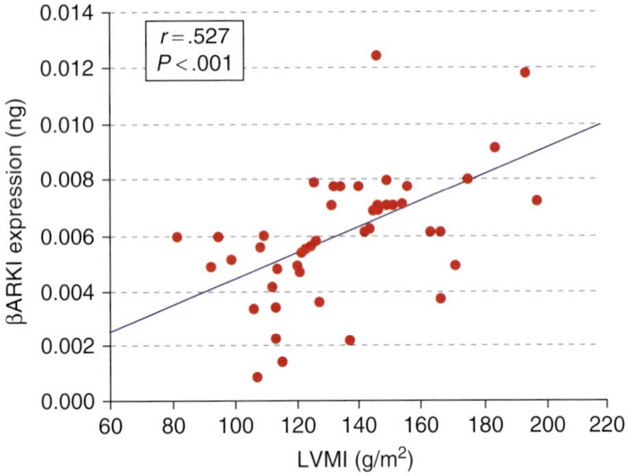

Fig. 7-23 Correlation between LVM and expression of β-adrenergic receptor kinase-1 (β-ARK1) in lymphocytes. (From Park SJ, Choi DJ, Kim CW. Hypertensive left-ventricular hypertrophy: relation to beta-adrenergic receptor kinase -1 (β-ARK1) in peripheral lymphocytes. *J Hypertens* 2004;22:1025–32.)

7. LVH and prognosis

A) Echocardiographic LVH

Animal study has shown that the transition from LVH to heart failure involves chronic β-receptor stimulation (73). Therefore, it is

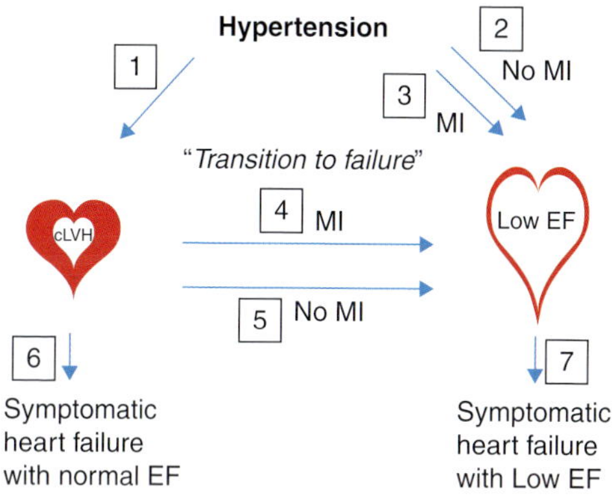

Fig. 7-24 Patients with concentric LVH (1) progress to heart failure with normal ejection fraction (EF) (unless with MI), while eccentric LVH (2) or cases of myocardial infarction (MI) (3) progress to heart failure with low EF. (From Drazner MH. The progression of hypertensive heart disease. *Circulation* 2011;123:327–34.)

not surprising that in man, pathological hypertrophy can lead on to heart failure (**Figure 7-14**) (41) and that eccentric LVH can lead to systolic heart failure with a low ejection fraction, and concentric LVH can lead on to diastolic heart failure with a normal ejection fraction (**Figure 7-24**) (38).

Early studies showed that in middle-aged hypertensives, a high LVM was associated with an increased relative risk of 3.52 for a future cardiovascular event, which was reduced to 1.38 if the LVH has been reversed by treatment (74). Others confirmed this (75), with concentric LVH having the worst prognosis (76). A 17-year follow-up of 7924 subjects showed that the presence of LVH, whether with hypertension or not, markedly increased the risk of cardiac death (**Figure 7-25**) (83). A large meta analysis indicated that patients with LVH had an increased risk of 2.3 of experiencing a future cardiovascular event, and an increased risk of 2.5 regarding all-cause mortality (77).

Although LVH persists in 20% of the subjects (78), physiological hypertrophy, occurring in athletes, usually regresses after long-term deconditioning. Therefore, it is possible that "Athletes Heart" is not entirely innocent (79): only long-term studies will answer the question.

B) ECG LVH

In middle-aged male hypertensives, 24% of those with echocardiographic LVH also had ECG LVH (80). In such patients, symptomatic and silent ischemia occur in about 50% of cases, with reversible

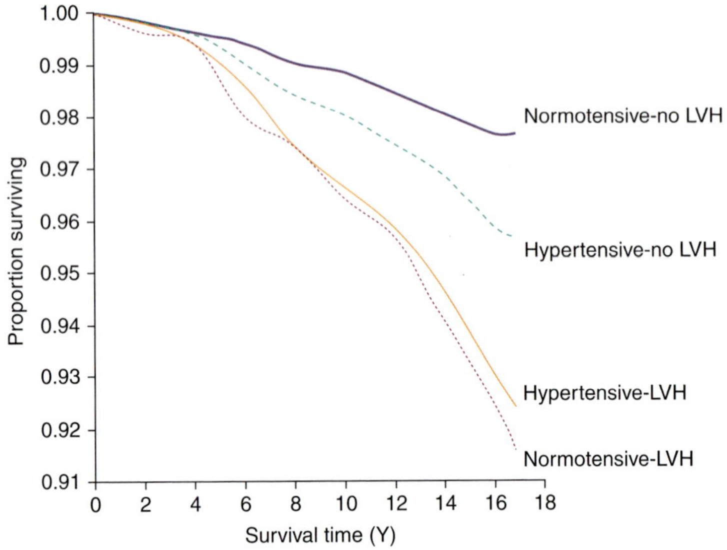

Fig. 7-25 The presence of LVH, with or without hypertension, markedly increases the risk of cardiac death. (From Brown DW, Giles WH, Croft JB. Left-ventricular hypertrophy as a predictor of coronary heart disease mortality and the effect of hypertension. *Am Heart J* 2000;140:848–56.)

thallium perfusion defects, even in the absence of coronary artery disease (80, 81). Subjects with ECG LVH and strain pattern (depressed S-T segment and inverted T-wave) have an increased relative risk of future ischemic heart disease of 4.1 (36). Reversal of these ECG changes reduces cardiovascular events and death (82). A 17-year follow-up study of 7924 subjects showed clearly the poor prognosis of subjects, with or without hypertension, with ECG LVH and strain pattern (83). A similar 15-year follow-up study of 15,792 subjects indicated that ECG LVH in men was a powerful predictor of coronary heart disease (CHD) events, whereas in women, ECG LVH predicted heart failure. The absence of ECG LVH is associated with a reduced risk of sudden death (85).

8. Effects of antihypertensive drug therapy upon LVH

A) General

All antihypertensive drugs are able to reverse LVH to a greater or lesser degree. A meta-analysis of the effects of all the main antihypertensive agents on LVM, posterior wall thickness, and interventricular septal thickness is shown in **Figure 7-26** (86).

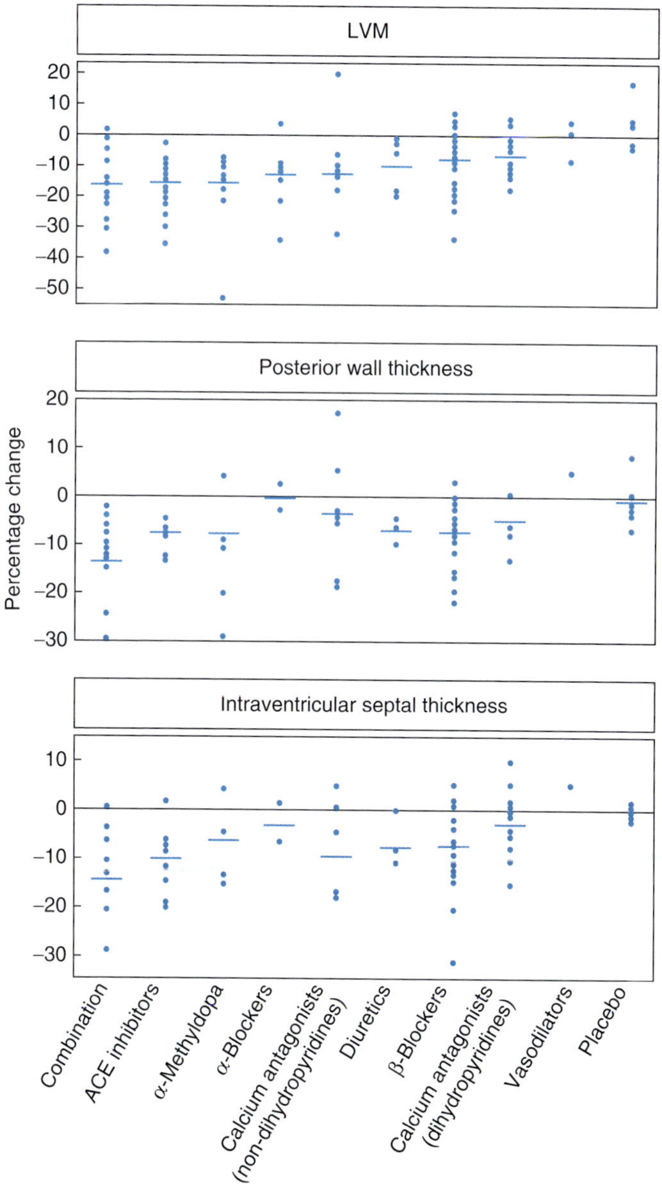

Fig. 7-26 Meta-analysis of the effects of antihypertensive drugs on LVM and thickness of posterior wall and interventricular septum. (From Cruickshank JM, Messerli FH. *Left-Ventricular Hypertrophy and Its Regression*. London: Science Press; 1992, p71–81.)

B) Diuretics

The effect of diuretics on LVM, posterior wall thickness, and interventricular septal thickness is shown in Figure 7-26 (86). However, this meta-analysis does not take age into account. In elderly patients with isolated systolic hypertension (SHEP study), diuretics were associated with 13% reduction in LVM versus a 6% increase on placebo, over a 3-year follow-up (**Figure 7-27**) (87).

In older/middle-aged subjects, diuretic therapy was effective in reducing LVM in those with a high baseline degree of LVH (88).

In younger/middle-aged hypertensives, when compared with atenolol, the diuretic moduretic was superior in reducing LVM (atenolol increased left ventricular internal diameter—LVID) but was significantly inferior in reducing posterior wall and interventricular septal thickness and relative wall thickness (**Figure 7-28**) (89).

In a randomized comparison of hydrochlorothiazide and enalapril, over 1 year, the ACEI was superior in decreasing LVM, posterior wall, and interventricular septal thickness (90). Hydrochlorothiazide was also inferior to lisinopril in regressing myocardial fibrosis (91). Also, a thiazide diuretic was equal to

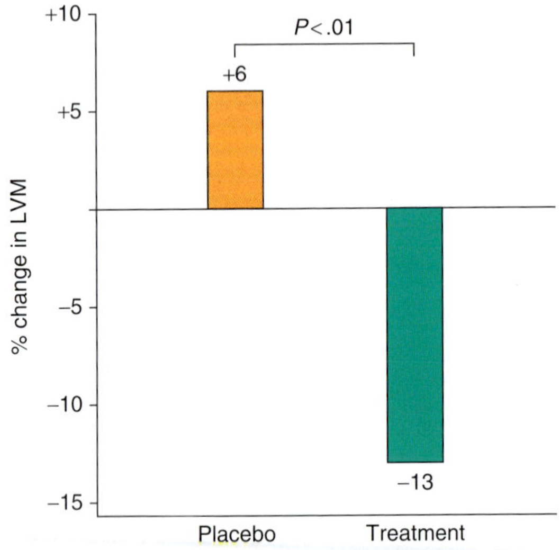

Fig. 7-27 SHEP – Effect of chlorthalidone ± atenolol and placebo upon LVM over 4.5 years. (From Ofili EO, Cohen JD, St Vrain JA, et al. Effect of treatment of isolated systolic hypertension on left-ventricular mass. *JAMA* 1998;279:778–80.)

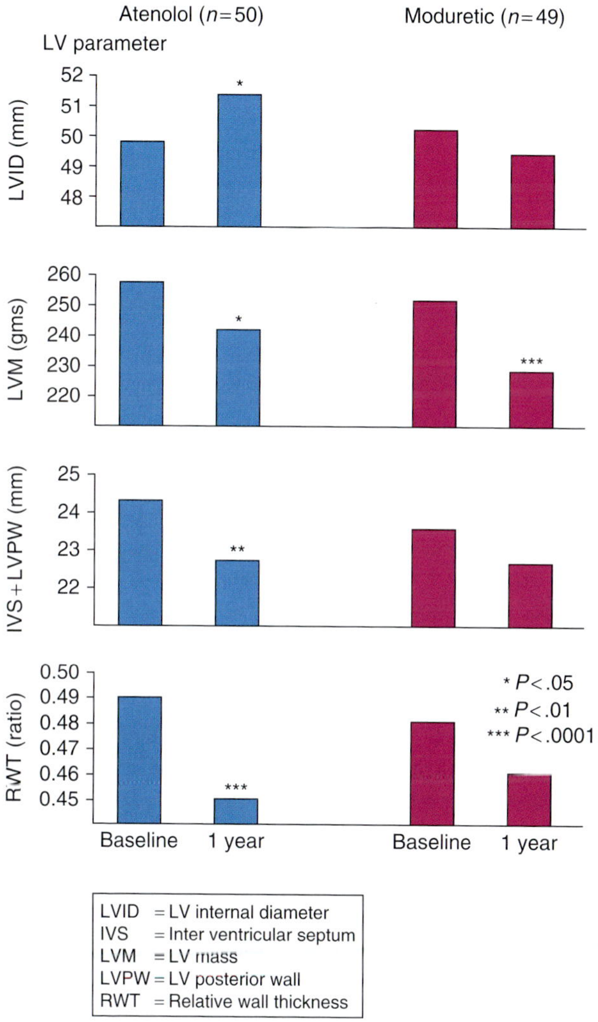

Fig. 7-28 Atenolol versus Diuretic in LVH (n = 99 diastolic hypertension). (From Otterstad JE, Foeland G, Soeyland AK, et al. Change in left-ventricular dimensions and systolic function in 100 mildly hypertensive men during one year's treatment with atenolol versus hydrochlorthiazide and amiloride (moduretic): a double-blind, randomized study. *J Int Med* 1992;231:493–501.)

the calcium antagonist isradipine in reducing septal wall thickness, but superior in reducing LVM (92). It should be added that all diuretics are not equally effective in reversing LVH; in a comparison of chlorthalidone and hydrochlorothiazide in 8012 middle-aged men, the former drug was the more effective in reversing ECG LVH (93).

C) BBs

More recent meta-analyses of treatment effects on LVM than that mentioned earlier (Figure 7-26) (86), also did not take age into account (94, 95). Accordingly, the position of BBs came bottom, and ARBs came top, of the list of drugs concerning efficacy in reversing increased LVM.

i) Young/middle-age (age < 60 years)

1. ECG LVH

In a 5-year follow-up of young/middle-aged moderate hypertensives on atenolol, ECG LVH was present in 28% at baseline, but in only 2% 5 years later, with significant reductions in "sum of S-V1 plus R-V5" and reversal of "T wave-inversion" in leads AVL or V5-6 (**Table 7-4**) (96). Thus, it was unexpected when, after a shorter time span of 18 months, atenolol had no effect on ECG LVH, in contrast to irbesartan which did (97).

TABLE 7-4 Over a 5.1-y follow-up of 129 hypertensives on atenolol-based therapy, there was a significant reversal of ECG LVH strain pattern as assessed by S-V1+R-V5 and T-wave inversion in leads 1, AVL, V5-6.

			Incidence of LVH		
Time of ECG record	Sum of S-V1 + R-V5 mm (range)	Height of R-AVL mm (range)	By S-V1 + R-V5 ≥ 35 mm n (%)	By R-AVL ≥ 12 mm n (%)	T-wave inversion in leads I, AVL V5 or V6 n (%)
1st visit	27.5 ± 0.77 (6.5–56.0)	7.15 ± 0.35 (0.0–20.0)	28 ± 5.1 (21.6)	14 ± 3.5 (11.2)	23 ± 4.4 (17.6)
Last visit (mean, 5.1 y after first visit)	22.2 ± 0.58* (5.3–37.5)	6.45 ± 0.32 (0.0–17.5)	2 ± 1.4* (1.6)	9 ± 2.9 (7.0)	10 ± 3.0** (7.8)

Abbreviations: ECG LVH, electrocardiographic left ventricular hypertrophy.
*P < .0001, **P = .014, versus first visit.
From Cruickshank JM, Messerli FH. *Left-Ventricular Hypertrophy and Its Regression*. London: Science Press; 1992, p71–81.

2. Echocardiographic LVH

In a study of 278 hypertensive patients randomized to either atenolol or the calcium blocker lacidipine and followed-up for 4 years, the BB reduced LVM by a significant 13.9%, compared with 12.5% with the calcium blocker (98). Others have confirmed this atenolol result (88). Thus, it was surprising that, in other studies, atenolol had no effect of LVM over 6–18 month period (97, 99, 100). Atenolol does not reduce the fibrotic component of LVH (101).

In a comparison between metoprolol and nebivolol (with β-3 ISA), the latter was more effective in reducing LV wall thickness, i.e. LV wall thickness is related to central pressures (102).

In a comparison of highly β-1 selective bisoprolol and the ACEI enalapril, over a 6-month period, bisoprolol was at least as effective as enalapril in reducing LVM, posterior wall thickness, and septal thickness (**Figure 7-29**) (103). Regression of LVM with bisoprolol

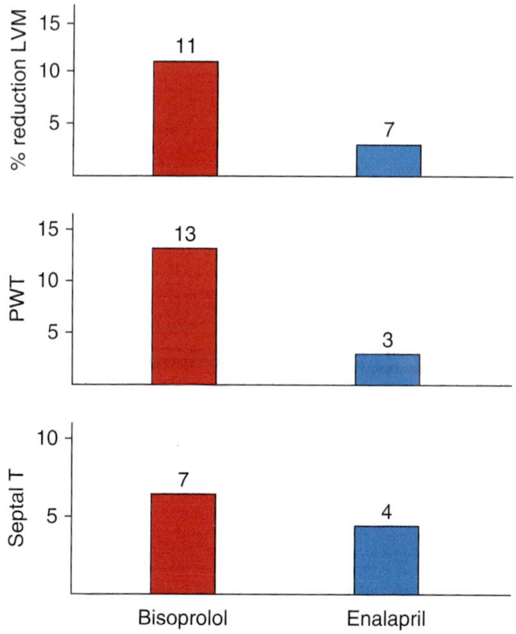

Fig. 7-29 Effect of bisoprolol and enalapril on LVH in 56 randomized hypertensives, mean age 50y, over a 6-mo period. (From Gosse P, Routaut R, Herreo G, et al. Beta-blockers versus ACE-inhibition in hypertension: effects on left-ventricular hyvpertrophy. *J Cardiovasc Pharmacol* 1990;16:S 145–50.)

is associated with a 22% increase in coronary flow reserve (CFR) (**Figure** 7-30) (104).

ii) Older hypertensives

1. ECG LVH

In the LIFE study, losartan was more effective than atenolol in reversing ECG LVH (105).

2. Echocardiographic LVH

In the Losartan Intervention For Endpoint reduction (LIFE) study, losartan was more effective than atenolol in reversing LVM (106). Atenolol was also inferior to the nondihydropyridine calcium blocker verapamil in reducing LVM in elderly hypertensives (107). Carvedilol, a BB with additional α-blocking action, was more effective than metoprolol in reducing LVM and improving CFR (108).

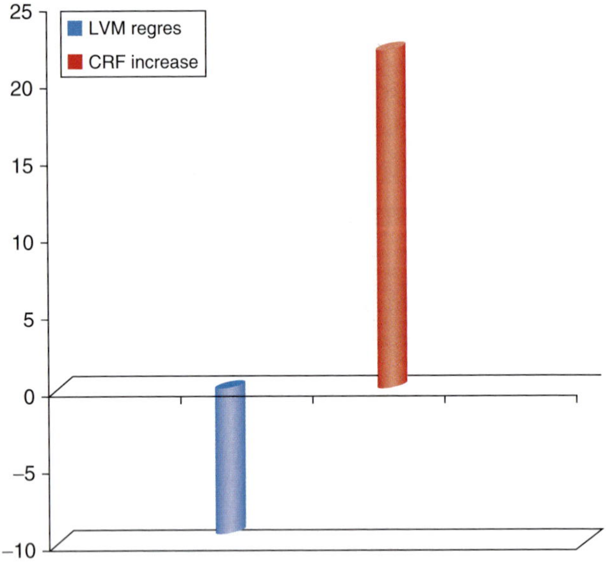

Fig. 7-30 Effect of bisoprolol over 1 year on LVM and coronary flow reserve (CFR) in 10 hypertensives + ischemic heart disease (IHD). (From Motz W, Vogt M, Scheler S, et al. Improvement of coronary flow reserve following regression of hypertrophy resulting from blood pressure lowering with a beta-blocker. *Dtsch Med Wochen* 1993;118:535–40.)

D) ACEIs

As illustrated earlier (Figure 7-26) (86), a meta-analysis (not taking age into account) showed that ACEIs came out well in terms of reversing LVM and reducing posterior wall and interventricular septal thickness.

i) Young/middle-aged hypertensives

As indicated earlier (88), in middle-aged hypertensives with marked LVH, captopril was, like atenolol and hydrochlorothiazide, superior to clonidine, diltiazem, and prazosin in reversing LVM. Enalapril was superior to hydrochlorothiazide in reversing LVM and reducing posterior wall and interventricular thickness (90). Lisinopril was also superior to hydrochlorothiazide in regressing myocardial fibrosis (91).

Compared with atenolol over 6 months, ramipril was superior in regressing LVM and reducing posterior wall and interventricular septal thickness (99); as was perindopril (100), which also was superior in increasing CFR. However, in a comparison between enalapril and highly β-1 selective bisoprolol, all the trends in regressing LVM and reducing posterior wall and septal thickness favored the BB (Figure 7-29) (103).

ii) Elderly

In the HOPE study (109), over 4.5 years, ramipril was superior to placebo in regressing and preventing ECG LVH, and this was linked to a reduced risk of death, myocardial infarction, stroke, and heart failure.

In a 2-year comparison of lisinopril and amlodipine (110), both drugs were similar in regressing LVM and improving diastolic function.

E) ARBs

In meta-analyses, not taking age into account, ARBs come out well in terms of regression of LVM (**Figure 7-31**) (94), and in reducing posterior wall and septal thickness.

i) Younger/middle-aged subjects

Vasodilator drugs, which reduce the magnitude of the reflected wave, for example, ARBs, ACEI, and calcium blockers, are effective

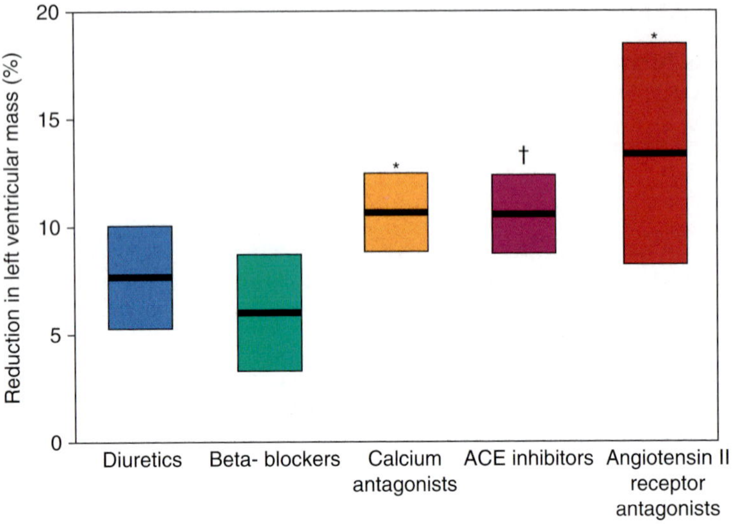

Fig. 7-31 Percent reduction of LVM by various antihypertensive agents. (From Klingbeil AU, Schneider M, Martus P, et al. A meta-analysis of the effects of treatment on left-ventricular mass in essential hypertension. *Am J Med* 2003;115:41–6.)

in regressing LVM (Figure 7-19) (59). In young subjects, over a 2-year period, candesartan was superior to placebo in regressing LVM (111).

In a comparison of atenolol and irbesartan, over an 18-month period, only the ARB reversed ECG LVH and echocardiographic LVH in those with high baseline values (97). Another comparison between atenolol and irbesartan produced a similar result (112). Also, in a comparison against atenolol, only losartan decreased myocardial collagen content (101).

A comparison between losartan and the renin-inhibitor aliskiren showed that both agents were equal in promoting LVM regression (113).

ii) Elderly

Telmisartan was superior to placebo in regressing ECG LVH and reducing new onset LVH by 37% (114). The effects of telmisartan were similar to those of the ACEI ramipril (114). In another comparison between the ARB eprosartan and the ACEI enalapril, the ACEI was best at regressing LVM (115).

In the LIFE study, losartan was superior to atenolol in regressing ECG LVH (105), although this advantage was less obvious in women (116). Losartan was also superior to atenolol in regressing LVM (106).

In Japanese hypertensive patients, valsartan was superior to amlodipine in regressing echocardiographic LVH (29).

F) Calcium Blockers

The effects of both dihydropyridine and nondihydropyridine calcium blockers on LVM and posterior wall/septal thickness are shown in Figure 7-26 (86). As vasodilators, they are effective in reducing the magnitude of the reflected wave, which is linked to central pressures and LV regression (Figure 7-19) (59). In meta-analyses, not taking age into account, calcium blockers are similar to ACEI and ARBs, but superior to BBs and diuretics, in regressing LVM (Figure 7-31) (94).

i) Nondihydropyridine

In middle-aged hypertensives, diltiazem was inferior to atenolol, captopril, and hydrochlorothiazide in regressing LVM over 1 year, but was effective in reducing posterior wall thickness (88). However, in the elderly, verapamil was superior to atenolol in regressing LVM (107).

ii) Dihydropyridine

As shown in Figure 7-26 (86), dihydropyridine calcium blockers appear to be similar to BBs in reducing LVM, but somewhat less effective in reducing wall and septal thickness.

In a 4-year study in middle-aged hypertensives, lacidipine and atenolol regressed LVM, posterior wall, and septal thickness to a similar extent (98). Nifedipine GITS was similar to enalapril in regressing LVM (117, 118). However, shorter acting dihydropyridines that markedly increase SNA, such as felodipine ER (118), are less effective in reversing LVH.

G) α-Blockers

Figure 7-26 (86) suggested that α-blockers were effective in regressing LVM, but less effective in reducing posterior wall and septal thickness. It might be expected that α-blockers would be effective in reversing LVH, as LVH is closely related to the early morning surge in BP, which is linked to high α-sympathetic stimulation (119). However, in middle-aged hypertensives, prazosin was less effective than captopril, hydrochlorthiazide, and atenolol in regressing LVM (88); and in middle-aged subjects, the α-blocker bunazosin was similar to metoprolol in regressing LVM, although the latter was superior in improving diastolic function (120).

In the elderly, doxazosin was superior to atenolol in regressing LVM (121) and is better than propranolol in reducing fibrosis in LVH (122).

9. Renal sympathetic denervation

In 46 resistant hypertensives, renal sympathetic denervation not only lowered BP over 6 months but also improved left ventricular (LV) diastolic function and diminished LVM (123).

10. Children

Essential hypertension is not uncommon in adolescents and is closely linked to obesity and an increased LVM (124).

In the Bogalusa Heart Study, a group of 12-year olds was followed-up for 24 years (125): 6.5% of the children developed LVH, with diastolic BP being closely related to concentric LVH, and obesity being linked to eccentric LVH. Having achieved young/middle-age (mean age: 36 years), the Bogalusa subjects with concentric LVH were noted to have a wide-P-P, increased arterial stiffness, and decreased arterial compliance (126). Also, in this study, black subjects appeared more susceptible than white subjects to BP-related adverse cardiac remodeling (**Figure 7-32**) (127).

ATHEROMA AND VASCULAR STRUCTURE

1. Pathogenesis of atheromatous plaque

Early atherosclerosis is characterized by the deposition of intracellular and extracellular lipids and by the appearance of macrophages and T-lymphocytes in the vessel intima, which eventually form fatty streaks (128). The flat, fatty streaks may be transformed into raised fibrolipid plaques and, ultimately, into a fibroatheroma comprising a core of extracellular lipid covered on the luminal side by a thick

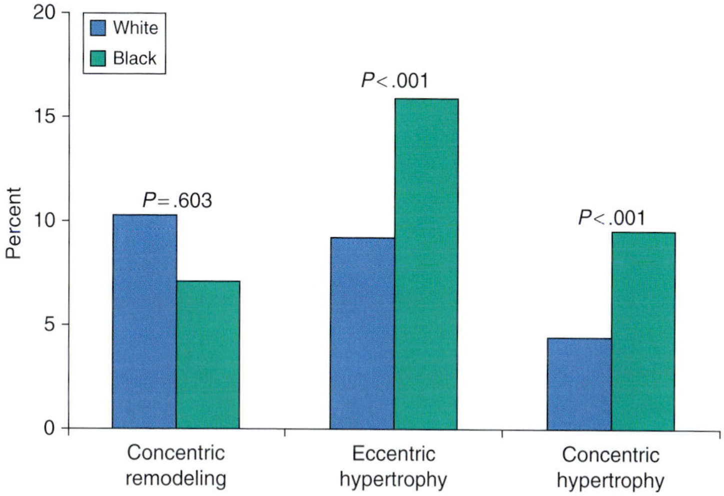

Fig. 7-32 Bogalusa Heart Study; in young/middle-aged population with raised BP, black subjects are at greater risk than white subjects of both concentric and eccentric LVH. (From Wang J, Chen W, Ruan L, et al. Differential effect of elevated blood pressure on left-ventricular geometry types in Black and White young adults in a community (from the Bogalusa Heart Study). *Am J Cardiol* 2011;107:717–22.)

fibrous cap. Such atheromataous plaques may achieve "vulnerable" status, and the various forms of vulnerable, unstable plaques are shown in **Figure 7-33**. The classic unstable plaque has a large lipid core, with increased accumulation of activated inflammatory cells that infiltrate the fibrous cap and induce substantial loss in both vascular smooth muscle-cells and collagen, leading to fibrous cap destabilization and disruption.

2. Stress, SNA, the renin-angiotensin system, and atheroma

Adrenaline and noradrenaline have been shown to precipitate the characteristic changes in the vascular wall of early atherogenesis (129) and to increase the atherogenetic uptake of low-density lipoprotein (LDL) (130). Psychosocial stress in monkeys induced coronary endothelial injury, prevented by chronic β-1 blockade (131). The stress-induced atheromatous lesions in monkeys were more extensive at higher heart rates (132) and were markedly reduced by

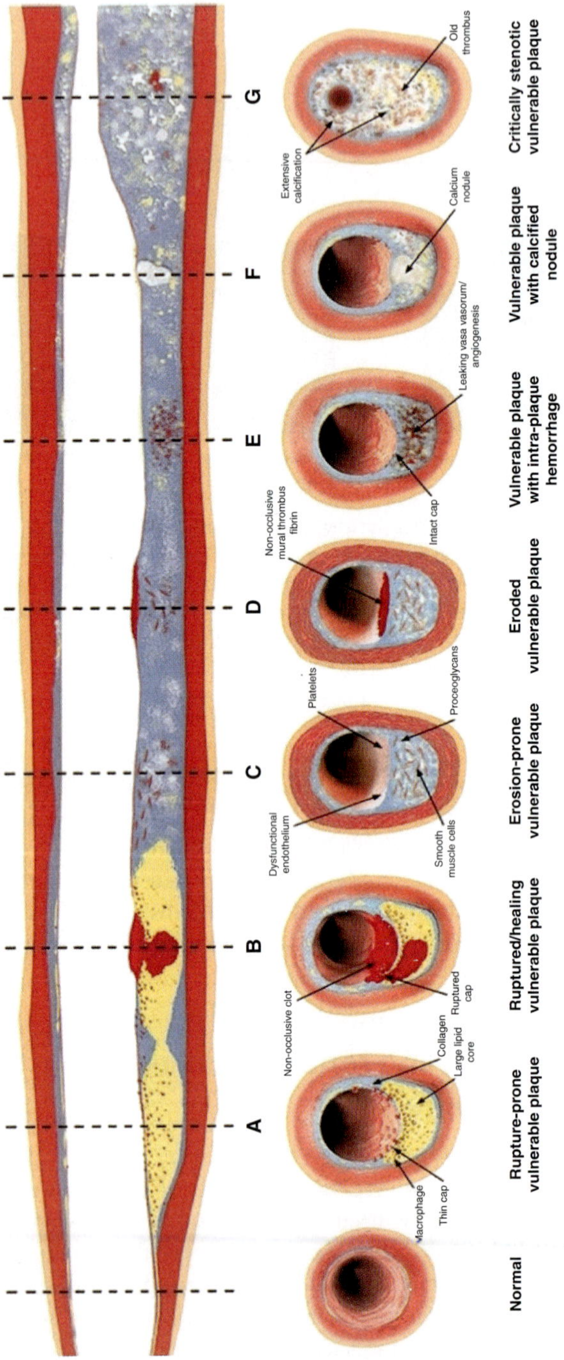

Fig. 7-33 Different Types of Vulnerable Plaque.

prior sinoatrial node ablation (133). Monocytes may be involved in the destabilization of atheromataous plaque by production of matrix metalloproteinases, and this process is encouraged by adrenaline and noradrenaline via β-stimulation (134).

There is evidence suggesting that the renin-angiotensin system may contribute to the inflammatory process within the vascular wall that is linked to the unstable plaque (135). High angiotensin II levels are linked to atherosclerotic plaques with signs of instability (136).

3. Endothelial shear stress, blood flow patterns, and atheroma

Animal study has shown that blood flow pattern is important regarding the site and degree of atheromataous plaque formation (137). **Figure 7-34** illustrates areas of lowered shear stress, increased shear stress, vortices with oscillatory shear stress, and undisturbed shear stress (laminar blood flow) (137). Laminar blood flow was associated with an absence of atheromataous plaque, oscillating flow with a high number of stable plaque lesions, and low shear stress

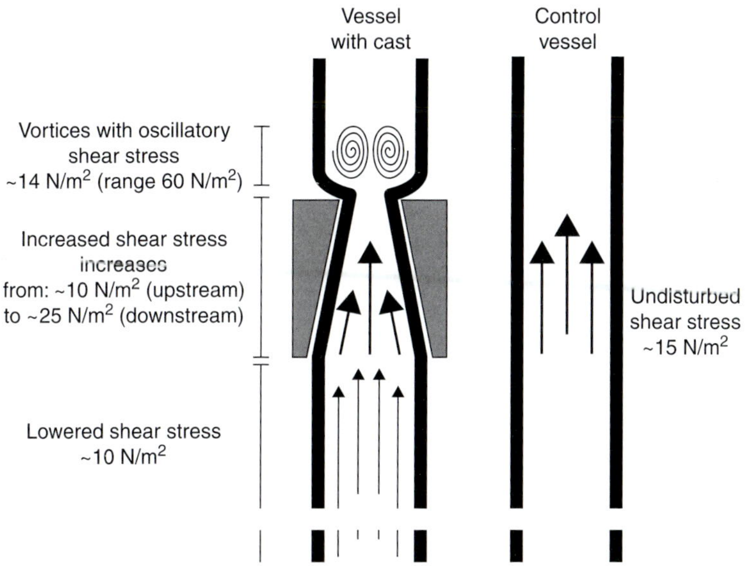

Fig. 7-34 Laminar flow and high shear stress on endothelial wall reduce the risk of atheromatous plaque formation. (From Cheng C, Temple D, van Haperen R, et al. Athersclerotic lesion size and vulnerability are determined by patterns of fluid shear stress. *Circulation* 2006;113:2744–53.)

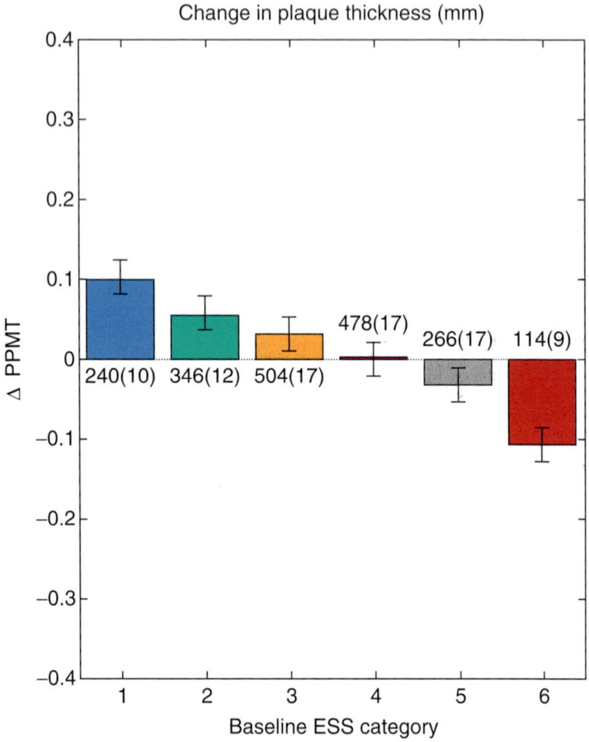

Fig. 7-35 Low ESS category is linked to increased plaque thickness. (From Stone PH, Coskun AU, Kinlay S, et al. Effect of shear stress on the progression of coronary artery disease, vascular remodeling and in-stent restonosis in humans. *Circulation* 2003;108:348–44.)

with a high number of vulnerable, unstable plaque lesions. Other studies have also shown that low endothelial shear stress (ESS) is linked to vulnerable atheromataous plaque (138), with high levels of metalloproteins that are linked to matrix breakdown (139). These animal data have been reproduced in humans undergoing a 6-month follow-up of in-stent restenosis, where low ESS forces were linked to increased plaque thickness as assessed by intracoronary ultra sound (**Figure 7-35**) (140).

An intravascular ultrasound study in 20 patients with coronary artery disease indicated that low shear forces were linked to greater plaque, and necrotic core, progression, whereas high shear forces encouraged transformation to a more vulnerable phenotype (141). Optimal shear forces (laminar flow) result in nitric oxide (NO) release within the endothelium (**Figure 7-36**) (142).

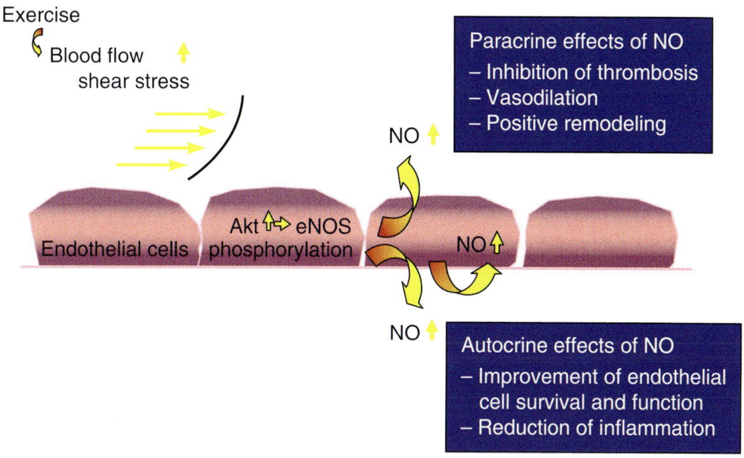

Fig. 7-36 Exercise and prevention of atheroma; via flow shear-force effects on endothelium; Akt, protein kinase B; eNOS, NO synthetase; and NO. nitric oxide. (From Dimmeler S, Zeiher AM. Exercise and cardiovascular health: get active to "AKTivate" your endothelial nitric oxide synthase. *Circulation* 2003;107:3152–8.)

4. Ways to achieve laminar blood flow and reduced endothelial damage/atheromataous plaque

Hydralazine, in contrast to propranolol, increased the likelihood of high velocity, turbulent flow patterns in patients with carotid stenosis (143). Accordingly, propranolol, in contrast to hydralazine, reduced the degree of atherosclerosis in rabbits that are fed on a high-cholesterol diet (144). A randomized, crossover study in patients with carotid stenosis (2 weeks per drug) showed that metoprolol, in contrast to nifedipine or captopril, achieved optimal laminar blood flow (145) (**Table 7-5**). Metoprolol and atenolol were shown to reduce the risk of endothelial damage in stressed monkeys (131). In patients who had undergone coronary angiography, high heart rates increased, and BBs reduced, the risk of plaque disruption (146) (**Table 7-6**).

5. Antihypertensive drugs and their effect on intima-medial thickness, atheromataous plaque volume, and plaque stability

A) Intima-medial thickness

Some studies indicate that carotid-wall intima-media thickness intima-media ratio (IMT), a presumed surrogate measure of atherosclerosis, is a predictor of future cardiovascular events (147). However, a recent

TABLE 7-5 Effect of antihypertensive agents on arterial flow-patterns in man

	Neutral	Turbulent flow	Laminar flow
Placebo	Yes	No effect	No effect
Hydralazine	No	Worse	No
Nifedipine	No	Worse	No
Captopril	Yes	No effect	No effect
Metoprolol	No	Diminished	Yes

From Spence JD. Effects of hydralazine versus propranolol on blood velocity patterns in patients with carotid stenosis. *Clin Sci* 1983;65:91–3; Spence JD, Perkins DG, Kline RL, et al. Hemodynamic modification of atherosclerosis. Effects of propranolol versus hydralazine in hypertensive, hyperlipidemic rabbits. *Athersclerosis* 1984;50:325–33; Spence JD. Effects of antihypertensive drugs on flow disturbance: nifedepine, captopril and metoprolol evaluated by quantitative spectral analysis of Doppler flow patterns in patients with carotid stenosis. *Clin Invest Med* 1994;17:319–25.

TABLE 7-6 In 106 patients who had 2 coronary angiograms over 6 mo, plaque disruption was significantly less frequent with BB usage and more common at high heart rates.

	OR (95% CI)	*P*
LVM > 270 g	4.92 (1.83–13.25)	.02
HR mean > 80 bpm	3.19 (1.15–8.85)	.02
BB use	0.32 (0.13–0.88)	.02
Wall thickness IVS	1.68 (0.57–9.91)	.06
PPF	1.81 (0.67–4.90)	.07
ACEIs	0.51 (0.19–1.34)	.06
Statins	0.42 (0.16–1.22)	.06

Abbreviations: ACEIs, angiotensin-converting enzyme inhibitor; CI, confidence interval; HR, IVS, LVM, left ventricular mass; PPF.

From Heidland VE, Strauer BE. Left ventricular muscle mass and elevated heart rate are associated with coronary plaque disruption. *Circulation* 2001;104:1477–82.

meta-analysis concludes that IMT progression, unlike a single measure of carotid IMT, is not a predictor of future cardiovascular events (149, 150).

In middle-aged patients with high cholesterol and on statins, a randomized study comparing placebo versus metoprolol succinate over 3 years showed that the BB significantly reduced the progression rate of carotid intima-media thickness (IMT) (**Figure 7-37**) (148). In a randomized comparison of atenolol and lacidipine in middle-aged hypertensive patients over 4 years, the calcium blocker was more effective in slowing the progression of carotid IMT (151).

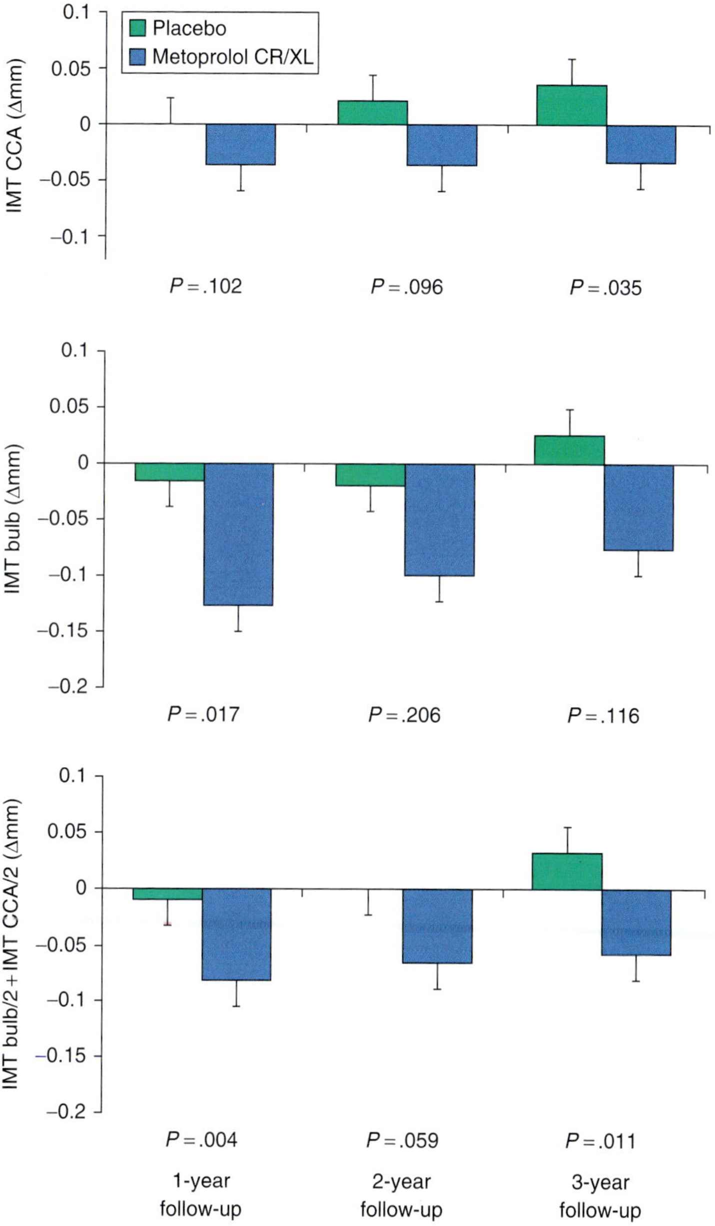

Fig. 7-37 Effect of metoprolol versus placebo on carotid IMT over 3 y in patients on statins. (From Wiklund O, Hulthe J, Wikstrand J, et al. Effect of controlled release/extended release metoprolol on carotid intima-medial thickness in patients with hypercholesterolemia. *Stroke* 2002;33:572–7.)

A randomized comparison between β-1 selective celiprolol and enalapril over a 9-month period revealed that carotid IMT was diminished equally by both drugs (152). A similar comparison between atenolol and the ARB olmesartan, indicated that both drugs decreased the IMT equally, although the ARB reduced the volume of larger atherosclerotic plaques at 2 years (153).

In hypertensives randomized to the sulphydryl ACEI zofenopril versus enalapril over 5 years, the former was more effective in slowing the progression of intima-medial thickness of the carotid artery (154). A 2-year comparison of lisinopril and amlodipine in elderly hypertensives showed that both drugs reduced the IMT equally (155). A 1-year randomized comparison between the ACEI quinapril and the ARB losartan in hypertensives revealed that quinapril reduced carotid IMT more effectively than losartan (156). In contrast, a comparison of losartan and enalapril in Japanese hypertensives showed that both drugs reduced carotid IMT equally (157).

In rabbits fed on a high-cholesterol diet, low-dose indapamide, but not hydrochlorothiazide, reduced the IMT (158). Not only does hydrochlorthiazide have no effect on IMT, but also it blocks the beneficial effects of the ACEI quinapril (159).

An overview of 16 double-blind, randomized trials revealed that all antihypertensive agents reduce IMT, but that calcium blockers were the best (160).

B) Intravascular ultrasound (atheromataous plaque volume)

A pooled analysis of 4 intravascular (coronary) ultrasonography trials in middle-aged subjects showed that in those patients receiving BBs (1154 of 1515 patients), over 1 year, there was a highly significant reduction in plaque volume versus placebo, the effect being about two-thirds of the effect of statins (**Figure 7-38**) (161). The BBs in this trial were mainly metoprolol and atenolol, and both drugs had a similar antiatheromatous effect, which was in part independent of changes in heart rate. The BB benefit is clearly a function of β-1 blockade.

Another randomized, placebo-controlled study in middle-aged, normotensive ischemic subjects showed that over a 2-year period, amlodipine and enalapril slowed the progression of coronary atheromatous plaque (**Figure 7-39**) (162) (not regression, as observed with BBs (161)). A placebo-controlled, randomized trial over 3 years in high-risk subjects showed that the ACEI perindopril had no effect on atheromataous plaque volume (163).

ARBs (losartan) have been shown to prevent aortic fatty streaks in monkeys fed atherogenic diets (164).

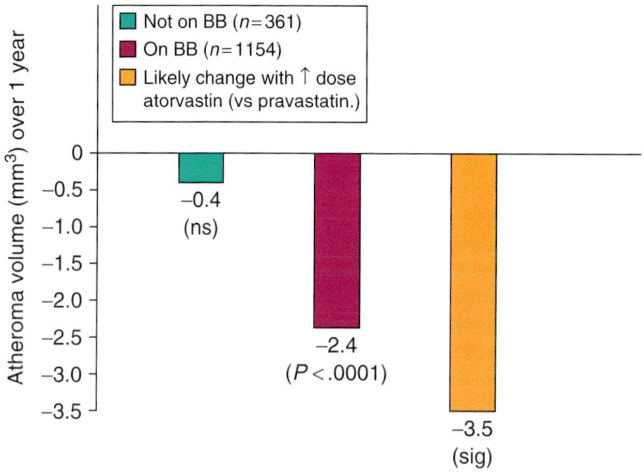

Fig. 7-38 Decrease in coronary atheromatous volume (mm³) by BBs over 1 year (independent of statins, ACEIs, other drugs, LDL Conc. HR). (From Sipahi I, Tuzcu M, Wolski KE, et al. Beta-blockers and progression of coronary atherosclerosis: pooled analysis of 4 intravascular ultrasonography trials. *Am Int Med* 2007;147:10–18.)

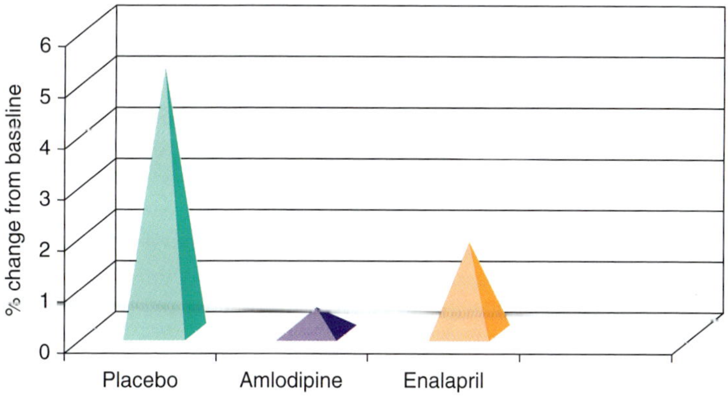

Fig. 7-39 CAMELOT study; effect of randomized placebo, amlodipine and enalapril on atheroma progression over 2 years in hypertensives with CHD. (From Nissen SE, Tuzcu M, Libby P, et al. Effect of antihypertensive agents on cardiovascular events in patients with coronary artery disease and normal blood pressure. The CAMELOT study: a randomized control trial. *JAMA* 2004;292:2217–26.)

C) Plaque stability

In a study of 110 patients who underwent two coronary angiograms over a 6-month period, it was noted that there was a significant

68% reduction in the risk of plaque disruption with a BB (partly linked to bradycardia), compared with a 49% trend with an ACEI (146) (Table 7-6). Modern techniques, such as intravascular optical coherence tomography (OCT), are able to identify plaques that will progress rapidly; these plaques have a high incidence of intimal laceration, large lipid pools with thin caps, and intraluminal thrombi (165, 166).

It is possible that ACEIs and ARBs (though plaque regression data are limited) may stabilize the plaque, possibly via nitric-oxide donation (128) or modifying the underlying inflammatory process (167, 168).

SUMMARY AND CONCLUSIONS

1. In essential hypertension, a major event such as death, myocardial infarction, stroke or heart failure, is invariably preceded by vital end-organ damage; this chapter concentrates on renal dysfunction, LVH, and the atheromataous plaque, as well as on the effect of antihypertensive drug therapy on these conditions.
2. Renal dysfunction is usually assessed by eGFR and albuminuria; a low eGFR denotes not only renal failure but also a poor prognostic sign for premature cardiovascular events and death.
3. There is a prevailing view that ACEIs and ARBs have renoprotective properties beyond blood pressure control, though combining these two classes of drugs can worsen renal function; the apparent advantage of ACEIs and ARBs over other drugs in protecting renal function largely disappears when BP differences are taken into account; renoprotection with ACEIs may wear-off over a 3-year period (in children).
4. In young/middle-aged subjects, nonselective BBs reduce renal blood flow and can diminish renal function; moderately β-1 selective BBs like atenolol and metoprolol have similar renoprotective effects as ACEIs; highly β-1 selective bisoprolol was at least as renoprotective as the ARB losartan over a 1-year period; additional α-blocking properties, for example, carvedilol, may endow a greater renoprotective action.
5. In large trials, for example, ALLHAT, both diuretics (chlorthalidone) and calcium blockers (amlodipine) were not inferior to ACEIs (lisinopril) in terms of renoprotection.
6. LVH can be assessed by either ECG (good specificity but poor sensitivity) or echocardiography; ECG being cheap and accessible and should be the first tool to detect LVH.

7. There is nonpathological and pathological LVH; the former, so-called "Athlete's-Heart," has only modest increases in LV wall and septal thickness, diastolic LV size, and has normal wall stress; pathological LVH relates to relative wall thickness (ratio of LV wall thickness to diastolic diameter) which, when increased, is termed concentric hypertrophy (with high-wall stress), and eccentric hypertrophy when relative wall thickness is not increased (with low-wall stress).
8. Concentric hypertrophy is strongly linked to BP, particularly central, levels (especially in the elderly), and eccentric hypertrophy is linked to volume overload and, importantly, neurohumoral factors; increased SNA can induce LVH in the absence of a raised BP (β-adrenergic receptor kinase-1 (β ARK-1) levels are raised), and high angiotensin II levels are linked to myocardial fibrosis.
9. ECG LVH, particularly with the "strain" pattern, is a strong predictor of future morbid and fatal cardiac ischemic events in men and heart failure in women; echocardiographic concentric hypertrophy has a poor prognosis, particularly for the development of diastolic (normal ejection fraction) heart failure; eccentric hypertrophy is linked particularly to systolic (low ejection fraction) heart failure; in general, echocardiographic LVH is associated with a 2.5–3.5-fold increased risk of a cardiovascular or fatal event.
10. Reversal of LVH is linked to an improved prognosis; diuretics are highly effective at reducing LVM in the elderly, but in younger/middle-aged hypertensives are inferior to BBs in reducing LV wall and septal thickness, and to ACEIs in reducing LVM, wall and septal thickness, and fibrosis.
11. BBs, in the younger/middle-aged hypertensives, reverse ECG LVH and strain; they are superior to diuretics in regressing posterior wall and septal thickness, and are similar to calcium antagonists in reversing LVM; high β-1 selectivity (bisoprolol) is at least as effective as ACEIs in reversing LVM and posterior wall and septal thickness, and in improving CFR; nebivolol (with β-3 ISA) was superior to metoprolol in reducing posterior wall thickness; BBs do not reduce LV wall fibrosis; in the elderly, BBs are relatively ineffective in reversing ECG and echocardiographic LVH, but with additional α-blocking activity (e.g., carvedilol) are effective in reducing LVM.
12. ACEIs are effective in regressing LVH in young/middle-aged hypertensives, and are superior to diuretics and moderately beta-1 selective atenolol but not highly β-1 selective bisoprolol,

in regressing LVH; in the elderly, ACEIs are effective in regressing both ECG and echocardiographic LVH, and are similar to calcium blockers in this respect.

13. ARBs, like ACEIs, reduced the magnitude of the reflected wave (from periphery), and are effective in young/middle-aged in regressing LVM, being superior to atenolol in this respect; in the elderly, ARBs are superior to atenolol in regressing ECG and echocardiographic LVH, but may be less effective than ACEIs; in Japanese hypertensives, ARBs are superior to calcium blockers in regressing LVH.
14. Nondihydropyridine calcium blockers appear to be inferior to BBs, ACEIs, and diuretics in reversing LVH in young/middle-aged subjects, but superior to BBs in the elderly; long acting dihydropyridine calcium blockers (in contrast to short acting, that increase SNA) reverse LVH to a similar extent as BBs and ACEIs in the young/middle aged; in the elderly, dihydropyridine calcium blockers may be inferior to ARBs in regressing LVH.
15. The α-blocker prazosin, in the young/middle-aged, was less effective than BBs, diuretics and ACEIs in regressing LVH, but bunazosin was similar to metoprolol in reversing LVH; in the elderly, α-blockers are superior to BBs in regressing LVH and reducing fibrosis.
16. Renal sympathetic denervation is effective in reversing LVH in resistant hypertensives.
17. Atheromatous plaque is characterized by the deposition of intracellular and extracellular lipids and by the appearance of macrophages and T-lymphocytes in the vessel wall intimal layer; an unstable plaque has a large lipid core with a high level of activated inflammatory cells that infiltrate the fibrous cap, leading to thinning, destabilization and disruption.
18. High heart rates and SNA (β-1 stimulation) are involved in the atherogenic process and in the development of the unstable plaque and its disruption; high angiotensin II activity is linked to the fibrous tissue content of the plaque and plaque instability.
19. Blood flow patterns determine where atheromataous plaque will develop, with low-shear stress and oscillatory patterns being linked to high levels of plaque development; laminar blood flow associated with low heart rates (β-1 blockade) is linked to an absence of atheromataous plaque.
20. A surrogate for the presence of atheromataous plaque is the carotid intima-medial thickness (IMT); in younger/middle-

aged hypertensives β-blockade, calcium blockers, ACEIs, and ARBs reduce the IMT; in the elderly, calcium antagonists, ACEIs, ARBs, and possibly the diuretic indapamide may be effective in reducing the IMT.

21. A more powerful technique in measuring actual atheromataous plaque volume is intravascular ultrasonography; by this methodology, β-1 blockade has been shown to actually regress plaque growth in middle-aged subjects after a 1-year period, in contrast to calcium blockers and ACEIs which only slow progression.
22. Plaque stability and absence of disruption are encouraged by BBs and low heart rates and to a lesser extent by ACEIs.

REFERENCES

1. Pickering GW. *High Blood Pressure*. 2nd ed. London: JA Churchill Ltd; 1968.
2. Ruilope LM, Bakris GL. Renal function and target organ damage in hypertension. *Eur Heart J* 2011;32:1599–604.
3. National Kidney Foundation. K/DOQI clinical practice guidelines for chronic kidney disease: evaluation, classification and stratification: part 5. Evaluation of laboratory measurement for clinical assessment of kidney disease. *Am J Kidney Dis* 2002;39(suppl 2): S1–S266.
4. De Jong P, Curhan GC. Screening, monitoring and treatment of albuminuria: public health perspectives. *J Am Soc Nephrol* 2006;17:2120–6.
5. Grassi G, Seravalle G, Dell'Oro R. Sympathetic activation in obesity. A non-innocent bystander. *Hypertension* 2010;56:338–40.
6. Mitchell GF. Increased aortic stiffness: and unfavourable cardiorenal connection. *Hypertension* 2004;43:151–3.
7. Weiner DE, Rifkin DE. Kidney function and the risk of cardiovascular disease. *BMJ* 2009;339:2–3.
8. Wright JT, Bakris G, Greene T, et al. Effect of blood pressure lowering antihypertensive drug class on progression of hypertensive kidney disease. Results from AASK Trial. *JAMA* 2002;288:2421–31.
9. Kurtz TW. False claims of blood pressure–independent protection by blockade of the renin angiotensin aldosterone system? *Hypertension* 2003;41:193–6.
10. Casas JP, Chua W, Loukogeorgakis S, et al. Effect of inhibitors of the renin-angiotensin system and other anti-hypertensive drugs on renal outcomes: systematic review and meta-analysis. *Lancet* 2005;366:2026–33.
11. Mann JF, Schmieder RE, McQueen M, et al. Renal outcomes with telmisartan, ramipril or both, in people at high vascular risk (the ONTARGET study). *Lancet* 2008;372:547–53.

12. The ESCAPE Trial Group. Strict blood pressure control and progression of renal failure in children. *N Engl J Med* 2009;361:1639–50.
13. Fugeno T, Hasebe N, Kikuche K. Evidence-based usefulness of calcium antagonists and ACEIs and ARBs for the primary and secondary prevention of major cardiovascular and renal events in patients with hypertension. *Clin Calcium* 2005;15:1695–708.
14. Mackinnon M, Leenen FH, Ruzicka M. Does ALLHAT change the management of hypertension in chronic kidney disease? *Curr Hypertens Rep* 2005;7:474–83.
15. Wright JT, Probstfield JL, Cushman WC, et al. ALLHAT findings revisited in the context of subsequent analyses, other trials and meta-analyses. *Arch Intern Med* 2009;169:832–42.
16. Imai E, Chan JC, Ito S, et al. Effects of olmesartan on renal and cardiovascular outcomes in type-2 diabetes with overt nephropathy: a multicentre, randomised placebo controlled study. *Diabetologia* 2011;54:2978–86.
17. Hiller H, Ito S, Izzo JL, et al. Olmesartan for the delay or prevention of microalbuminuria in type 2 diabetes. *N Engl J Med* 2011;364:907–17.
18. Nakamura A, Imaizumi A, Yanagawa Y, et al. Beta-2 adrenoceptor activation attenuates endotoxin–induced acute renal failure. *J Am Soc Nephrol* 2004;15:316–25.
19. Wilkinson R. Beta-blockers and renal function. *Drugs* 1982;23:195–206.
20. Zacharias FJ. Long-term clinical experience with atenolol. Royal Society of Medicine, International Congress and Symposium Series No 19. 1979;19:75–91.
21. UK Prospective Diabetes Study Group. Efficacy of atenolol and captopril in reducing risk of macrovascular and microvascular complications in type-2 diabetes:UKPDS39. *BMJ* 1998;317:713–20.
22. Parinello G, Paterna S, Torres D, et al. One year renal and cardiac effect of bisoprolol versus losartan in recently diagnosed hypertensive patients. *Clin Drug Investig* 2009;29:591–600.
23. Bakris GL, Fonseca V, Katholi RE, et al. Differential effects of beta-blockers on albuminuria in patients with type 2 diabetes. *Hypertension* 2005;46:1309–15.
24. Hart PD, Bakris GL. Should beta-blockers be used to control hypertension in people with chronic kidney disease? *Semin Nephrol* 2007;27:555–64.
25. Lewis EJ, Hunsicker LG, Clarke WR, et al. Renoprotective effect of the angiotensin receptor antagonist irbesartan in patients with nephropathy due to type-2 diabetes. *N. Engl J Med* 2001;345:851–60.
26. Ruggenenti P, Perna A, Loriga G, et al. Blood pressure control for reno-protection in patients with non-diabetic chronic renal disease (REIN-2): multicentre, randomised, controlled trial. *Lancet* 2005;365:939–46.
27. Agodoa LY, Appel L, Bakris GL, et al. Effect of ramipril vs amlodipine on renal outcomes in hypertensive nephrosclerosis. *JAMA* 2001;285:2719–28.

28. Ruggenenti P, Fassi A, Ilieva AP, et al. Preventing microalbuminuria in type-2 diabetes. *N Engl J Med* 2004;351:1941–51.
29. Narumi H, Takano H, Shindo S, et al. Effects of valsartan and amlodipine on cardiorenal protection in Japanese hypertensive patients. *Hypertens Res* 2011;34:62–9.
30. Bidani AK, Griffin KA. Pathophysiology of hypertensive renal damage. Implications for therapy. *Hypertension* 2004;44:595–601.
31. Schrier RW, Estacio RO, Esler M, et al. Effects of aggressive blood pressure control in normotensive type-2 diabetic patients on albuminuria, retinopathy and strokes. *Kidney Int* 2002;61:1086–97.
32. Miall WE, Greenberg G. *Mild Hypertension, is there Pressure to Treat?* Cambridge: Cambridge University Press; 1987, p146–7.
33. Wilhelmsen L, Berglund G, Elmfeldt D, et al. Beta-blockers versus diuretics in hypertensive men: main results from the HAPPHY Trial. *J Hypertens* 1987;5:561–72.
34. SHEP Cooperative Research Group. Prevention of stroke by antihypertensive drug treatment in older persons with isolated systolic hypertension. *JAMA* 1991;265:3255–64.
35. Goldman MJ. *Principles of clinical electrocardiography*. Canada: Lange Medical Publication; 1970, p100.
36. Larsen CT, Dahlin J, Blackburn H et al. Prevalence and prognosis of ECG left ventricular hypertrophy, S-T segment depression and negative T-wave. *Europ Heart J* 2002;23:315–24.
37. de Simone G, Izzo R, Trimarco B. Left ventricular hypertrophy: old marker, new problems and new possibilities. *J Hypertens* 2011;29:480–2.
38. Drazner MH. The progression of hypertensive heart disease. *Circulation* 2011;123:327–34.
39. Lieb W, Xanthakis V, Sullivan LM, et al. Longitudinal tracking of LVM over the adult life course. Framingham offspring Study. *Circulation* 2009;119:3085–92.
40. Morita H, Larson MG, Barr SC, et al. Single-gene mutations and increased left-ventricular wall thickness in the community. The Framingham Heart Study. *Circulation* 2006;113:2697–705.
41. Hill JA, Olson EN. Cardiac plasticity. *New Engl J Med* 2008;358: 1370–80.
42. Dorn II GW. The fuzzy logic of physiological cardiac hypertrophy. *Hypertension* 2007;49:962–70.
43. Douglas PS, O'Toole ML, Katz SE, et al. Left-ventricular hypertrophy in athletes. *Am J Cardiol* 1997;80:1384–8.
44. Pluim BM, Zwinderman AH, van der Laase A, et al. The athletes heart. *Circulation* 1999;100:336–44.
45. Pluim BM, Lamb HJ, Kayser HW, et al. Functional and metabolic evaluation of the athlete's heart by magnetic resonance imaging and dobutamine stress magnetic resonance spectroscopy. *Circulation* 1998;97:666–72.
46. Sugishita Y, Iida K, Ohtsuka S, et al. Ventricular wall stress revisited. A keystone of cardiology. *Jpn Heart J* 1994;35:577–87.

47. Sugishita Y, Iida K, Yukisada K. Mechanical and non-mechanical factors in hypertensive hypertrophy, their clinical roles. *Jpn Circ J* 1990;54:568–74.
48. Sugishita Y, Iida K, Yukisada K, et al. Classification of hypertrophied hearts in essential hypertension: evaluation by LV wall stress and adrenergic response. *Br Heart J* 1988;59:244–52.
49. Calentano A, Palmieri V, Esposito n, et al. Inappropriate left-ventricular mass in normotensive and hypertensive patients. *Am J Cardiol* 2001;87:361–3.
50. Chinali M, De Marco M, D'Addeo G, et al. Excessive increase in left-ventricular mass identifies hypertensive subjects with clustered geometric and functional abnormalities. *J Hypertens* 2007;25:1073–8.
51. Jennings LR, McMullen JR. Left-ventricular hypertrophy: beyond the image and defining human cardiac phenotype in hypertension. *J Hypertens* 2007;25:941–7.
52. Carabello BA. Understanding coronary blood flow. *Circulation* 2006;113:1721–2.
53. Schafer S, Kelm M, Mingers S, et al. Left-ventricular remodeling impairs coronary flow reserve in hypertensive patients. *J Hypertens* 2002;20:1431–7.
54. Conen D, Zeller A, Pfisterer M, et al. Usefulness of B-Type natriuretic peptide and C-reactive protein in predicting the presence or absence of left-ventricular hypertrophy in patients with systemic hypertension. *Am J Cardiol* 2006;97:249–52.
55. Verdecchia P, Schillaci G, Borgioni C, et al. Prevalent influence of systolic over pulse pressure on left-ventricular mass in essential hypertension. *Europ Heart J* 2002;23:658–65.
56. Bliziotis IA, Destounis A, Stergiou GS. Home versus ambulatory and office blood pressure inpredicting target organ damage in hypertension: a systematic review and meta-analysis. *J Hypertens* 2012;30:1289–99.
57. Roman MJ, Okin PM, Kizer JR, et al. Relations of central and brachial blood pressure to left-ventricular hypertrophy and geometry: the Strong Hear Study. *J Hypertens* 2010;28:384–8.
58. Zhang Y, Li Y, Ding F-H, et al. Cardiac structure and function in relation to central blood pressure components in Chinese. *J Hypertens* 2011;29:2462–8.
59. Hashimoto J, Westerhof BE, Westerhof N, et al. Different role of wave reflection magnitude and timing on left-ventricular mass reduction during antihypertensive treatment. *J Hypertens* 2008;26:1017–24.
60. Marcus R, Krause L, Weder AB, et al. Sex-specific determinants of increased left-ventricular mass in the Tecumseh Blood Pressure Study. *Circulation* 1994;90:928–36.
61. Rider OJ, Petersen SE, Francis JM, et al. Ventricular hypertrophy and cavity dilatation in relation to body mass index in women with uncomplicated obesity. *Heart* 2011;97:203–8.

62. Karason K, Sjostrom L, Wallentin I, et al. Impact of blood pressure and insulin on the relationship between body fat and left-ventricular structure. *Eur Heart J* 2003;24:1500–5.
63. Palmieri V, de Simone G, Arnett DK, et al. Relation of various degrees of body mass index in patients with systemic hypertension to left ventricular mass, cardiac output and peripheral resistance. *Am J Cardiol* 2001;88:1163–8.
64. Cabassi A, Dancelli S, Pattoneri P, et al. Characterisation of myocardial hypertrophy in prehypertensive spontaneously hypertensive rats: interaction between adrenergic and nitrosative pathways. *J Hypertens* 2007;25:1719–30.
65. Levick SP, Murray DB, Janicki JS, et al. Sympathetic nervous system modulation of inflammation and remodelling in the hypertensive heart. *Hypertension* 2010;55:270–6.
66. Lambert E, Sari CI, Dawood T, et al. Sympathetic nervous system activity is associated with obesity-induced subclinical organ damage in young adults. *Hypertension* 2010;56:351–8.
67. Burns J, Sivananthan MV, Balls S, et al. Relationship between central sympathetic drive and magnetic resonance imaging-determined left-ventricular mass in essential hypertension. *Circulation* 2007;115:1999–2005.
68. Strand AH, Gudmundsdotir H, Os I, et al. Arterial plasma noradrenaline predicts left-ventricular mass independently of blood pressure and body build in men who develop hypertension over 20 years. *J Hypertens* 2006;24:905–13.
69. Kelm M, Schafer S, Mingers S, et al. Left ventricular mass is linked to cardiac noradrenaline in normotensive and hypertensive patients. *J Hypertens* 1996;14:1357–64.
70. Zoccali C, Mallamici F, Tripepi G, et al. Norepinephrine and concentric hypertrophy in patients with end-stage renal disease. *Hypertension* 2002;40:41–6.
71. Park SJ, Choi DJ, Kim CW. Hypertensive left-ventricular hypertrophy: relation to beta-adrenergic receptor kinase -1 (beta ARK1) in peripheral lymphocytes. *J Hypertens* 2004;22:1025–32.
72. Kurdi M, Booz GW. New take on the role of angiotensin II in cardiac hypertrophy and fibrosis. *Hypertension* 2011;57:1034–8.
73. Veliotes DG, Woodiwiss AJ, Deftereos DA, et al. Aldosterone receptor blockade prevents transition to cardiac pump dysfunction induced by beta-adrenoceptor activation. *Hypertension* 2005;45:914–20.
74. Muiesan ML, Salvetti M, Rizzoni D, et al. Association of change in left ventricular mass with prognosis during long-term antihypertensive treatment. *J Hypertens* 1995;13:1091–5.
75. Verdecchia P, Schillaci G, Borgioni C, et al. Prognostic significance of serial changes of left-ventricular mass in essential hypertension. *Circulation* 1998;97:48–54.

76. Ghali JK, Liao Y, Cooper RS. Influence of left-ventricular geometric patterns in prognosis in patients with and without coronary artery disease. *J Am Coll Cardiol* 1998;31:1635–40.
77. Vakali BA, Okin PM, Devereux RB. Prognostic implications of left-ventricular hypertrophy. *Am Heart J* 2001;141:334–41.
78. Pelliccia A, Maron BJ, De Luca R, et al. Remodeling of left-ventricular hypertrophy in elite athletes after long-term deconditioning. *Circulation* 2002;105:944–9.
79. McCann GP, Muir DF, Hillis WS. Athletic left-ventricular hypertrophy: long-term studies are required. *Eur Heart J* 2000;21:351–3.
80. Otterstad JE, Davies M, Ball SG, et al. Left-ventricular hypertrophy and myocardial ischaemia in hypertension. The Thames Study. *Eur Heart J* 1993;14:1622–8.
81. Pringle SD, Dunn FG, Tweddle AC, et al. Symptomatic and silent myocardial ischaemia in hypertensive patients with left-ventricular hypertrophy. *Br Heart J* 1992;67:377–82.
82. Okin PM, Devereux RB, Jern S, et al. Regression of electrocardiographic left-ventricular hypertrophy during antihypertensive treatment and the prediction of major cardiovascular events. *JAMA* 2004;292:2343–9.
83. Brown DW, Giles WH, Croft JB. Left-ventricular as a predictor of coronary heart disease mortality and the effects of hypertension. *Am Heart J* 2000;140:848–56.
84. Desai CS, Ning H, Lloyd-Jones DM. Competing cardiovascular outcomes associated with electrocardiographic left ventricular hypertrophy. *Heart* 2012;98:330–4.
85. Wachtell K, Okin PM, Olsen MH, et al. Regression of electrocardiographic left-ventricular hypertrophy during antihypertensive therapy and reduction of sudden death. The LIFE Study. *Circulation* 2007;116:700–5.
86. Cruickshank JM, Messerli FH. *Left-Ventricular Hypertrophy and its Regression*. London: Science Press; 1992, p71–81.
87. Ofili EO, Cohen JD, St Vrain JA, et al. Effect of treatment of isolated systolic hypertension on left-ventricular mass. *JAMA* 1998;279: 778–80.
88. Gottdiener JS, Reda DJ, Massie BM, et al. Effect of single-drug therapy on reduction of left-ventricular mass in mild to moderate hypertension. *Circulation* 1997;95:2007–14.
89. Otterstad JE, Foeland G, Soeyland AK, et al. Change in left-ventricular dimensions and systolic function in 100 mildly hypertensive men during one year's treatment with atenolol vs hydrochlorthiazide and amiloride (moduretic): a double-blind, randomised study. *J Int Med* 1992;231: 493–501.
90. Dahlof B, Hansson L. Regression of left-ventricular hypertrophy in previously untreated essential hypertension: different effects of enalapril and hydrochorthiazide. *J Hypertens* 1992;10:1513–24.

91. Brilla CG, Funck RC, Rupp H. Lisinopril-mediated regression of myocardial fibrosis in patients with hypertensive heart disease. *Circulation* 2000;102:1388–93.
92. Papademetriou V, Gottdiener JS, Narayan P, et al. Hydrochlorthiazide is superior to isradipine for reduction of left-ventricular mass. *J Am Coll Cardiol* 1997;30:1802–8.
93. Ernst ME, Neaton JD, Grimm RH, et al. Long-term effects of chlorthalidone versus hydrochlorothiazide on electrocardiographic left-ventricular hypertrophy in multiple Risk Factor Intervention Trial. *Hypertension* 2011;58:1001–7.
94. Klingbeil AU, Schneider M, Martus P, et al. A meta-analysis of the effects of treatment on left-ventricular mass in essential hypertension. *Am J Med* 2003;115:41–6.
95. Fagard RH, Celis H, Thijs L, et al. Regression of left-ventricular mass by antihypertensive treatment. A meta-analysis of randomised comparative trials. *Hypertension* 2009;54:1084–91.
96. Cruickshank JM, Higgins TJ, Pennert K, et al. The efficacy and tolerability of antihypertensive treatment based on atenolol in the prevention of stroke and the regression of left-ventricular hypertrophy. *J Hum Hypertens* 1987;1:87–93.
97. Schneider MP, Klingbeil AU, Delles C, et al. Effect of irbesartan versus atenolol on left-ventricular mass and voltage. *Hypertension* 2004;44:61–6.
98. Agabiti-Rosei E, Trimarco B, Muiessan ML, et al. Cardiac structural and functional changes during long-term antihypertensive treatment with lacidipine and atenolol in the European Lacidipine Study on Atherosclerosis (ELSA). *J Hypertens* 2005;23:1091–8.
99. Agabiti-Rosei E, Ambrosioni E, Dal Palu C, et al. ACE inhibitor ramipril is more effective than beta-blocker atenolol in reducing left-ventricular mass in hypertension. *J Hypertens* 1995;13: 1325–34.
100. Buus NH, Bottcher M, Jorgensen CG, et al. Myocardial perfusion during long-term angiotensin-converting enzyme inhibition or beta-blockade in patients with essential hypertension. *Hypertension* 2004;44:465–70.
101. Cuilla MM, Paliotti R, Esposito A, et al. Different effects of antihypertensive therapies based on losartan or atenolol on ultra sound and biochemical markers of myocardial fibrosis. *Circulation* 2004;110:552–7.
102. Kampus P, Serg M, Kals J, et al. Differential effects of nebivolol and metoprolol on central aortic pressure and left-ventricular wall thickness. *Hypertension* 2011;57:1122–8.
103. Gosse P, Routaut R, Herreo G, et al. Beta-blockers vs ACE-inhibition in hypertension: effects on left-ventricular hypertrophy. *J Cardiovasc Pharmacol* 1990;16:S145–50.
104. Motz W, Vogt M, Scheler S, et al. Improvement of coronary flow reserve following regression of hypertrophy resulting from

blood pressure lowering with a beta-blocker. *Dtsch Med Wochen* 1993;118:535–40.

105. Okin PM, Devereux RB, Jern S, et al. Regression of electrocardiographic left-ventricular hypertrophy by losartan versus atenolol. *Circulation* 2003;108:684–90.
106. Devereux RB, Dahlof B, Gerdts E, et al. Regression of hypertensive left-ventricular hypertrophy by losartan compared to atenolol. LIFE Trial. *Circulation* 2004;110:1456–62.
107. Schulman SP, Weiss JL, Becker LC, et al. The effects of antihypertensive therapy on left-ventricular mass in elderly patients. *N Engl J Med* 1990;322:1350–6.
108. Xiaozhen H, Yun Z, Mei Z, et al. Effect of carvedilol on coronary flow reserve in patients with hypertensive left-ventricular hypertrophy. *Blood Pressure* 2010;19:40–7.
109. Matthew J, Sleight P, Lonn E, et al. Reduction of cardiovascular risk by regression of electrocardiographic markers of left-ventricular hypertrophy by the antiotensin-converting enzyme inhibitor ramipril. *Circulation* 2001;104:1615–21.
110. Terpstra WF, May JF, Swit AJ, et al. Long-term effects of amlodipine and lisinopril on left-ventricular mass and diastolic function in elderly, previously untreated hypertensive patients: the ELVERA trial. *J Hypertens* 2001;19:303–9.
111. Skov K, Eiskjaer H, Hansen HE, et al. Treatment of young subjects at high familial risk of future hypertension with an angiotensin receptor blocker. *Hypertension* 2007;50:89–95.
112. Malmqvist K, Kahan T, Edner M, et al. Comparison of actions of irbesatran versus atenolol on cardiac repolarisation in hypertensive left-ventricular hypertrophy. *Am J Cardiol* 2002;90:1107.
113. Solomon SD, Appelbaum E, Manning WJ, et al. Effect of the direct renin inhibitor aliskiren, the angiotensin receptor blocker losartan, or both on left-ventricular mass in patients with hypertension and left-ventricular hypertrophy. *Circulation* 2009;119:530–7.
114. Verdecchia P, Sleight P, Mancia G, et al. Effects of telmisartan, ramipril and their combination on left ventricular hypertrophy in individuals at high risk. *Circulation* 2009;120:1380–9.
115. Diamond JA, Gharavi A, Roychoudhury D, et al. Effect of long-term eprosartan versus enalapril antihypertensive therapy on left-ventricular mass and coronary flow reserve in stage I-II hypertension. *Curr Med Res Opin* 1999;15:1–8.
116. Okin PM, Gerdts E, Kjeldsen SE, et al. Gender differences in regression of electrocardiographic left-ventricular hypertrophy during antihypertensive therapy. *Hypertension* 2008;52:100–6.
117. Devereux RB, Palmieri V, Sharpe N, et al. Effects of once daily angiotensin-converting enzyme inhibition and calcium channel blockade-based antihypertensive treatment regimens on left-ventricular hypertrophy and diastolic filling in hypertension. *Circulation* 2001;104:1248.

118. Leenen FH, Meyers MG, Joyner CD, et al. Differential effects of once daily antihypertensive drugs on blood pressure, left-ventricular mass and sympathetic activity: nifedepine GITS versus felodipine-ER versus enalapril. *Can J Cardiol* 2002;18:1285–93.
119. Palatini P, Grassi G. The morning blood pressure surge: a dynamic and challenging concept. *J Hypertens* 2011;29:2316–9.
120. Schobel HP, Langenfeld M, Gatzka C, et al. Treatment and post-treatment effects of alpha-versus beta-receptor blockers on left-ventricular structure and function in essential hypertension. *Am Heart J* 1996;132:1004–9.
121. Barrios V, Escobar C, Tomas JP, et al. Comparison of the effects of doxazosin and atenolol on target organ damage in adults with type-2 diabetes mellitus and hypertension in the CARDHIAC study. *Clin Ther* 2008;30:98–107.
122. Perlini S, Palladini G, Ferrero I, et al. Sympathectomy or doxazosin, but not propranolol, blunt myocardial interstitial fibrosis in pressure-overload hypertrophy. *Hypertension* 2005;46:1213–8.
123. Brandt MC, Mahfoud F, Reda S, et al. Renal sympathetic denervation reduces left ventricular hypertrophy and inproves cardiac function in patients with resistant hypertension. *J Am Coll Cardiol* 2012;59:901–9.
124. Lurbe E. Hypertension and target organ damage in children and adolescents. *J Hypertens* 2007;25:1998–2000.
125. Toprak A, Wang H, Chen W, et al. Relation of childhood risk factors to left-ventricular hypertrophy (eccentric or concentric) in relatively young adulthood (from the Bogalusa Heart Study). *Am J Cardiol* 2008;101:1621–5.
126. Toprak A, Reddy J, Chen W, et al. Relation of pulse pressure and arterial stiffness to concentric left-ventricular hypertrophy in young men (from the Bogalusa Heart Study). *Am J Cardiol* 2009;103:978–84.
127. Wang J, Chen W, Ruan L, et al. Differential effect of elevated blood pressure on left-ventricular geometry types in Black and White young adults in a community (from the Bogalusa heart Study). *Am J Cardiol* 2011;107:717–22.
128. Herman AG, Moncada S. Therapeutic potential of nitric oxide donors in the prevention and treatment of atherosclerosis. *Europ Heart J* 2005;26:1945–55.
129. Hauss WH, Bauch HJ, Schulte H. Adrenaline and noradrenaline as possible chemical mediators in the pathogenesis of arteriosclerosis. *Am NY Acad Sci* 1990;598:91–101.
130. Born GY. Recent evidence for the involvement of catecholamines and of macrophages in atherosclerotic processes. *Ann Med* 1991;23:569–72.
131. Skantze HB, Kaplan J, Pettersson K, et al. Psychosocial stress causes endothelial injury in cynomolgus monkeys via beta-1 adrenoceptor activation. *Atherosclerosis* 1998;136:153–61.

132. Manuck SB, Kaplan JR, Adams MR, et al. Effects of stress and the sympathetic nervous system on coronary artery atherosclerosis in the cynomolgus macaque. *Am Heart J* 1988;116:328–33.
133. Beere PA, Glagov S, Zarins CK. Experimental atherosclerosis at the carotid bifurcation on the cynomolgus monkey. Localisation, compensatory enlargement, and the sparing affect of lowered heart rate. *Atheroscler thromb* 1992;12:1245–53.
134. Speidl WS, Toller WG, Kaun C, et al. Catecholamines potentiate LPS-induced expression of MMP-1 and MMP-9 in human monocytes and in the human monocytic cell-line U937. *FASEB J* 2004;18:603–5.
135. Schieffer B, Schieffer E, Hilfiker-Kleiner D, et al. Expression of angiotensin II and interleukin-6 in human coronary atherosclerotic plaques. *Circulation* 2000;101:1372–8.
136. Tedgui A, Mallat Z. *Hypertension*: a novel regulator of adaptive immunity in atherosclerosis? Hypertension 2004;44:257–8.
137. Cheng C, Temple D, van Haperen R, et al. Athersclerotic lesion size and vulnerability are determined by patterns of fluid shear stress. *Circulation* 2006;113:2744–53.
138. Chatzizisis YS, Jonas M, Coskun AV, et al. Prediction of the localisation of high-risk coronary atherosclerotic plaques on the basis of low endothelial shear stress. *Circulation* 2008;117:993–1002.
139. Chatizizisis YS, Baker AB, Sukhova GK, et al. Augmented expression and activity of extracellular matrix-degrading enzymes in regions of low endothelial shear stress colocalize with coronary atheromata with thin fibrous caps in pigs. *Circulation* 2011;123:621–30.
140. Stone PH, Coskun AU, Kinlay S, et al. Effect of shear stress on the progression of coronary artery disease, vascular remodelling and in-stent restonosis in humans. *Circulation* 2003;108:348–44.
141. Samady H, Eshtehardi P, McDaniel MC, et al. Coronary artery wall shear stress is associated with progression and transformation of atheroschlerotic plaque and arterial remodelling in patients with coronary artery disease. *Circulation* 2011;124:779–88.
142. Dimmeler S, Zeiher AM. Exercise and cardiovascular health: get active to "AKTivate" your endothelial nitric oxide synthase. *Circulation* 2003;107:3152–8.
143. Spence JD. Effects of hydralazine versus propranolol on blood velocity patterns in patients with carotid stenosis. *Clin Sci* 1983;65:91–3.
144. Spence JD, Perkins DG, Kline RL, et al. Hemodynamic modification of atherosclerosis. Effects of propranolol vs hydralazine in hypertensive, hyperlipidemic rabbits. *Athersclerosis* 1984;50:325–33.
145. Spence JD. Effects of antihypertensive drugs on flow disturbance: nifedepine, captopril and metoprolol evaluated by quantitative spectral analysis of Doppler flow patterns in patients with carotid stenosis. *Clin Invest Med* 1994;17:319–25.

146. Heidland UE, Strauer BE. Left ventricular muscle mass and elevated heart rate are associated with coronary plaque disruption. *Circulation* 2001;104:1477–82.
147. Polak JF, Pencina MJ, Pencina KM, et al. Carotid-wall intima-thickness and cardiovascular events. *N Engl J Med* 2011;365:213–21.
148. Wiklund O, Hulthe J, Wikstrand J, et al. Effect of controlled release/extended release metoprolol on carotid intima-medial thickness in patients with hypercholesterolemia. *Stroke* 2002;33:572–7.
149. Lorenz MW, Polak JF, Kavousi M, et al. Carotid intima-media thickness progression to predict cardiovacsular events in the general population (the PROG-IMT collaborative project): a meta-analysis of individual participant data. *Lancet* 2012;379:2053–62.
150. Nambi V, Pedroza C, Kao LS. Carotid intima-media thickness and cardiovascular events. *Lancet* 2012;379:2028–30.
151. Zanchetti A, Bond G, Hennig M, et al. Calcium antagonist lacidipine slows down progression of asymptomatic carotid atherosclerosis (ELSA). *Circulation* 2002;106:2422–7.
152. Boutouyrie P, Bussy C, Tropeano AI, et al. Local pulse pressure and regression of arterial wall hypertrophy during antihypertensive treatment. CELIMENE study. The celiprolol intima-media enalapril study. *Arch Mal Coer Vaiss* 2000;93:911–15.
153. Stumpe KO, Agabiti-Rosei E, Zielinski T, et al. Carotid-intima thickness and plaque volume changes following 2-year angiotensin II-receptor blockade. *Therapeutic Adv Cardiov Dis* 2007;1:97–106.
154. Napoli C, Briezzese G, Ignarro LJ, et al. Long-term treatment with sulfhydryl angiotensin-converting enzyme inhibition reduces carotid intima-media thickening and improves the nitric oxide/oxidative stress pathways in newly diagnosed patients with mild to moderate primary hypertension. *Am Heart J* 2008;156:1154.
155. Terpstra WF, May JF, Smit AJ, et al. Effects of amlodipine and lisinopril on intima-media thickness in previously untreated, elderly hypertensive patients. *J Hypertens* 2004;22:1309–16.
156. Uchiyama-Tanaka Y, Mori Y, Kishimoto N, et al. Comparison of the effects of quinapril and losartan on carotid intima-media thickness in patients with mild-moderate hypertension. *Kidney Blood Press Res* 2005;28:111–6.
157. Sonada M, Asyagi T, Takanaka K, et al. A one-year study of the antisclerotic effects of the angiotensin-II receptor blocker losartan in hypertensive patients. A comparison with angiotensin-converting enzyme inhibitors. *Int Heart J* 2008;49:95–103.
158. Lebrillant E, Roulet MJ, Robert R, et al. Study of antiatherogenic properties of indapamide in a pharmacological model. *J Cardivasc Pharmacol* 1993;22(6):S53–6.
159. Fonseca FA, Ihara SS, Izar MC, et al. Hydrochorthiazide abolishes the anti-atherosclerotic effect of quinapril. *Clin Exp Pharmacol Physiol* 2003;30:779–85.

160. Cuspidi C, Negri F, Guidici Y, et al. Effects of antihypertensive drugs on carotid intima-media thickness: focus on angiotensin II receptor blockers. A review of randomised, controlled trials. *Integr Blood Press Control* 2009;2:1–8.
161. Sipahi I, Tuzcu M, Wolski KE, et al. Beta-blockers and progression of coronary atherosclerosis: pooled analysis of 4 intravascular ultrasonography trials. *Am Int Med* 2007;147:10–18.
162. Nissen SE, Tuzcu M, Libby P, et al. Effect of antihypertensive agents on cardiovascular events in patients with coronary artery disease and normal blood pressure. The CAMELOT study: a randomised control trial. *JAMA* 2004;292:2217–26.
163. Rodriguez–Granillo G, de Winter S, Bruining N, et al. Effect of perindopril on coronary remodelling: insights from a multicentre, randomised study. *Eur Heart J* 2007;28:2326–31.
164. Strawn WB, Chappell MC, Dean RH, et al. Inhibition of early atherogenesis by losartan in monkeys with diet-induced hypercholesterolemia. *Circulation* 2000;101:1586–93.
165. Uemura S, Ishigami K, Soeda T, et al. Thin-cap fibroatheroma and murochannel findings in optical coherence tomography correlates with subsequent progression of coronary atheromataous plaques. *Eur Heart J* 2012;33:78–85.
166. Radu MD, Falk E. In search of vulnerable features of coronary plaques with optical coherence tomography. *Eur Heart J* 2012;33:9–12.
167. Schoenhagen P, Sipahi I. Arterial remodelling: an independent pathophysiological component of atherosclerotic disease progression and regression. Insight from serial pharmacological intervention trials. *Eur Heart J* 2007;28:2299–300.
168. Benndorf RA, Boger RH. Pleiotropic effects of telmisartan: still more to come? *J Hypertens* 2008;26:854–6.

Hard Endpoint Studies

CHAPTER 8

GENERAL ASPECTS

1. Relationship between treated hypertension and cardiovascular events

An early overview of 17 randomized trials indicated that a 5 6 mm Hg reduction in diastolic blood pressure (DBP) reduced stroke risk by 38% and coronary heart disease (CHD) risk by 16% (1). A follow-up of that overview (2), now including 29 randomized trials, concluded that all drug groups were equivalent in reducing major cardiovascular (CV) events and that larger reductions of blood pressure (BP) lead to larger reductions of risk (**Figure 8-1**), whatever the age group (3) or sex (4).

In hypertensive patients with diabetes, a meta-analysis of 31 intervention trials (5) showed that a decrease in systolic blood pressure (SBP) and DBP correlated with reduction in the risk of stroke but not myocardial infarction (**Figures 8-2** and **8-3**) (5).

Even in high-risk, middle-aged patients without hypertension, a meta-analysis of 25 high-quality trials showed that antihypertensive therapy resulted in significant reductions in stroke (22%), myocardial infarction (20%), heart failure (29%), and all-cause death (13%)

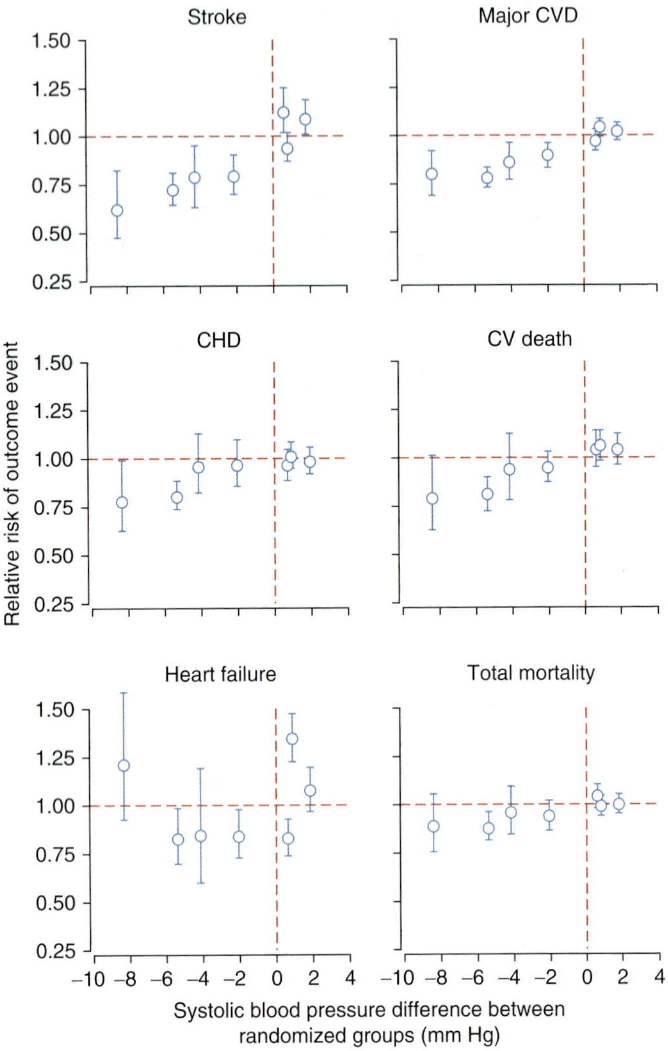

Fig. 8-1 Effects of decrease in treated SBP on major vascular outcomes and death. (From Blood Pressure Lowering Treatment Trialists' Collaboration. Effect of different regimens to lower blood pressure on major cardiovascular events in older and hunger people. *BMJ* 2008;336:1121–3.)

(6). Thus, there is a possible case for treating high-risk patients, for example, patients with diabetes with prehypertension (7).

Some (8) go even further and recommend that BP should be lowered in everyone over a certain age, rather than measuring it in everyone and treating it in some!

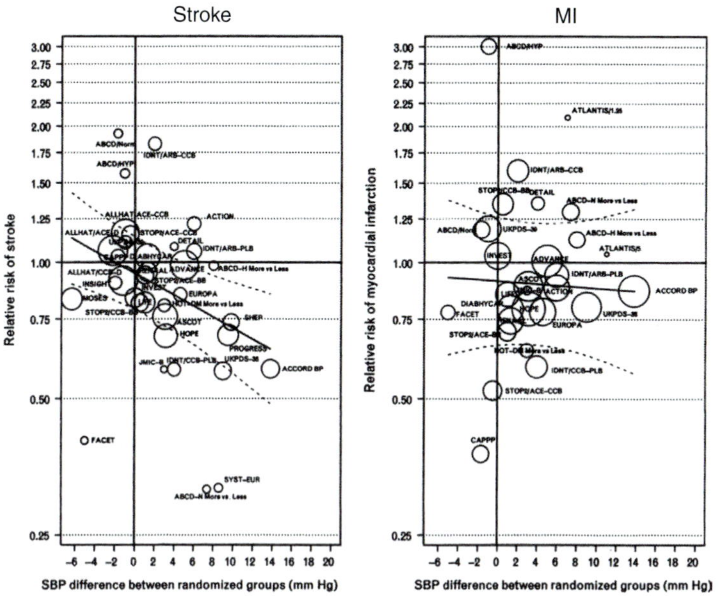

Fig. 8-2 Effects of lowering SBP upon stroke and MI (myocardial infarction) in 73,913 patients with diabetes; strong relationship with stroke but not MI. (From Reboldi G, Gentile G, Angeli F, et al. Effects of intensive blood pressure reduction on myocardial infarction and stroke in diabetes. *J Hypertens* 2011;29:1253–69.)

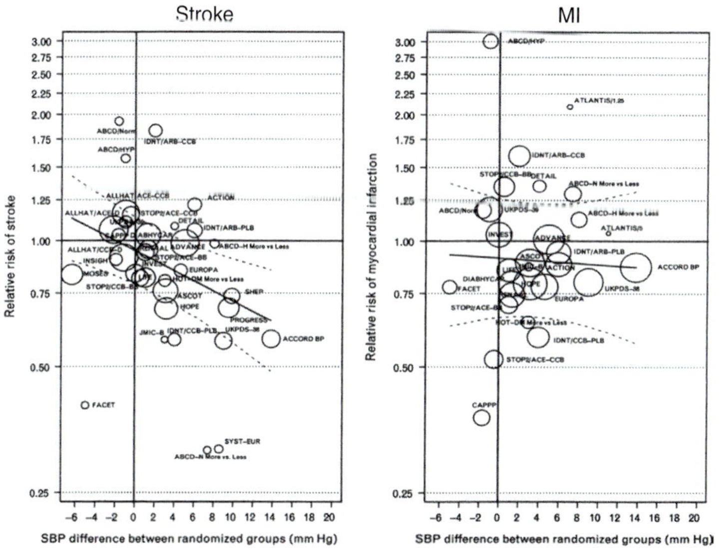

Fig. 8-3 Effects of lowering DBP upon stroke and MI in 73,913 diabetics; strong relationship with stroke but not MI. (From Reboldi G, Gentile G, Angeli F, et al. Effects of intensive blood pressure reduction on myocardial infarction and stroke in diabetes. *J Hypertens* 2011;29:1253–69.)

2. How far to lower blood pressure?

Although European Guidelines recommend to lower SBP to less than 140 mm Hg, there is scant evidence to support this recommendation (9).

In the Systolic Hypertension in the Elderly Program (SHEP) study (10), involving elderly patients with isolated systolic hypertension, within the active treatment group (vs. placebo) only, a 5 mm Hg decrease in DBP resulted in a significant 14% increase in stroke risk and an 8% increase in coronary heart disease risk, but reassuringly treated patients did not perform worse than patients receiving placebo in terms of cardiovascular disease (CVD) events.

In elderly Japanese patients with isolated systolic hypertension, there was no significant reduction in a composite of CV events in those randomized to strict BP control (achieved BP = 142/77 mm Hg) (11). In contrast, a randomized study of 9711 Chinese middle-aged/elderly patients showed that tighter control of SBP (138 mm Hg), versus less tight (142 mm Hg), resulted in a significant reduction in the primary endpoint of stroke, all CV events, and all deaths (12).

In high-risk patients (n=25,620) with mild hypertension and diabetes or vascular disease, the ONTARGET study showed that over 5 years, reducing the BP from a baseline of 142/80 mm Hg by 6.4/4.3 mm Hg on angiotensin-converting-enzyme inhibitor (ACEI) or angiotensin receptor blocker (ARB), and 9.5/6.3 mm Hg on the combination of ACEI/ARB, resulted in a primary composite outcome that was the same in all 3 groups, but a higher adverse reaction count in the combination group (13). The results of the Action to Control Cardiovascular Risk in Diabetes (ACCORD) Study Group in elderly patients with type 2 diabetes agreed with these results (14). Patients were randomized to achieve a SBP of less than 140 or less than 120 mm Hg. Achieved SBPs were 133.5 and 119.3 mm Hg, and after a mean follow-up of 4.7 years, there was no difference in primary composite outcome of fatal and nonfatal major CV outcomes, although nonfatal stroke was significantly reduced in the lower SBP group (**Figure 8-4**).

Thus, guideline's advice to reduce SBP to less than 130 mm Hg is not supported, to date, by the data.

3. What about the J-curve phenomenon?

A) Diastolic BP—Retrospective data

In 1978, a re-analysis of the Framingham database revealed that during an 18-year period of observation, a DBP of below about 90 mm Hg was associated with an increased risk of a CV event (15).

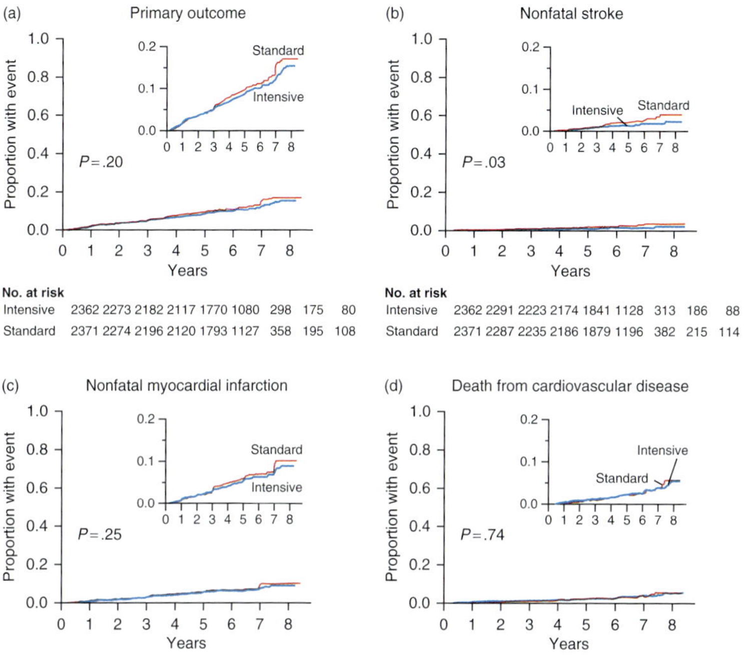

Fig. 8-4 ACCORD study: in 4733 high-risk patients with type 2 diabetes randomized to targeted SBP < 140 versus. 120 mm Hg, there was no reduction in fatal and nonfatal major CV events in the lower SBP group (SBP = 119.3 mm Hg) vs. the higher SBP group (133.5 mm Hg). (From The ACCORD Study Group. Effects of intensive blood-pressure control in type 2 diabetes mellitus. *N Engl J Med* 2010;362:1575–85.)

This observation was soon confirmed, but the increased risk was confined to myocardial infarction (16). This J-curve phenomenon was shown, by Cruickshank, to be confined to hypertensives with myocardial ischemia, and the J-point was about 85 mm Hg DBP (**Figure 8-5**); there was no J-curve for stroke (17). The Framingham Group confirmed that the J-curve for DBP and myocardial infarction was confined to those with coronary artery disease (18). Several other studies confirmed these observations (19), and were explained based on dramatically diminished (or absent) coronary flow reserve in the presence of severe narrowing of the coronary arteries, particularly in the presence of LVH or high heart rates (20) (**Figure 8-6**). In the very elderly subjects (mean age 85 years) with CVD, there was a diastolic J-point of about 70 mm Hg, below which there was an increase in CV and overall mortality (21).

It should be noted that, unlike the brain, in the coronary circulation, oxygen extraction is maximal at rest, so that lowering DBP below the level of autoregulation can lead to myocardial ischemia (22).

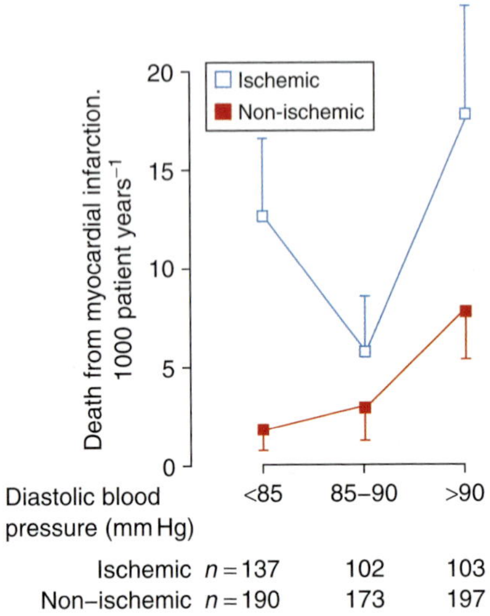

Fig. 8-5 In 902 moderate/severe hypertensives treated for 6 years, in those with CAD, there was a J-curve relationship between DBP and death from MI, with a J-point at 84 mm Hg. (From Cruickshank JM, Thorp JM, Zacharias FJ. Benefits and potential harm of lowering high blood pressure. *Lancet* 1987;1:581–4.)

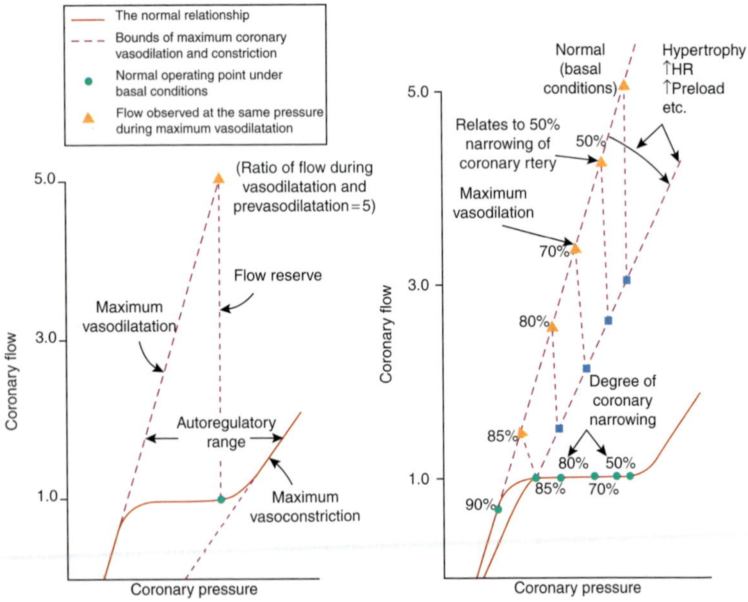

Fig. 8-6 Relationship between coronary pressure and flow; coronary flow reserve is about 5, but approaches 0 with atheromatous narrowing of 85%–90%. (From Klocke FJ. Measurements of coronary flow reserve: defining pathophysiology versus making decisions about patient care. *Circulation* 1987;76:1183–9.)

B) Diastolic BP—prospective data (HOT Study)

All the above studies were retrospective and were thus vulnerable to "reverse causality," that is, is the J-curve due to established disease leading to low DBP and increased risk? Thus, a prospective study was required, and that study was the HOT study (23).

The HOT study was performed in 18,790 hypertensives (mean age 61.5 years), and the conclusion was that intensive lowering of BP with felodipine was not harmful. However, no details were given on the 3080 hypertensives with ischemic heart disease. Fortunately, these data eventually came to light (**Figure 8-7** and **Tables 8-1** and **8-2**) (24). The relationship between myocardial infarction and target DBP was J-shaped for the ischemic group, but not for the nonischemic group. Aiming to lower DBP to less than 80 mm Hg, compared with less than 85 mm Hg, was associated with a 22% increase in the risk of a myocardial infarction. In contrast, there was no J-curve relationship between stroke and DBP in the ischemic group.

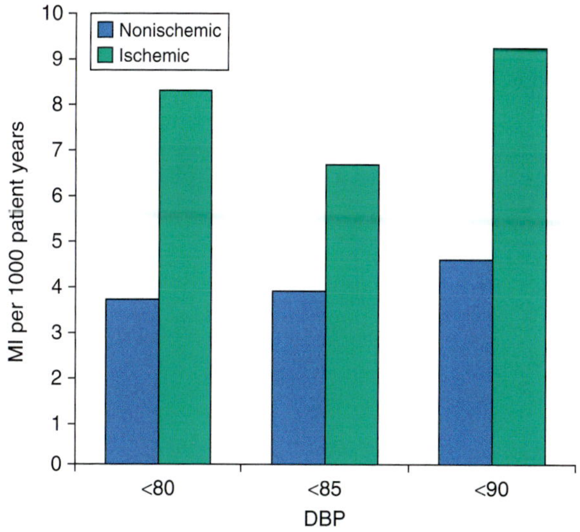

Fig. 8-7 HOT study; in this prospective J-curve study in 18,790 hypertensives, 3080 hypertensives with CAD displayed a J-curve relationship between DBP and total MI, with a J-point at about 83 mm Hg. (From Cruickshank JM. Antihypertensive treatment and the J-curve. *Cardiovascular Drugs Ther* 2000;14:373–9.)

TABLE 8-1 HOT study; note in patients with IHD, there is a J-curved relationship between treated DBP and MI

Group	Target DBP (mm Hg)	*n*	Base SBP/DBP (mm Hg)	Achieved SBP/DBP (mm Hg)	All MI + silent MI		
					Events/1000 patient-years	Comparison	RR
Non-IHD	≤90	5245	169/105	143/85	4.7	90 vs. 85	1.13
	≤85	5228	169/105	141/83	4.1	85 vs. 80	1.07
	≤80	5237	169/105	139/81	3.9	90 vs. 80	1.21
With IHD	≤90	1019	174/106	146/85	9.3	90 vs. 85	1.37
	≤85	1036	173/106	144/83	6.8	85 vs. 80	0.82
	≤80	1025	173/106	143/81	8.3	90 vs. 80	1.12

Abbreviations: DBP, diastolic blood pressure; IHD, ischemic heart disease; MI, myocardial infarction; SBP, systolic.
From Cruickshank JM. Antihypertensive treatment and the J-curve. *Cardiovascular Drugs Ther* 2000;14:373–9.

TABLE 8-2 HOT study; note in patients with IHD, there is no J-curve relationship between DBP and stroke

					All MI + silent MI		
Group	Target DBP (mm Hg)	*n*	Base SBP/DBP (mm Hg)	Achieved SBP/DBP (mm Hg)	Events/1000 patient-years	Comparison	RR
Non-IHD	≤90	5245	169/105	143/85	3	90 vs. 85	0.73
	≤85	5228	169/105	141/83	4.1	85 vs. 80	1.17
	≤80	5237	169/105	139/81	3.5	90 vs. 80	0.85
With IHD	≤90	1019	174/106	146/85	9.3	90 vs. 85	1.18
	≤85	1036	173/106	144/83	7.9	85 vs. 80	1.48
	≤80	1025	173/106	143/81	5.3	90 vs. 80	1.75

DBP—diastolic blood pressure; IHD, ischemic heart disease; MI, myocardial infarction; SBP, systolic blood pressure; RR, relative risk.
**P* value for trend = .046
From Cruickshank JM. Antihypertensive treatment and the J-curve. *Cardiovascular Drugs Ther* 2000;14:373–9.

C) Systolic BP—retrospective data

The International Verapamil-Trandolopril Study (INVEST), in elderly patients with systolic hypertension and coronary artery disease, showed that, unlike with DBP, there was no J-curve phenomenon for SBP and primary outcome (all-cause death and myocardial infarction) in older patients with hypertension and coronary artery disease (**Figure 8-8**) (25). Also, there was no increase in stroke risk at low BPs in this study (25). The group of patients with an increased risk of stroke at lower BPs are those with bilateral severe (>70%) carotid stenosis (26).

In a 5-year follow-up of hypertensive patients with coronary artery disease (Treating to new Targets trial) (27), a J-curve relationship between coronary events (but not stroke) for both SBP and DBP was noted, with an optimal BP of 146/81.4 mm Hg.

In older, high-risk patients with type 2 diabetes (ONTARGET) (28), there was a J-curve relationship (nadir about 130 mm Hg) between SBP and all outcomes except stroke (**Figure 8-9**). Similarly, in the INVEST study (29), in patients with both coronary heart disease and type 2 diabetes, there was an increased risk of all-cause mortality at lower treated SBPs (**Figure 8-10**). In a 5-year follow-up of 5788 middle-aged patients with vascular disease, BP less than 143/82 mm Hg was associated with an increase in vascular events (30).

A recent re-analysis of the LIFE study (31), involving a 4.6-year follow-up of 9193 high-risk (ECG-LVH), older (mean age 66 years) hypertensives, produced some remarkable results. A multivariate Cox analysis revealed that an in-treatment SBP of 131–140 mm Hg was associated with significant reduction in the risk of stroke and myocardial infarction. However, an achieved SBP of less than or equal to 130 mm Hg had no significant impact on stroke, myocardial infarction, and composite endpoint, but was associated with a nonsignificant 32% increase in CV mortality and a significant 37% increase in all-cause death (**Figure 8-10a**)., To rule out early deaths due to underlying illness, an analysis of all-cause deaths after 2 years of follow-up was carried out, using 5 mm Hg SBP cutoff increments (**Figure 8-10b**). It is apparent that a lower SBP, up to a cutoff point of 135 mm Hg or less, remained associated with a significant increased all-cause mortality risk, and it was not until a SBP of at least 155 mm Hg was used as a cutoff point that lower SBP became associated with a lower mortality risk (Figure 8-10b).

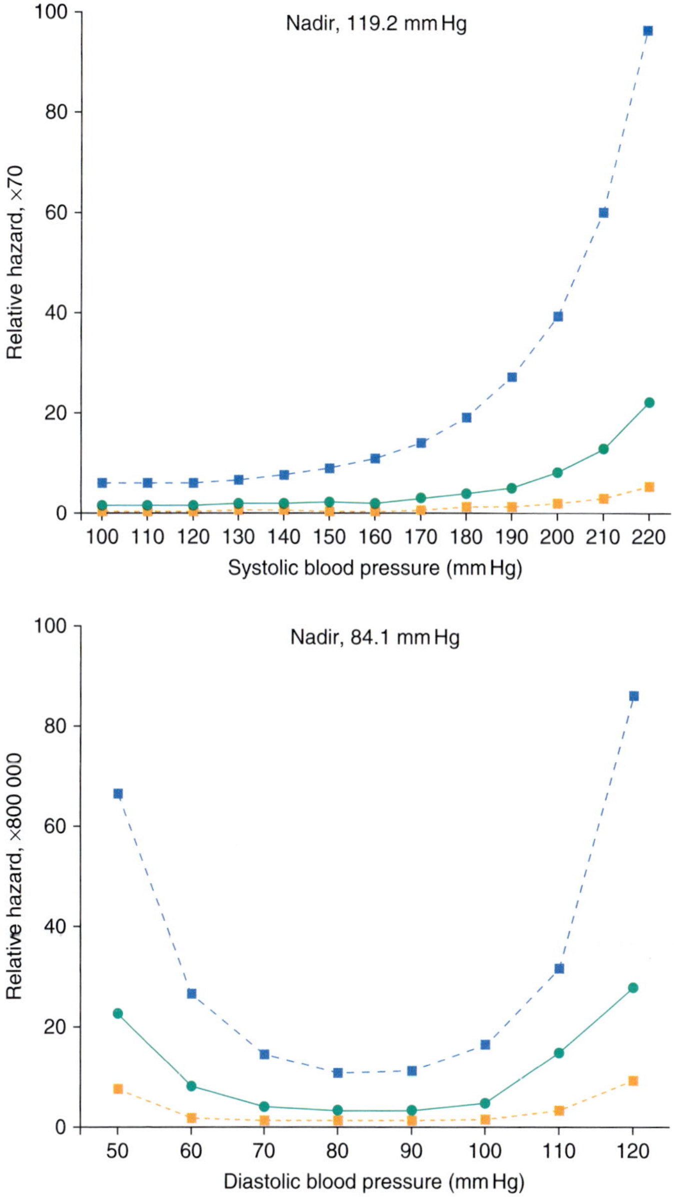

Fig. 8-8 INVEST study: in 22,576 elderly hypertensives with CAD, unlike DBP, there is no J-curve relationship between SBP and all-cause death and MI.

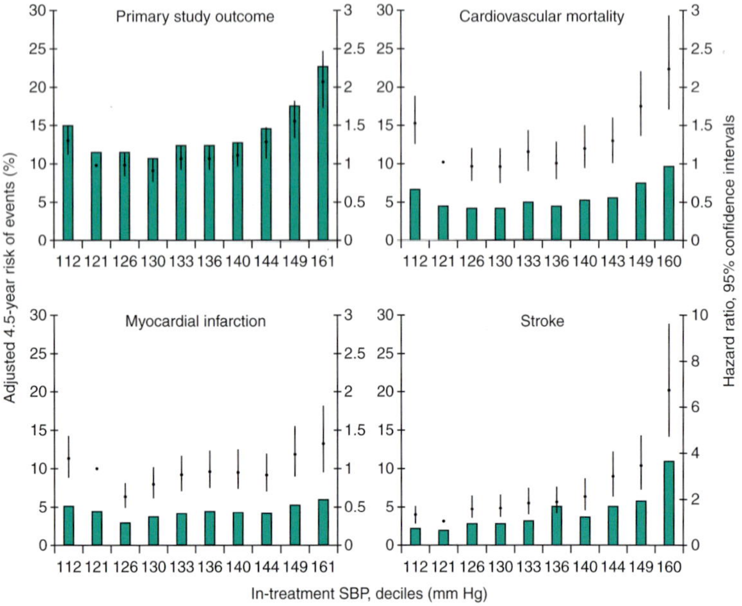

Fig. 8-9 ONTARGET study: in 25,588 high-risk elderly patients, there was a J-curve relationship between SBP and all outcomes except stroke, with a J-point at 125–130 mm Hg. (From Sleight P, Redon J, Verdecchia P, et al. Prognostic value of blood pressure in patients with high vascular risk in the Ongoing Telmisartan Alone and in combination with Ramipril Global Endpoint Trial study (ONTARGET). *J Hypertens* 2009;27:1360–9.)

DOES IT MATTER HOW BLOOD PRESSURE IS LOWERED?

1. Reducing dietary sodium

There has been no large, prospective, hard endpoint study to assess the possible benefits, or harm, of lowering raised BP by low-sodium diets. There is a great need for such a study, as there are worries that, in view of the ability of low-sodium diets to increase plasma renin, aldosterone, and noradrenaline levels, CV endpoints may be adversely affected (32). Certainly in mice a low salt diet provoked a vascular inflammatory response and atherogenesis, which was blocked by ACE-inhibition (33).

One controlled study (34) did indicate that a low-sodium diet, versus a randomized control, reduced CV events by a significant 25%. A meta-analysis of outcome trials indicated a significant 20% reduction in CV events in those exposed to low-sodium diets (**Figure 8-11**) (35).

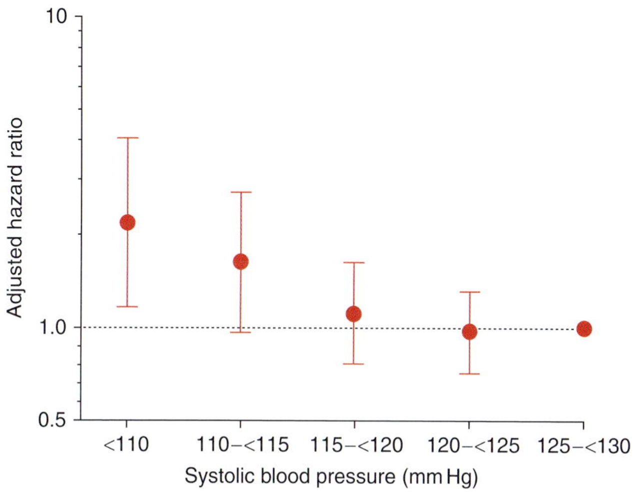

Fig. 8-10 INVEST study: in the 6400 patients with both CAD and diabetes, there was a J-curve relationship between SBP and all-cause mortality with a J-point at about 125 mm Hg. (From Cooper-Dehoff RM, Gong Y, Handberg EM, et al. Tight blood pressure control and cardiovascular outcomes among hypertensive patients with diabetes and coronary artery disease. *JAMA* 2010;304:61–8.)

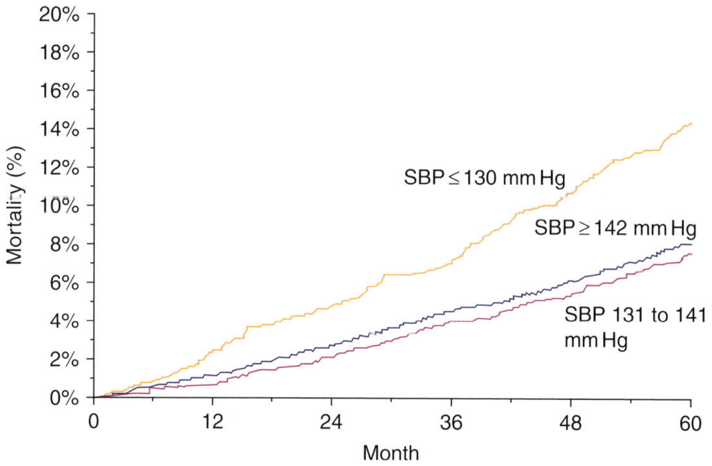

Fig. 8-10a LIFE study; Kaplan–Meier survival curves over 5 years, showing that treated SBP of 130 mm Hg or less was associated with significant increase (37%) in all-cause death. (From Okin PM, Hille DA, Kjeldsen SE, et al. Impact of lower achieved blood pressure on outcomes in hypertensive patients. *J Hypertens* 2012;30:802–10.)

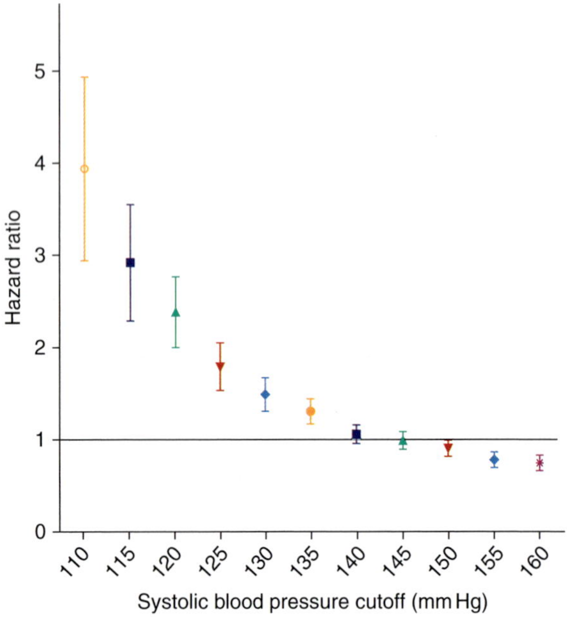

Fig. 8-10b LIFE study: hazard ratios of all-cause death according to treated SBP by 5 mm Hg cutoff points; SBPs of ≤ 135 mm Hg are associated with a significant excess of all-cause death. (From Okin PM, Hille DA, Kjeldsen SE, et al. Impact of lower achieved blood pressure on outcomes in hypertensive patients. *J Hypertens* 2012;30:802–10.)

Study*	Reduced-salt		Control		Relative risk (95% CI)
	Events	Total	Events	Total	
TOHP I	17	321	32	311	0.51 (0.29–0.91)
TOHP II	71	938	80	935	0.88 (0.65–1.20)
Morgan	6	34	5	33	1.16 (0.39–3.45)
TONE	36	322	46	331	0.80 (0.53–1.21)
Total	**130**	**1615**	**163**	**1610**	**0.80 (0.64–0.99)**

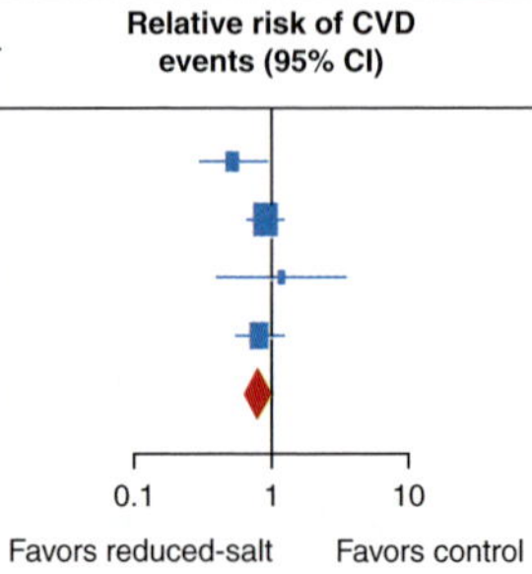

Fig. 8-11 Meta-analysis of cardiovascular events in salt-reduction trials in normotensive and hypertensive individuals. (From He FJ, MacGregor GA. Salt reduction lowers cardiovascular risk: a meta-analysis of outcome trials. *Lancet* 2011;378:380–2.)

Others have called for caution (36), based on the results of the National Health and Nutritional Examination SurveyI (NHANESI) study (37), that suggested sodium intake was inversely associated

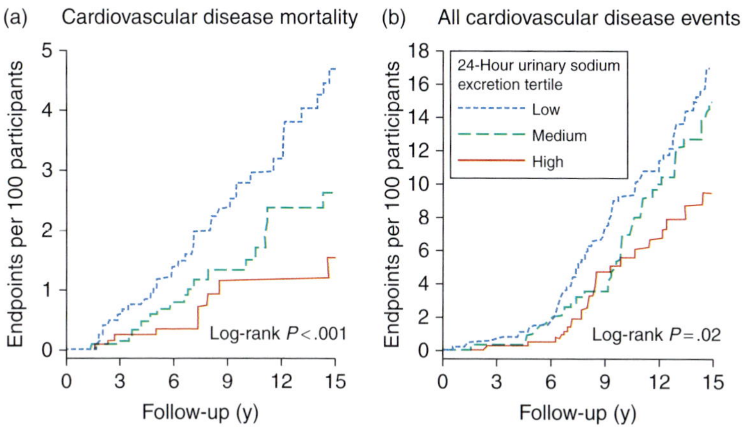

Fig. 8-12 In 3681 subjects (no CVD) followed up for 7.9 years, lower urinary sodium excretion was linked to significantly higher CVD mortality. (From Stolarz-Skrzypek K, Kuznetsova T, Thijs L, et al. Fatal and non-fatal outcomes, incidence of hypertension, and blood pressure changes in relation to urinary sodium excretion. *JAMA* 2011;305:1777–85.)

with all-cause and CVD mortality. Further concern arose from a study suggesting that lower sodium excretion (implying low-sodium intake) was associated with high CVD mortality (**Figure 8-12**) (38).

A possible explanation for disagreements on the pros and cons of low-sodium diets is the existence of a J-curve relationship between sodium excretion and CV events (**Figure 8-13**) (39). The J-curve is associated with CV deaths, myocardial infarction, and heart failure, but not stroke. Higher potassium excretion was associated with a reduced risk of stroke. Low-sodium/high-potassium diets have been linked to marked reductions in CV mortality (40).

2. Antihypertensive drugs

A). Diuretics

i) Young/middle-aged diastolic hypertensives

The first randomized, placebo-controlled study in middle-aged hypertensives was the Australian Mild Hypertension Study (41), which showed that in those randomized to the diuretic, there was a significant 45% reduction in stroke, but zero effect on fatal and nonfatal myocardial infarctions (**Figure 8-14**).

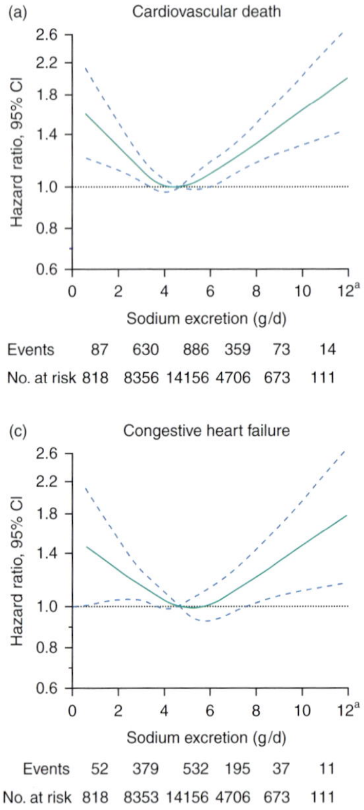

Fig. 8-13 In 28,880 subjects followed up for 4.5 years, there was a J-shaped relationship between urinary sodium excretion and CV events. (From O'Donnel MJ, et al., 2011 (39).)

A similar result was obtained in the large (n = 17,354), MRC trial of mild hypertension (**Figure 8-15**) (42), with no reduction in myocardial infarction (number one killer, 3 times more common than stroke) in the diuretic group versus placebo; in that study, transmural infarctions (pathological Q-waves on ECG) were significantly more common on diuretic therapy compared with β-blocker therapy (**Figure 8-15a**) (43).

Of even greater concern was the result from the Oslo study in middle-aged men (44), where compared with randomized nontreatment, diuretic therapy caused a significant increase in myocardial infarction (**Figure 8-16**). As pointed out in Chapter 6, thiazide-type diuretics increase sympathetic nerve activity, and this may well be the reason why diuretics reduced stroke risk (related to level of BP) but

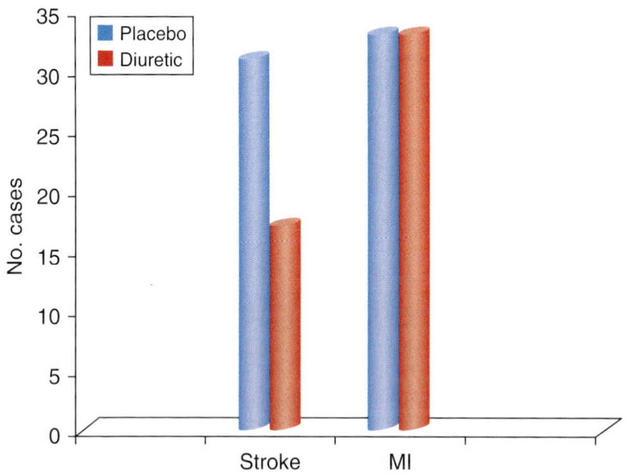

Fig. 8-14 Australian Mild Hypertension study—diuretic vs. placebo in 3427 hypertensives (mean age 50 years): diuretics prevent stroke but not MI. (From Report by the Management Committee. The Australian therapeutic trial in mild hypertension. *Lancet* 1980;1:1261–7.)

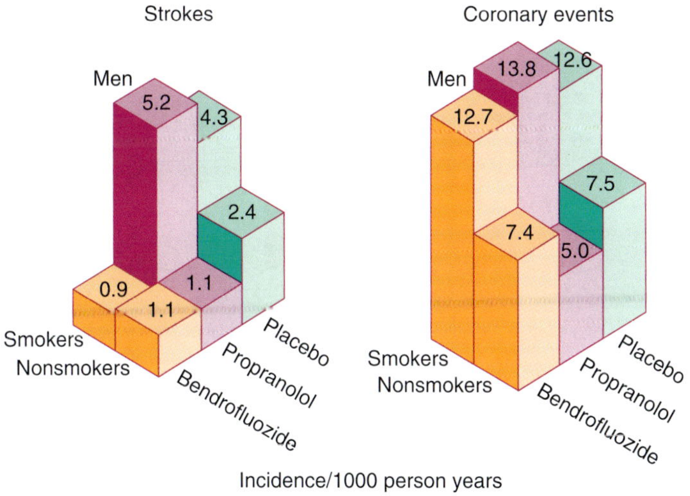

Fig. 8-15 MRC mild hypertension study (1985); diuretics reduce stroke but not coronary events.

not the risk of myocardial infarction (related to level of sympathetic nerve activity, see Chapter 5), in younger patients with sensitized β-receptors.

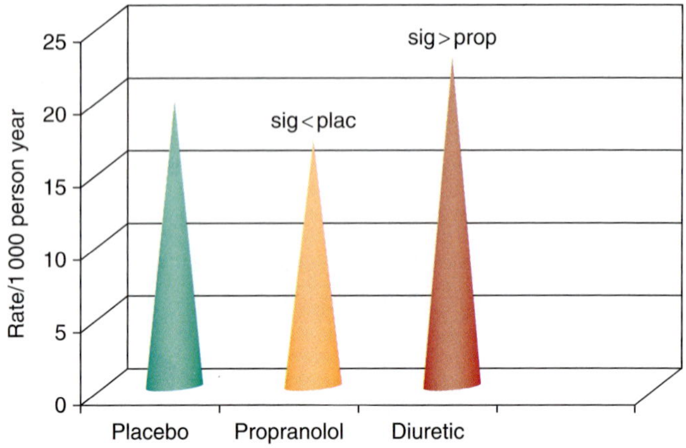

Fig. 8-15a MRC mild hypertension study (n = >17,000); propranolol prevents Q-wave MI.

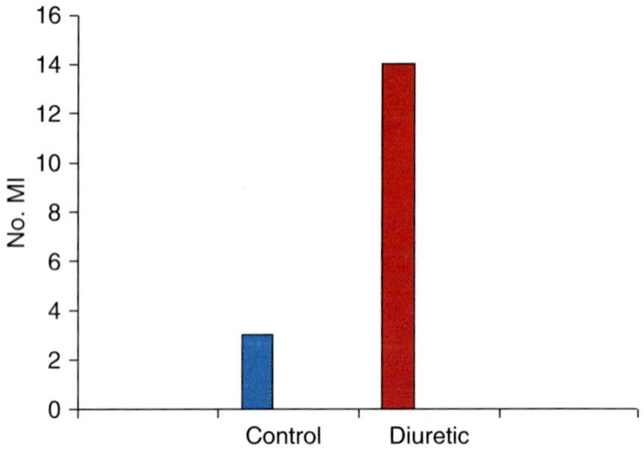

Fig. 8-16 Oslo study; 785 mildly hypertensive men, age 40–49 years, randomized to control or hydrochlorothiazide over 5.5 years; diuretics increase the risk of MI. (From Leren P, Helgeland A. Coronary heart disease and the treatment of hypertension. Some Oslo Study Data. *Am J Med* 1986;80:3–6.)

ii) Elderly systolic hypertensives

Placebo-controlled Studies

There are three classic placebo-controlled studies involving diuretics. First, the SHEP study (45), where 4736 elderly (mean age 71 years) subjects with isolated systolic hypertension were randomized to either placebo or chlorthalidone 12.5–25 mg (atenolol was second-line drug) and

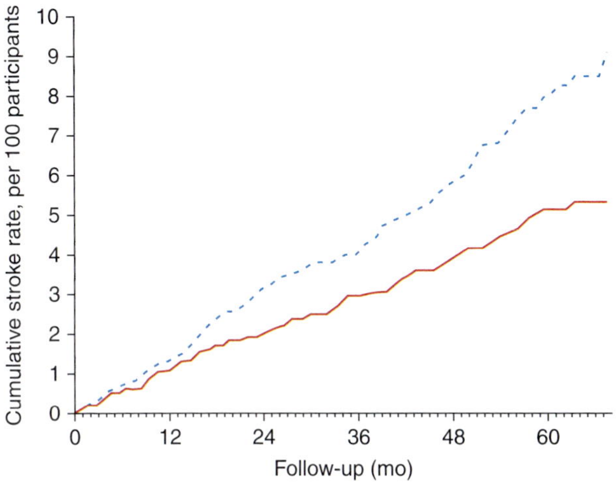

Fig. 8-17 SHEP study (1991); in 4736 elderly patients with isolated systolic hypertension, chlorthalidone (vs. placebo) reduced stroke risk by a significant 36%.

followed up for 4.5 years. Stroke was reduced by 36% (**Figure 8-17**), and (unlike in younger diastolic hypertensive) there was a significant 27% reduction in fatal and nonfatal coronary events. Heart failure was also reduced significantly (46), to a tune of 81% reduction in those with a history of myocardial infarction. After 5 years, all patients went onto active therapy, and at 22 years of follow-up, CV death was still significantly lower in those originally randomized to chlorthalidone (47).

Second, the MRC elderly trial (48), involving 4396 older hypertensives (mean age 70 years), where the randomized diuretic was hydrochlorothiazide 25–50 mg and amiloride 2.5–5.0 mg, compared with randomized placebo or atenolol. After 7-year follow up, stroke was reduced by a significant 31% (**Figure 8-17a**), and (even better than SHEP) coronary events were reduced by a massive significant 44% versus placebo (**Figure 8-18**).

Third, the Hypertension in the Very Elderly Trial (HYVET) study was performed in the very old subjects (older than 80 years) (49). In this study of 3845 very elderly hypertensives, the slow-release diuretic indapamide 1.5 mg, with or without, the ACEI perindopril, was compared with placebo over 2 years. The beneficial results of the diuretic are shown in **Figure 8-22**, where there is a 21% reduction in the risk of all-cause death, a 30% reduction in stroke, and a 64% reduction in heart failure. Thus, aiming to achieve a BP of 150/80 mm Hg in the very elderly subjects is highly beneficial, with the benefit appearing within 1 year (50).

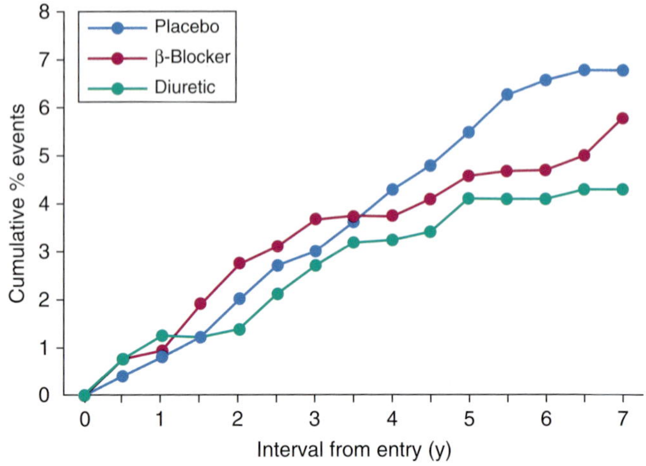

Fig. 8-17a MRC elderly study (1992): in 4396 elderly hypertensives followed up for 7 years, only the diuretic (not atenolol) significantly reduced stroke vs. placebo.

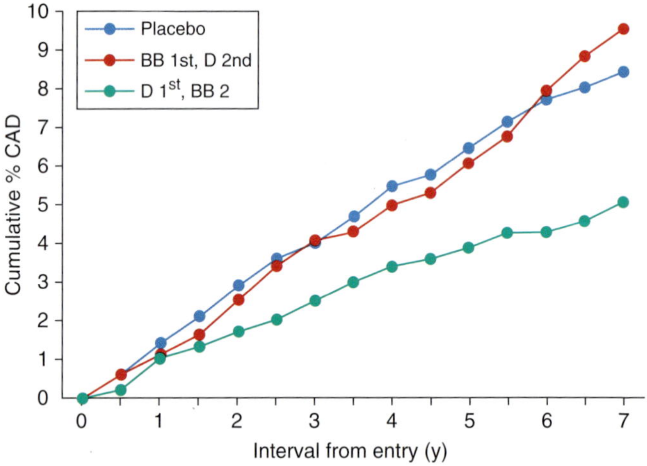

Fig. 8-18 MRC elderly study (1992)—after 7 years follow-up, only the diuretic (not atenolol) significantly reduced the risk of CAD vs. placebo by 44%.

Versus calcium blocker

In the Intervention as a Goal in Hypertension Treatment (INSIGHT) study (51) with 6321 elderly hypertensives, hydrochlorothiazide 25 mg and amiloride 2.5 mg was compared with nifedipine GITS 30 mg over 4 years. Atenolol was a second-line therapy in both arms. Both drugs were similar in reducing CV and cerebrovascular events.

The massive ALLHAT study (52) in 33,357 older hypertensives (mean age 67 years) compared chlorthalidone 12.5–25 mg with the calcium blocker amlodipine 2.5–10 mg, and the ACEI lisinopril 10–40 mg, over a 7-year period. The cumulative event rates for all-cause mortality, stroke, coronary heart disease, and heart failure are shown in **Figure 8-19**. All 3 drugs were similar,

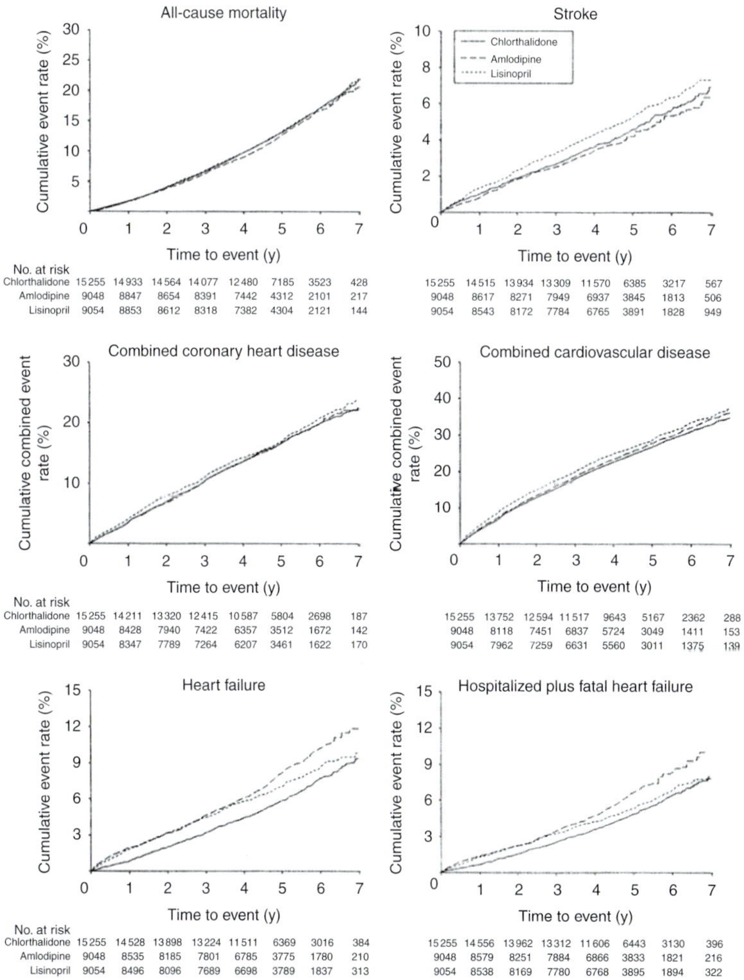

Fig. 8-19 ALLHAT study (2002): 33,357 older hypertensives were randomized to chlorthalidone, amlodipine, and lisinopril; after 4.9 years follow-up, all were similar in reducing CV events, except for heart failure where amlodipine was inferior.

except in heart failure prevention, where chlorthalidone was the best. Indeed, the diuretic was the best in preventing systolic heart failure and better than amlodipine and doxazosin in preventing diastolic heart failure (**Figure 8-20**) (53). Prevention of heart failure is important, as once heart failure develops, the outlook is grim (54). In the ALLHAT Study, the diuretic chlorthalidone was particularly beneficial in black patients, especially in prevention of heart failure (55).

Versus ACEI

The results of the ALLHAT study have been described earlier. In the Second Australian National Blood Pressure Study Group study (56) in 6083 elderly (mean age 72 years) hypertensives over 4.2 years, the diuretic hydrochlorothiazide was inferior to the ACEI enalapril, in preventing CV endpoints and death in men, but not in women (**Figure 8-21**). It is a matter for conjecture as to what the results would have been had chlorthalidone, or indapamide, been the chosen as diuretic, or amiloride (potassium sparing) had been added to the hydrochlorothiazide.

Versus β-blockers

In the MRC elderly study (48), atenolol 50 mg was compared with placebo and diuretic (hydrochlorothiazide and amiloride). The results have been described earlier, where the diuretic, but not the β-blocker, differed significantly from placebo on the prevention of stroke and myocardial infarction (**Figures 8-17a** and **8-18**).

Final thoughts on diuretics

Results of large meta-analyses, which conclude that "low-dose diuretic is the most effective first-line treatment for preventing the occurrence of CVD morbidity and mortality" (57), should have restricted their comments to the elderly, as there is no evidence that diuretics prevent myocardial infarction in young/middle-aged, diastolic hypertensives. In the young/middle-aged diastolic hypertensive subjects, there is no desensitization of β-receptors, and high sympathetic nerve activity is linked to an increased risk of myocardial infarction (see Chapter 5). Hence, drugs that lower BP, but increase sympathetic nerve activity, that is, diuretics, dihydropyridine calcium blockers, and ARBs, reduce stroke risk, but do not reduce the risk of myocardial infarction in the younger/middle-aged diastolic hypertensives. In the elderly systolic hypertensives

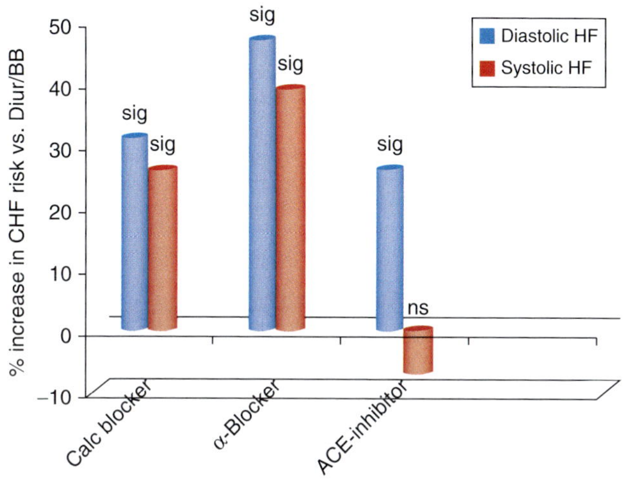

Fig. 8-20 Superiority of Diur/BB combination in the prevention of systolic and diastolic CHF vs. calcium blocker and α-blocker, and diastolic CHF vs. ACEI, in elderly hypertension. ALLHAT 2008.

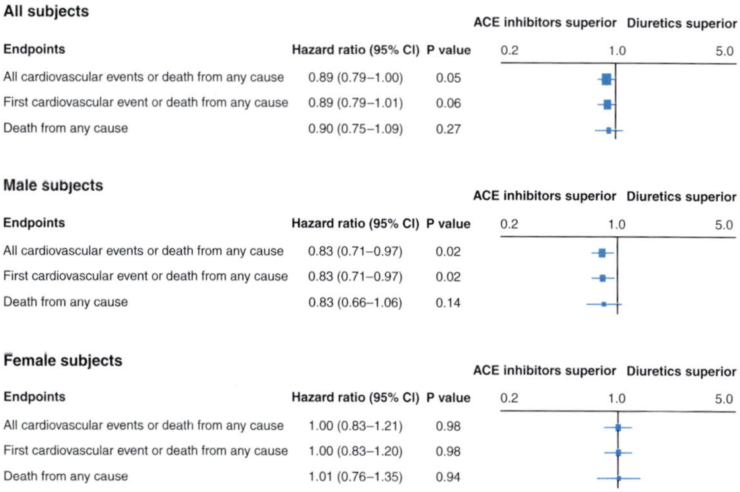

All subjects

Endpoints	Hazard ratio (95% CI)	P value
All cardiovascular events or death from any cause	0.89 (0.79–1.00)	0.05
First cardiovascular event or death from any cause	0.89 (0.79–1.01)	0.06
Death from any cause	0.90 (0.75–1.09)	0.27

Male subjects

Endpoints	Hazard ratio (95% CI)	P value
All cardiovascular events or death from any cause	0.83 (0.71–0.97)	0.02
First cardiovascular event or death from any cause	0.83 (0.71–0.97)	0.02
Death from any cause	0.83 (0.66–1.06)	0.14

Female subjects

Endpoints	Hazard ratio (95% CI)	P value
All cardiovascular events or death from any cause	1.00 (0.83–1.21)	0.98
First cardiovascular event or death from any cause	1.00 (0.83–1.20)	0.98
Death from any cause	1.01 (0.76–1.35)	0.94

Fig. 8-21 In 6083 elderly hypertensives randomized to enalapril or hydrochlorothiazide over 4.2 years, the ACEI was superior in reducing CV events and death in men but not women. Second Australian National BP Study Group 2003.

with β-receptor desensitization and stiff arteries, clearly a different "set of hemodynamic rules" apply, concerning the pathophysiology of myocardial infarction; now, the risk of myocardial infarction is clearly linked to central BP levels.

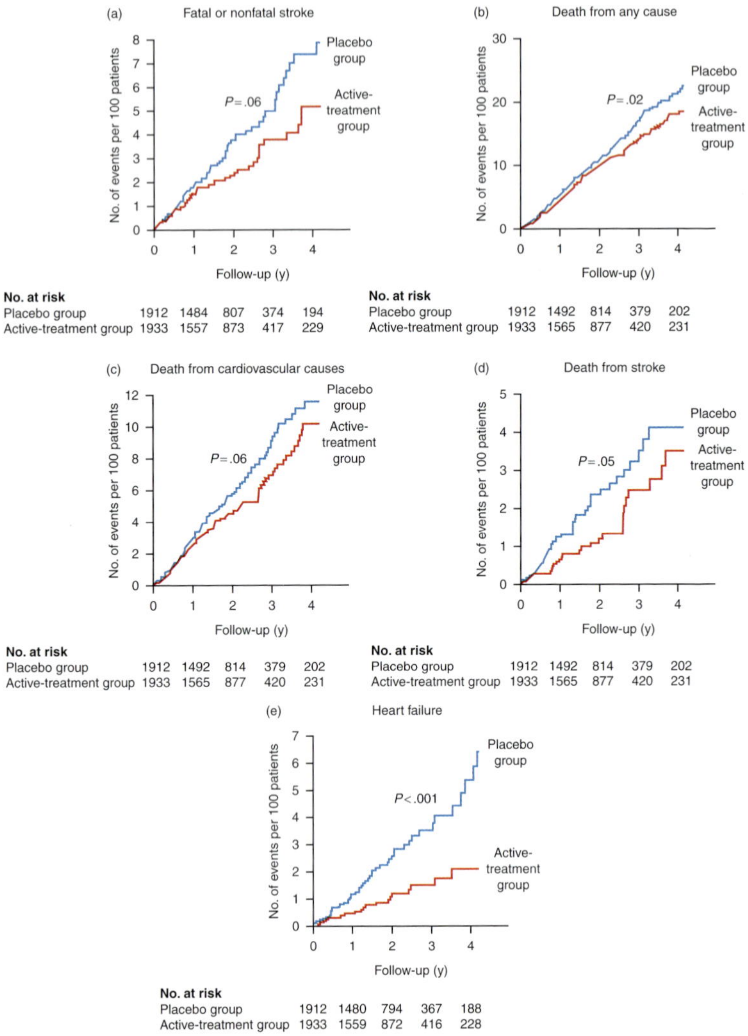

Fig. 8-22 HYVET study: in 3845 very old (mean age 84 years) hypertensives, indapamide ± perindopril was superior to placebo in preventing CV endpoints. (From Beckett NS, Peters R, Fletcher AE, et al. Treatment of hypertension in patients 80 years of age or older. *N Engl J Med* 2008;358:1887–98.)

Maybe it is time to stop using the generic term "diuretics," as there is growing evidence suggesting that classic thiazide diuretics, like hydrochlorothiazide, are less effective in lowering BP than chlorthalidone, indapamide, and aldosterone receptor blockers (58, 59). It is therefore not entirely surprising that a recent meta-analysis indicated that chlorthalidone id superior to hydrochlorthiazide in reducing the risk of heart failure and cardiovascular events (64)".

There is also the "hypokalemia problem" to consider. The ALLHAT study (60) showed that hypokalemia (potassium < 3.5 mmol/L) was associated with a 21% increase in mortality, but even more worrying was that hyperkalemia (potassium > 5.4 mmol/L), linked mainly to ACEIs, was associated with a 58% increase in CV events. Thus, management of potassium homeostasis is important regarding outcome (61), particularly as hydrochlorothiazide-induced low potassium levels are linked to high glucose levels (**Figure 8-22a**) (62). This problem can be avoided by the use of potassium-sparing diuretics like amiloride (62). However, some consider that "chemical diabetes," compared with true diabetes, is not dangerous (63).

Finally, another major advantage of first-line diuretic therapy in the elderly hypertensives is the fact that diuretics reduce the risk of hip fracture (65) and that this benefit disappears within 4 months of stopping therapy (66).

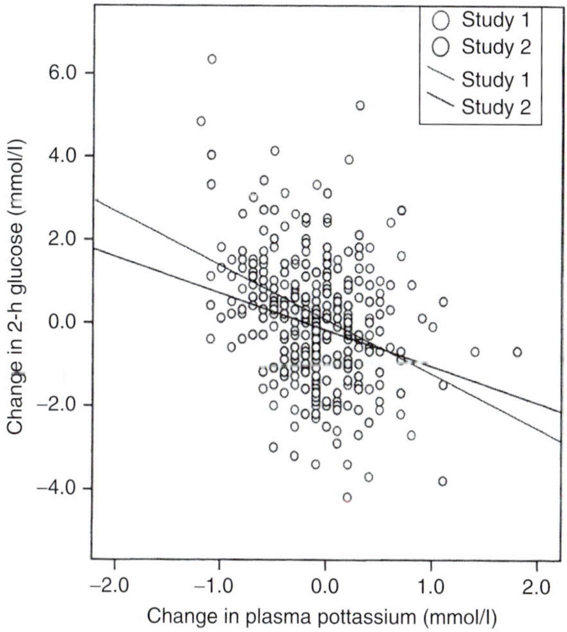

Fig. 8-22a Inverse correlation with change in plasma potassium over 4 weeks, with the change in 2-hour glucose. (From Stears AJ, Woods SH, Watts MA, et al. A double-blind, placebo-controlled, cross-over trial comparing the effects of amiloride and hydrochlorothiazide on glucose tolerance in patients with essential hypertension. *Hypertension* 2012;59:934–42.)

B). β-blockers

i) Young/middle-aged hypertensives without CHD

There are 4 major hard endpoint studies in the young/middle-aged, which involve β-blockers (**Table 8-3**), being the MRC study with nonselective propranolol (42), the International Prospective Primary Prevention Study in Hypertension (IPPPSH) study with nonselective oxprenolol (67), the Metoprolol Atherosclerosis Prevention in Hypertension (MAPHY) study with moderately β-1 selective metoprolol (68), and the UKPDS study with moderately β-1 selective atenolol (69).

The best way of viewing β-blocker risk/benefits in these studies is to take the smoking interaction into account. Figure 8-15 shows clearly that, in the MRC study on nonselective propranolol, compared to placebo, reduced stroke risk by 54% and coronary risk by 33%, but only in nonsmokers (42). This smoking interaction was also noted in the IPPPSH and MAPHY studies. It is apparent in **Figure 8-23** (70) that, compared with placebo or diuretics, the β-blockers reduced the risk of myocardial infarction (3 times more common than stroke) by 30%–45% in nonsmokers, a benefit negated, or reversed, in smokers (see later for explanation).

In the UKPDS study, (54b) the smoking issue was not addressed (23% were smokers). However, the trends in reducing the risk of all 7 primary endpoints (vs. less tight control of BP), and the secondary endpoint of heart failure, over a 9-year follow-up period, all favored the β-blocker atenolol over the ACEI

TABLE 8-3 Hard endpoint studies involving first-line β-blockers

Studies involving first-line BBs	Mean age (y)	P-P (mm Hg)
Young/middle-aged (<60 y)		
IPPPSH (52)	52	65
MRC (35)	51	63
MAPPHY (53)	52	59
UKPDS (54)	56	65
Elderly (60 + y)		
MRC Elderly (40)	70	94
HEP (56)	69	97
LIFE (57)	67	76
ASCOT (58)	63	70

Abbreviations: P-P, pulse pressure.

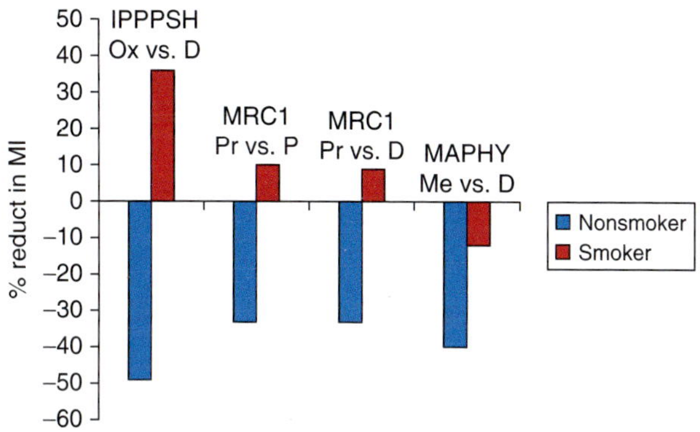

Fig. 8-23 β-Blocker/smoking interaction (MI) in young/middle-age hypertensives: the 30%–50% reduction in myocardial infarction (MI) by β-blocker vs. placebo or diuretic in nonsmokers is negated in smokers. (From Cruickshank JM. Don't β-blockers still have a role in hypertension? *BMJ* 2011;343;759.)

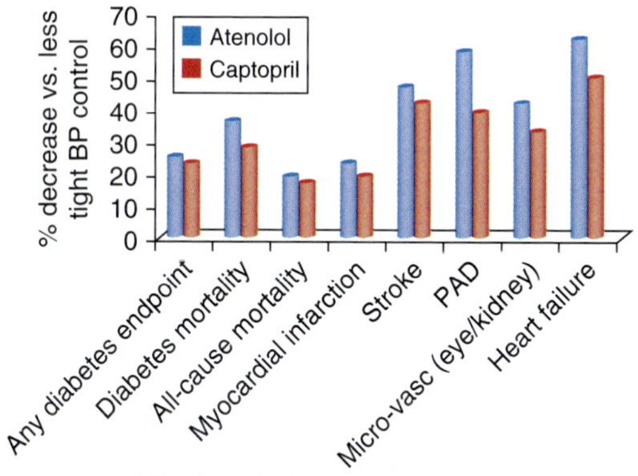

Fig. 8-24 UKPDS—the trends in reduction of all primary endpoints favor atenolol vs. captopril when compared with less tight BP control (diff = 10/5 mm Hg) over 10-year follow-up. (From *UKPDS* 39 1998 (54).)

captopril (**Figure 8-24**) (70). Notable was the absence of "special" renoprotective properties of the ACEI as seen in the microvascular (eye/kidney) columns. Also, the 50% reduction in stroke risk by atenolol (vs. less tight control of BP) refutes the commonly held view that β-blockers are relatively ineffective in reducing the frequency of strokes (relevant to elderly systolic hypertensives only). A 20-year follow-up of the UKPDS patients (**Figure 8-25**) (71) revealed that the earlier trends favoring atenolol persisted, but

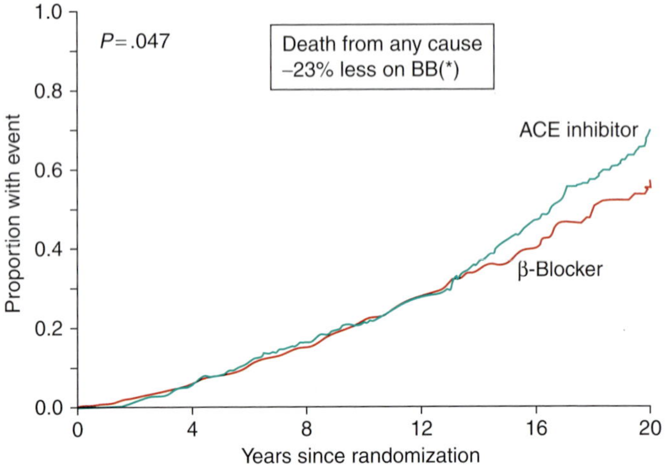

Fig. 8-25 UKPDS study: after g y 20 years follow-up, death from any cause was reduced by a significant 23% in those randomized to atenolol vs. captopril. (From Holman RR, Paul SK, Bethel MA, et al. Long-term follow-up after tight control of blood pressure in type-2 diabetes. *N Engl J Med* 2008;359:1565–76.)

for all-cause-death, there was now a significant 23% reduction in those originally randomized to the β-blocker group. Thus, in the one and only comparison between a β-blocker and an ACEI, the β-blocker performed well.

The European Lacidipine Study on Athersclerosis (ELSA) study (72) in 2334 middle-aged hypertensives revealed no difference between atenolol and the calcium blocker lacidipine in reducing CV events. Also, a placebo-controlled study in 793 middle-aged mild hypertensive, examining the effect of metoprolol CX/XL 25 mg OD on carotid intima-medial thickness, incidentally revealed that over the 3-year follow-up period, the β-blocker significantly reduced the risk of any CV event (73).

ii) Young/middle-aged hypertensives with CHD

The Total Ischemic Burden Bisoprolol Study (TIBBS) (74) involved 330 middle-aged patients with mild hypertension and stable coronary heart disease. Patients were randomized to either highly β-1 selective bisoprolol 10–20 mg once daily or slow-release nifedipine 20–40 mg twice daily. Bisoprolol was not only superior in decreasing the number of transient ischemic episodes on 48 hour Holter monitoring, but after 1-year follow-up, event-free survival was also significantly better (**Figure 8-25a**).

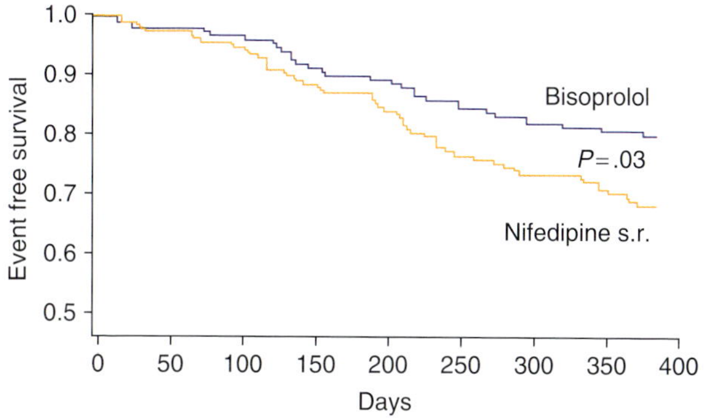

Fig. 8-25a TIBBS study: 307 CAD patients with mild hypertension; bisoprolol significantly superior to SR nifedipine in improving event-free survival (death, M.I. hospitalization). (From Von Armin T, 1995 (74).)

iii) Elderly systolic hypertensives

Without coronary heart disease

There are 4 such studies (48, 75–77), and in all 4 studies, the β-blocker atenolol performed relatively poor versus placebo and diuretic—MRC elderly study (48), randomized nontreatment—Hypertension trial in Elderly Patients (HEP) study (75), the ARB losartan—LIFE study (76), and the calcium antagonist amlodipine—Anglo-Scandinavian Cardiac Outcomes Trial (ASCOT) study (77) (**Table 8-4**) (78). The poor performance of atenolol (in the MRC elderly study), versus placebo and diuretic therapy, in reducing stroke risk (Figure 8-17a) and coronary risk (Figure 8-18) has already been shown. In the MRC elderly study, there was a powerful atenolol/smoking interaction (**Figure 8-26**), present whether atenolol was given as either first- or second-line drug. First-line atenolol (second-line diuretic), in non-smokers, reduced CV events versus placebo by a modest 16%, and this was massively negated in smokers (38% increase vs. placebo): Atenolol given as second-line drug to first-line diuretic therapy in nonsmokers was linked to a significant 40% reduction in CV events versus placebo, converted to a mere 8% reduction in smokers.

With coronary heart disease

The INVEST study (79) compared atenolol and the nondihydro-pyridine calcium blocker verapamil in 22,576 elderly hypertensives with coronary artery disease, over a 5-year period. Both drugs were similar in reducing CV events (**Figure 8-27**), unless there was a history of heart failure, in which case atenolol was superior. In patients

TABLE 8-4 First-line β-blockers (atenolol) perform poorly in elderly hypertension (wide pulse -pressure)

Trial	β-Blocker	Mean age (y)	Initial BP (mm Hg)	Pulse-Pressure (mm Hg)	Result
MRC elderly	Atenolol (vs. placebo vs. diuretic)	70	185/91	94	Only first-line diuretics differed from placebo in stroke prevention; diuretic superior to first-line atenolol in reducing coronary events
HEP	Atenolol (vs. non-treatment)	69	196/99	97	Significant reduction in stroke but no effect on coronary events by atenolol
LIFE	Atenolol (vs. losartan)	67	174/98	76	Losartan superior to atenolol in reducing cardiovascular mortality and nonfatal and fatal stroke
ASCOT	Atenolol ± diuretic (vs. amlodipine ± perindopril)	63	164/94	70	Amlodipine ± perindopril was superior to atenolol ± diuretic in reducing all-cause mortality and all coronary and stroke endpoints

From JM Cruickshank. Are we misunderstanding beta-blockers? *Int J Cardiol* 2007;120:10–27.

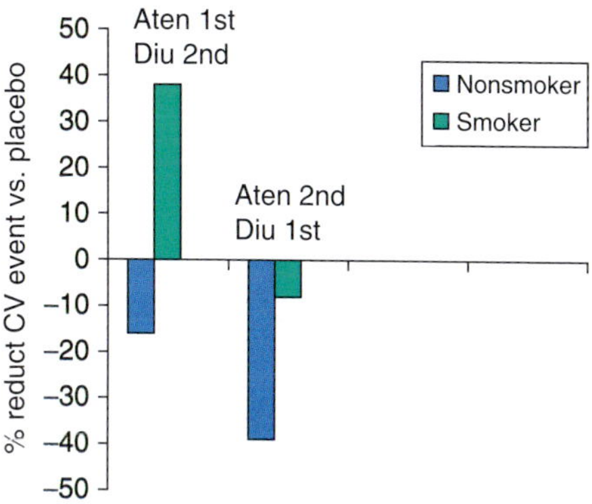

Fig. 8-26 BB/smoking interaction re CV event prevention vs. placebo in the MRC-elderly study; presents whether atenolol was given as first- or second-line drug. (From Cruickshank JM. Don't β-blockers still have a role in hypertension? *BMJ* 2011;343;759.)

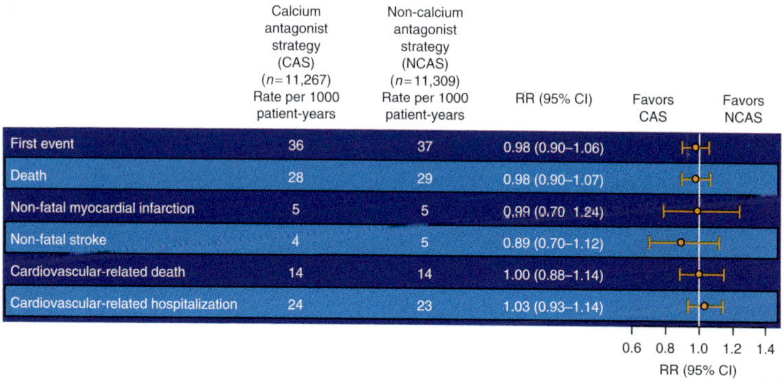

Fig. 8-27 The INVEST study—$n = 22{,}576$ hypertensives with CHD, mean age 66 years, randomized to verapamil/ACEI or atenolol/thiazide-based treatment. Equal effects on primary and secondary endpoints (but verapamil/ACE combination less effective in subjects with CCF). (From Pepine CJ, Handberg EM, Cooper-Dehoff RM, et al. A calcium antagonist vs. non-calcium antagonist hypertension treatment strategy for patients with coronary artery disease (INVEST). *JAMA* 2003;290:2805–16.)

with a history of myocardial infarction, both drugs were similar in reducing CV events (80).

It is worth noting that, like thiazide-type diuretics, β-blockers have been associated with a significant 23% reduction in bone fractures, probably via stimulation of osteoblast activity (81). The reduction in fracture rate is 29% when combined with diuretics (81).

iv) β-blockers and chronic obstructive airways disease

Although β-blockers should generally not be given to asthmatic patients with reversible airways disease, this is not the case with patients with chronic obstructive airways disease (COPD), where the airways obstruction is fixed. A study in 5977 COPD cases indicated that patients on a β-blocker experienced a 22% reduction in all-cause mortality (82). It has been suggested that in such cases, β-blockers may have a direct bronchoprotective effect, possibly via anti-inflammatory and mucous resolving actions (83).

v) How to explain the β-blocker/smoking interaction

An appreciation of the differing β-1:β-2 selectivity ratios in man is important (**Figure 8-28**) (84). This is relevant in the context of the 2- to 3-fold increase in plasma adrenaline (epinephrine) concentration during the smoking of a cigarette, lasting for at least 30 minutes (**Figure 8-29**). There are data to suggest that smoking induces a chronic increase in sympathetic nerve activity (**Figure 8-29a**) (86). In the presence of high adrenaline levels,

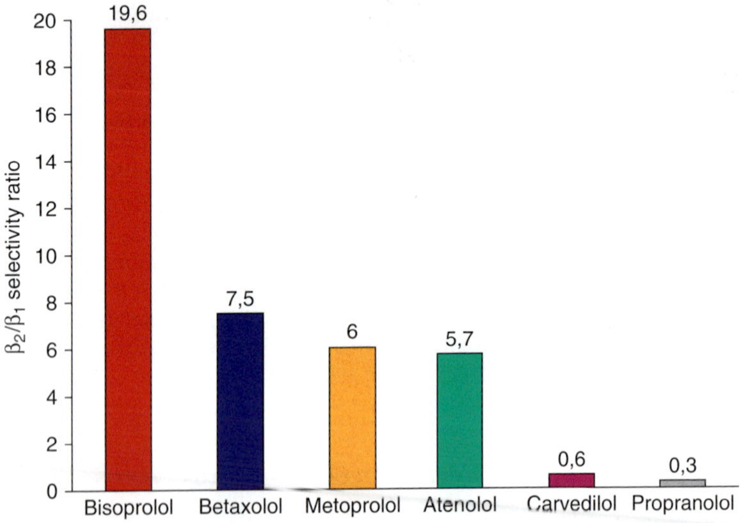

Fig. 8-28 β-1/2 Selectivity ratios at human β-receptors in vitro. (From Smith C, Teitler M. β-blocker selectivity at cloned human β-1 and β-2 adrenergic receptors. *Cardiovasc Drugs Ther* 1999;13:123–6.)

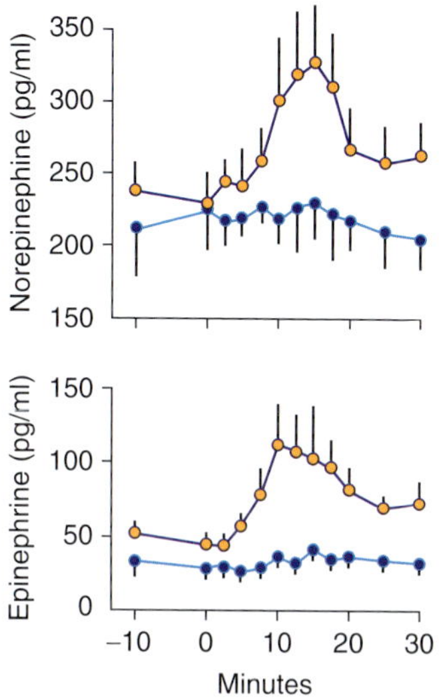

Fig. 8-29 Effect of smoking (dark blue) and sham-smoking on plasma catecholamines. (From Cryer PE, Hammond MW, Satiago JV, et al. Norepinephrine and epinephrine release and adrenergic mediation of smoking-associated hemodynamic and metabolic events. *N Engl J Med* 1976;295:573–7.)

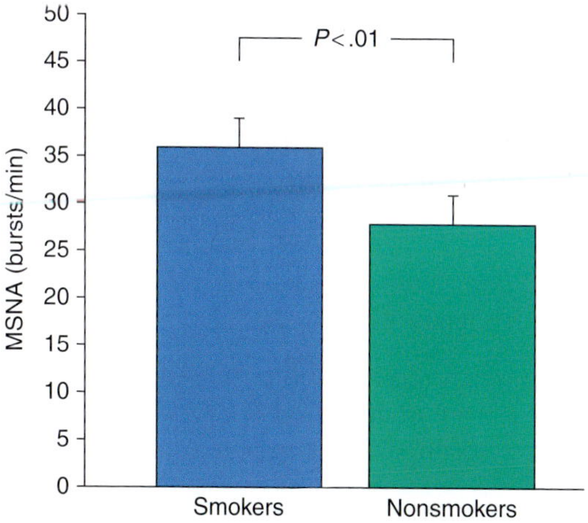

Fig. 8-29a Smoking is associated with chronic sympathetic nerve activation (MSNA) in hypertension. (From Hering D, Kucharska W, Kara T, et al. Smoking is associated with chronic sympathetic activation in hypertension. *Blood Pressure* 2010;19:152–5.)

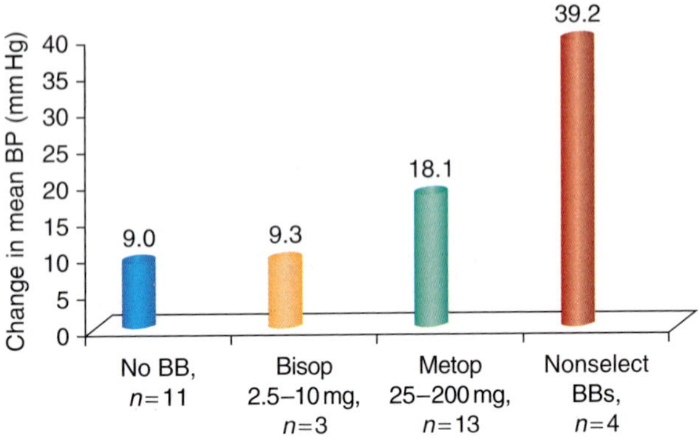

Fig. 8-30 Perioperative interaction between adrenaline and β-blockers: hypertensive blockers: response with nonselective/poorly selective BBs. (From Tarnow J, Muller RK. Cardiovascular effects of low-dose epinephrine infusions in relation to the extent of pre-operative β-blockade. *Anaesthesiology* 1991;74:1035–43.)

nonselective, and to a lesser extent moderately β-1 selective, β-blockers induce a marked hypertensive response (**Figure 8-30**) (87). This is due to the unbridled α-constrictor effect in the presence of β-1 and β-2 blockade. This can be avoided by high β-1 selectivity (bisoprolol) that preserves β-2 stimulation-induced vasodilation, resulting in the canceling out the effects of α-vasoconstriction (Figure 8-30). Thus, a patient smoking, say 20 cigarettes a day, treated with a nonselective, or moderately selective, β-blocker would be experiencing a BP possibly considerably higher than pretreatment levels for most of the day. Such a potentially dangerous situation could be avoided by use of a highly β-1 selective β-blocker.

vi) Explaining anti-β-blocker sentiment in the treatment of hypertension, and why it is misplaced

There has been much recent antiblocker sentiment as regards their role in the treatment of hypertension. As atenolol has been the β-blocker most associated with negative results in the elderly, some of the criticism has been specifically antiatenolol (88, 89, 90), and some specifically to β-blockers as a class, as first-line treatment in the elderly (91). However, the criticism has mostly been against β-blockers in general (92–98), with the final insult coming from the

UK NICE-Committee (99), where β-blockers have completely disappeared as a recommended therapy for uncomplicated hypertension in young/middle-aged subjects (ACEIs and ARBs are favored). This NICE-committee stance was questioned by Cruickshank (100) (see Chapter 10), and the reply was that β-blockers are not cost effective (101).

Most of the critical papers did not take age into account. When age is taken into account (102), it is readily apparent that in patients younger than 60 years, β-blockers are significantly superior to placebo in reducing death/stroke/myocardial infarction, with a positive trend in the elderly (**Figure 8-31**). In comparison with other drugs, in those younger than 60 years, there was a trend favoring β-blockers, but in those older than 60 years β-blockers were significantly less effective in reducing death/stroke/myocardial infarction (**Figure 8-32**).

But most important of all, none of the critics take into account the β-blocker–smoking interaction. Had they done so, it would have been patently evident that in young/middle-aged nonsmoking diastolic hypertensives, comprising about 75% of the total, nonselective/moderately selective β-blockers reduce the frequency of myocardial infarction by 30%–45% compared to randomized placebo or diuretics (Figure 8-23) (70). No other class of antihypertensive agent can rival this efficacy in the young/middle-age hypertensive subject. It is also worth noting that the β-blocker/smoking/adrenaline hypertensive interaction can be avoided by the use of a highly β-1 selective agent, for example, bisoprolol (Figure 8-30) (that also avoids metabolic disturbance and cost effective aspects in the treatment of drug-induced type 2 diabetes). Finally, in the one and only BB/ACEI comparison (UKPDS), atenolol was significantly superior to captopril in reducing all-cause death after 20-year follow-up (see above) (Figure 8-25).

Some of the critics suggest that β-blockers with vasodilatory properties, for example, carvedilol (additional α-blocking properties) and nebivolol (has β-3 ISA), might be preferable. However, the α-blocking properties of carvedilol are no longer evident after 4 months therapy, that is, tachyphylaxis (103). The result is to render carvedilol as a simple nonselective β-blocker. A similar tachyphylactic phenomenon has been noted with doxazosin (104). Indeed, with prazosin, the α-blocking properties are massively attenuated only after 24 hours (105).

In the one and only hard endpoint study with nebivolol, the Seniors Heart Failure study (106), there was no significant

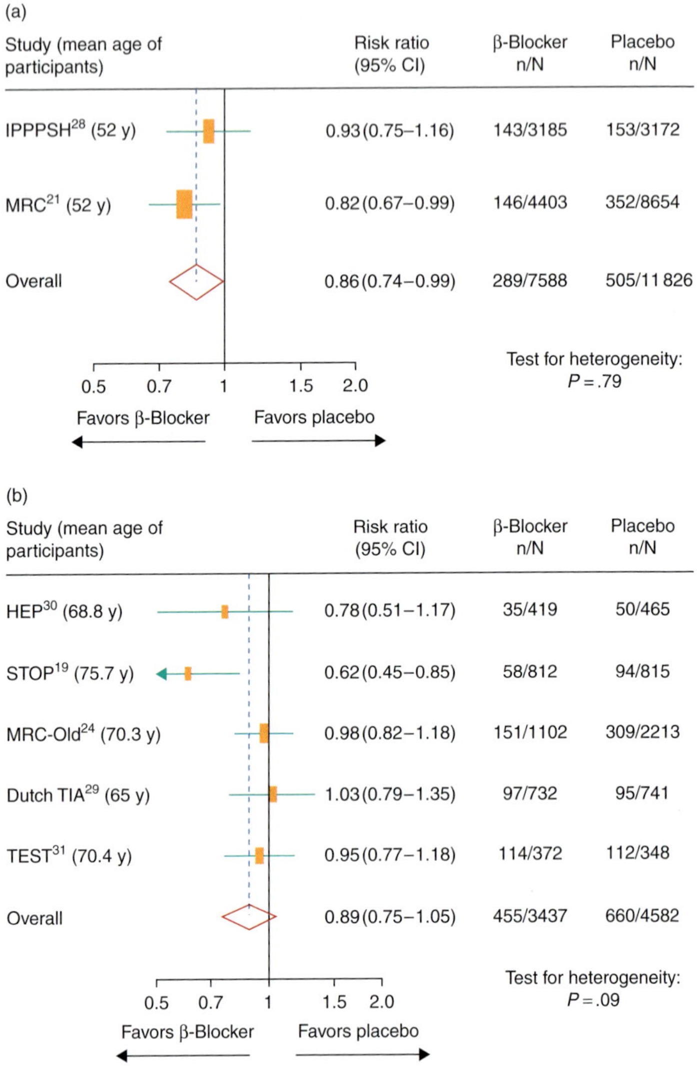

Fig. 8-31 Effect of BBs on death/stroke/MI vs. placebo in younger (<60 years) (a) and older (b) hypertensives. (From Khan N, MacAlister FA. Re-examining the efficacy of β-blockers for the treatment of hypertension: a meta-analysis. *Canadian MAJ* 2006;174:1737–42.)

reduction in all-cause death, which compares unfavorably with the significant 35% reduction in all-cause death with non-ISA β-blockers like metoprolol, carvedilol, and bisoprolol (70). The

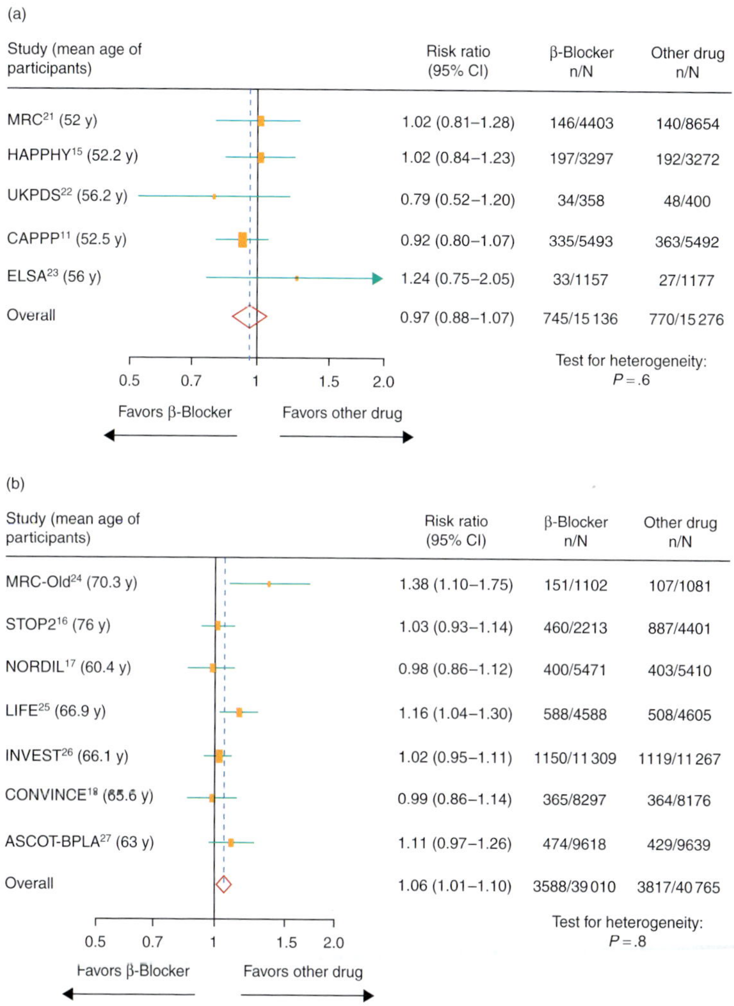

Fig. 8-32 β-blockers and reduction of death/stroke/MI vs. other drugs in hypertension in relation to age (a, young; b, old). (From Khan N, MacAlister FA. Re-examining the efficacy of β-blockers for the treatment of hypertension: a meta-analysis. *Canadian MAJ* 2006;174:1737–42.)

nitric oxide released via β-3 ISA appears to be harmful to the vulnerable heart; L-arginine (substrate for NO synthase) significantly increases the death rate, versus placebo, in postmyocardial infarction cases (107). vii) Beta-blockers reduce the risk of cancer.

Psychological stress may play an etiological role, and this could be partly mediated by noradrenaline and adrenaline (108). In several experimental cancer models beta-adrenergic receptors have been detected on tumor or stromal cells, and they may be linked to the metastasic process (109).

There is thus the exciting prospect that beta-blockade could be a novel adjuvent to existing anti-cancer strategies. In non-estrogen-responsive breast cancer the arachidonic acid cascade is under the control of beta-receptors (110), which may explain the significantly improved relapse-free survival with beta-blockade in such cases (111).

Beta-blockers, but not other anyihypertensive drugs, markedly reduce the risk of disease progression with melanoma (112).

Cell proliferation in smoking-induced non-small cell lung cancer is reversed by propranolol (113).

In pancreatic cancer, beta-2 blockade supresses invasion and proliferation, while beta-1 blockade also supressed invasion (114).

Beta-blockers may prevent prostatic cancer (115), and benefit patients with prostatic cancer requiring androgen deprivation therapy (i).

C) ACE inhibitors

i) Young/middle-aged diastolic hypertensives

The UKPDS study comparing atenolol or captopril, versus less tight control of BP, has already been described (Figure 8-24) (69, 70). The trends in reduction of all 7 primary endpoints (including stroke and microvascular renoprotection) versus less tight control of BP, favored the β-blocker. At 20 years of follow-up (71), the trends favoring the β-blocker over the ACEI persisted, but now, for all-cause death, strengthened, resulting in a significant 23% reduction in favor of the β-blocker group (Figure 8-25).

The Appropriate Blood Pressure Control in Diabetes (ABCD) Study (117) in middle-aged hypertensives with type 2 diabetes compared, over 5 years, the effects of enalapril and nisoldipine, a calcium channel blocker of the dihydropyridine class. There was a significantly higher incidence of fatal and nonfatal myocardial infarction in the calcium blocker group (**Figure 8-33**). Of possible relevance could be, as addressed in Chapter 6, the increase in sympathetic nerve activity/heart rate by dihydropyridine calcium blockers.

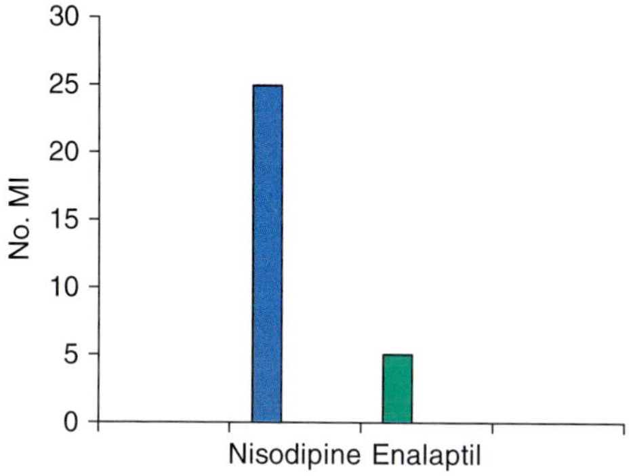

Fig. 8-33 ABCD study; in middle-aged hypertensives with diabetes randomized to enalapril or nisoldipine, there was a significant increase in MI in the CB group. (From Estacio RO, Jeffers BW, Hiatt WR, et al. The effect of nisoldipine as compared with enalapril on cardiovascular outcomes in patients with non-insulin-dependent diabetes and hypertension. *N Engl J Med* 1998;338:645–52.)

The Captopril Prevention Project study (118), in 10,985 middle-aged hypertensives, compared captopril and conventional treatment (diuretic or β-blocker). There was no difference between the groups in preventing CV mortality and morbidity, and the excess of strokes in the ACEI group was explained by a higher BP in that group.

ii) Older subjects

In the Healthy Outcomes through Patient Empowerment (HOPE) study in 9297 high-risk, older patients with pre/mild hypertension, ramipril was randomized versus placebo over a 5-year period (119). The ACEI reduced the composite endpoint of myocardial infarction, stroke, and CV death by a significant 22%. The ACEI benefits were particularly evident in the 3577 diabetics (**Figure 8-34**) (120), and albuminuria was reduced significantly. The benefits noted on ramipril treatment were still present at 7 years follow-up (121). Similar results to HOPE were seen in the European trial On the reduction of cardiac events with Perindopril in stable coronary Artery disease (EUROPA) study (122), involving perindopril versus placebo, in patients with stable coronary artery disease.

As already shown, in the Second Australian Trial (56) involving 6083 elderly hypertensives, enalapril was compared with hydrochlorothiazide over a 4-year period; the ACEI was superior in

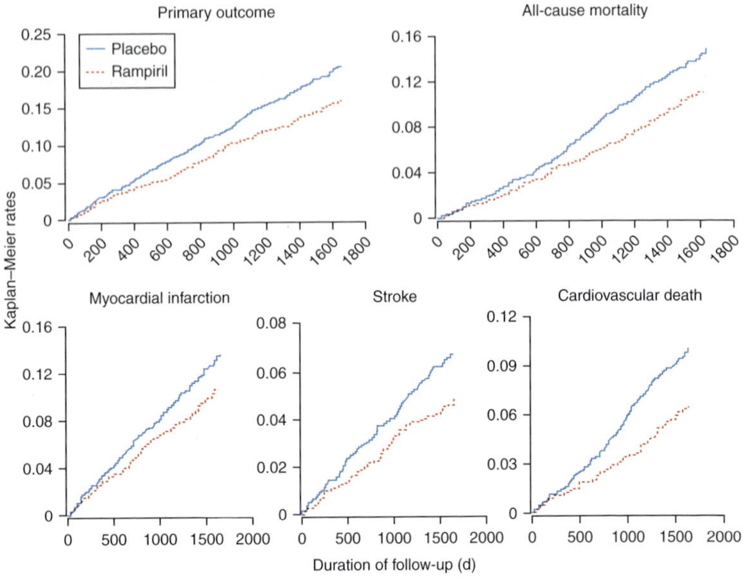

Fig. 8-34 HOPE Study Investigators. MICRO–HOPE study: effect of ramipril on CV endpoints and death in diabetics. (From Heart Outcomes Prevention Evaluation (HOPE) Study Investigators. Effects of ramipril on cardiovascular and microvascular outcomes in people with diabetes mellitus: results of the HOPE Study and MICRO– HOPE Substudy. *Lancet* 2000;355:253–9.)

preventing CV events and deaths. The choice of diuretic might be relevant, as shown in the ALLHAT study (52), where chlorthalidone was the chosen diuretic. As indicated earlier, in this massive study of 33,357 elderly hypertensives, comparing chlorthalidone, lisinopril, and amlodipine, after 7 years, the cumulative event rates were similar for all 3 drugs, except for heart failure prevention, where the diuretic was best (Figure 8-19). In the prevention of systolic heart failure, the diuretic was better than the ACEI, but not so with diastolic heart failure (Figure 8-20) (53).

In the ONTARGET study (13), involving 25,500 high-risk elderly subjects with mild hypertension, the ACEI ramipril was equal to the ARB telmisartan in reducing the composite CV endpoint. The combination of the 2 drugs did not improve outcome, but important adverse reactions such as hypotensive symptoms, syncope, and renal dysfunction were increased.

There has been some debate regarding the efficacy of ACEI in preventing stroke. Certainly, in the Perindopril Protection Against Recurrent Stoke Study (PROGRESS) (123), involving poststroke patients, compared to randomized placebo, perindopril alone did not prevent further stroke after 3 years of follow-up; only the combination of the ACEI and the diuretic indapamide was associated with reduction of stroke risk. In a meta-analysis (124), it was concluded that although ACEIs reduced stroke risk, the degree was somewhat less than for calcium blockers (**Figure 8-35**), the reverse being true to coronary heart disease prevention (**Figure 8-35a**).

D) Angiotensin receptor blockers

i) Young/middle-aged hypertensives

In 577 Chinese/Japanese patients with type 2 diabetes with overt nephropathy, randomized to either placebo or olmesartan over 3.2 years, there was an excess of CV deaths, 10 versus 3, in those randomized to the ARB (125). In that study, olmesartan did not improve renal outcomes, and there was 9.2% versus 5.3% excess of hyperkalemia in the ARB group.

In a study of 4447 patients with type 2 diabetes and prehypertension, the participants were randomized to either placebo or olmesartan over 3.2 years (126); it was revealed that the ARB significantly increased the risk of CV death in subjects with and without a history of coronary heart disease, and also increased the risk of sudden death and death from myocardial infarction (**Figure 8-36**).

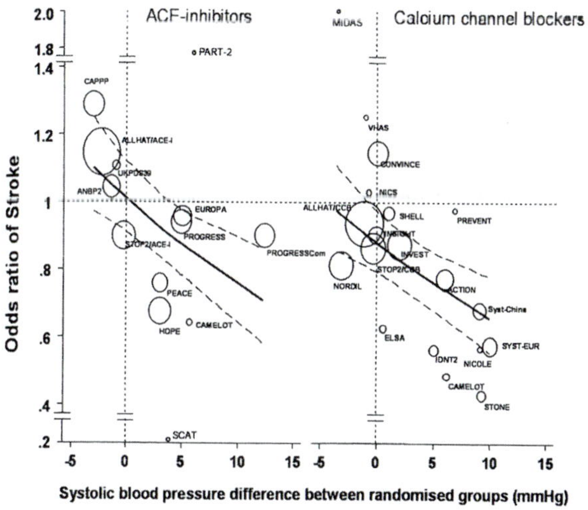

Fig. 8-35 Calcium blockers are more effective than ACC inhibitors at reducing the risk of stroke. (From Verdecchia P, Reboldi G, Angeli F, et al. Angiotensin-converting enzyme inhibitors and calcium channel blockers for coronary artery disease and stroke prevention. *Hypertension* 2005;46:386–92.)

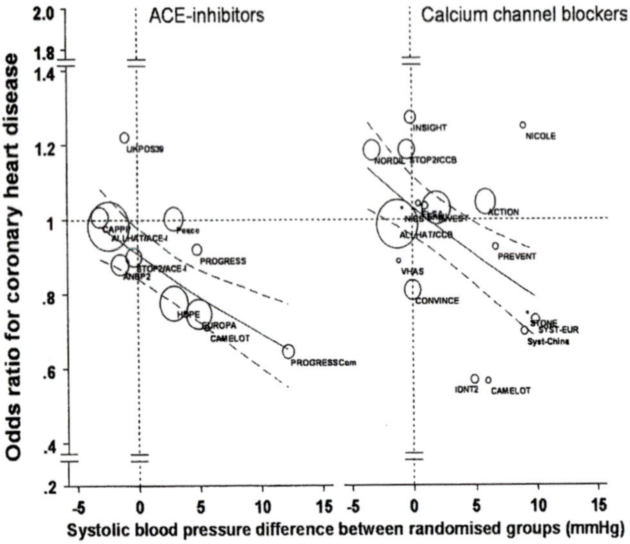

Fig. 8-35a ACEIs are more effective than calcium blockers in reducing the risk of MI. (From Verdecchia P, Reboldi G, Angeli F, et al. Angiotensin-converting enzyme inhibitors and calcium channel blockers for coronary artery disease and stroke prevention. *Hypertension* 2005;46:386–92.)

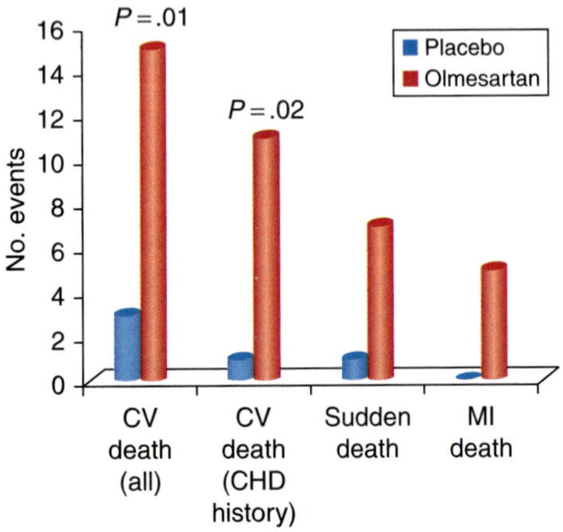

Fig. 8-36 Olmesartan vs. placebo (randomized) in 4447 patients with type 2 diabetes mellitus, mean age 57 years, mean BMI 31, BP 136/81, over 3.2 years: the ARB significantly increased the risk of CV endpoints and death. (From Haller H, Ito S, Izzo JL, et al. Olmesartan for the delay or prevention of microalbuminuria in type-2 diabetes. *N Engl J Med* 2011;364:907–17.)

ii) Elderly hypertensives

As already referred to in the LIFE study (76), losartan was compared to atenolol in 1323 elderly patients with isolated systolic hypertension. The ARB was generally superior to the β-blocker (**Figure 8-37**), although there was no difference in the risk of myocardial infarction. The advantage of losartan over atenolol was particularly notable in diabetics (127).

The Telmisartan Randomised AssessmeNt study in ACEinNtolerant subjects with cardiovascular Disease (TRANSCEND) Trial (128) involved 5926 high-risk patients intolerant to ACEIs, who were randomized to either placebo or telmisartan, over a four-and-a-half-year period. The ARB had no effect on the primary composite endpoint (in spite of a BP 4.0/2.0mm Hg lower), but there were trends toward fewer strokes and myocardial infarctions in the ARB group.

Another placebo-controlled study in 9306 high-risk mild hypertensives, the so-called the Nateglinide And Valsartan in Impaired Glucose Tolerance Outcomes Research (NAVIGATOR) trial (129), also revealed no differences between the ARB valsartan and placebo in the reduction of CV events.

The Valsartan Antihypertensive Long-term Use Evaluation trial (VALUE) study, in 15,245 high-risk hypertensives, compared valsartan and the calcium blocker amlodipine over a 4.2-year period (130). The main outcome of cardiac disease did not differ between the groups, and the trend toward fewer strokes and the significantly fewer myocardial infarctions with the calcium blocker

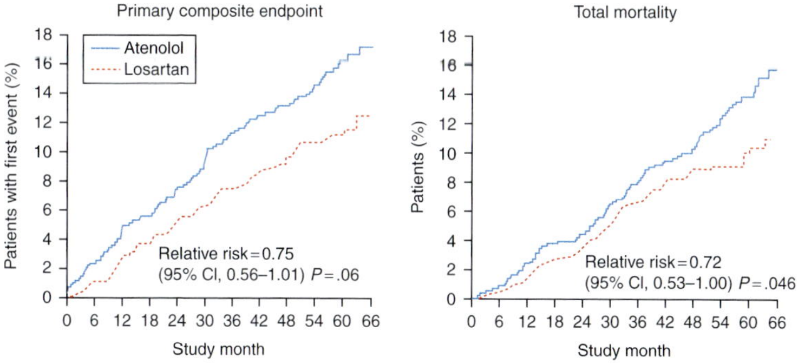

Fig. 8-37 LIFE study; in elderly hypertensives, losartan is superior to atenolol in reducing the risk of the primary composite and death. (From Kjeldsen SE, Dahlof B, Devereux RB, et al. Effect of losartan on cardiovascular morbidity and mortality in patients with isolated hypertension and left-ventricular hypertrophy. *JAMA* 2002;288:1491–8.)

could have been well due to lower BP values. A further 2 studies on Japanese hypertensives (131, 132), one with glucose intolerance (98a), showed that valsartan and amplodipine did not differ in their ability to reduce the primary endpoint (131). However, there was an excess of heart failure cases in the amlodipine group, and an excess of myocardial infarctions in the valsartan group (132).

The ONTARGET study (13), as already mentioned, revealed no significant differences between telmisartan and ramipril.

A study in Japanese hypertensives with coronary disease compared candesartan with non-ARB standard therapy over 4.2 years (133), and showed no difference in the primary endpoint/first major adverse CV event, although there were strong trends favoring non-ARB treatment in reducing total and CV death and myocardial infarction. A similar study in Japanese high-risk hypertensive patients, but involving valsartan, over 3 years concluded that the ARB was best at preventing CV events (134). However, the advantage was in stroke prevention, and in the first year of the study, the SBP was 2 mm Hg lower in the ARB group.

Two placebo-controlled studies in the poststroke period, one involving telmisartan (135) and the other candesartan (136), revealed no benefit from ARB treatment; indeed a poor outcome was increased by a significant 17% with candesartan.

iii) Do ARBs increase the risk of myocardial infarction?

Unlike ACEIs, ARBs increase the concentration of angiotensin II (137), and also increase sympathetic nerve activity in younger subjects (55). As pointed out in Chapter 5, increased sympathetic nerve activity, cyclic AMP concentration, and β-receptor density, are closely linked to an increased risk of myocardial infarction, but not stroke, in young/middle-aged hypertensives.

Although ACEIs tend to decrease sympathetic nerve activity (see Chapter 6, refs 136–138, 154), the picture for ARBs is mixed. ARBs decreased sympathetic activity in older patients (Chapter 6, ref 156) (131), whereas it was increased in younger/middle-aged patients (Chapter 6, refs 162, 158, Figure 6-37).

Accordingly, a lively debate has ensued regarding ARBs and the risk of myocardial infarction. Meta-analyses involving older hypertensives have indicated that ARBs reduce the risk of myocardial infarction equally with ACEIs (138) and other drugs (139). However, others have concluded that ARBs may increase the risk of myocardial infarction (140). It has been pointed out that in 9 of the 11 hard endpoint studies involving ARBs, there was an excess of

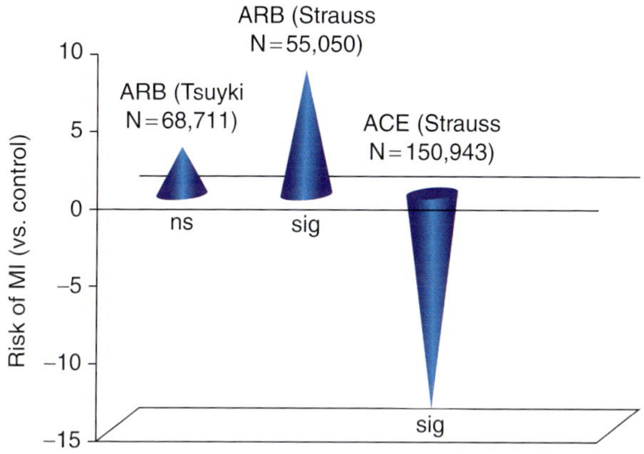

Fig. 8-37a Relative risk of MI in meta-analyses of ARB and ACEIs. (From Strauss and Hall, *Lancet* 2007 (146).)

myocardial infarctions in those allocated to the ARB (141). Thus, there was a significant 8% excess of myocardial infarcts with ARBs compared to a significant 14% reduction with ACEIs (**Figure 8-37a**) (142). Others have emphasized the significant excess of myocardial infarcts associated with ARBs (143).

The above debate has evolved firmly in favor of those who are concerned about ARBs, with the publication of 2 recent placebo-controlled studies in young/middle-aged subjects with type 2 diabetes (125, 126), where there was a marked excess of CV deaths (92), including sudden death and death due to myocardial infarction (Figure 8-36) (126). Moreover, a recent meta-analysis of 158,998 hypertensive patients involved in randomised trials, comparing the effects of ACEIs and ARBs upon all-cause mortality, revealed a significant 10% reduction with ACEIs compared to no effect of ARBs (this difference was significant) (144).

E) Calcium blockers

i) Young/middle-aged hypertensives

Without coronary heart disease

As has already been mentioned, in the ELSA study (72), atenolol and lacidipine reduced CV events to a similar degree in 2334 middle-aged hypertensives over a 4-year period.

In the ABCD study (117), where nisoldipine was compared to enalapril over a 5-year period, there was a significant excess of fatal and nonfatal myocardial infarctions in the calcium blocker group (Figure 8-33). The possible role of calcium blocker-induced increases in sympathetic nerve activity (Chapter 6) was addressed.

With coronary heart disease

Also addressed earlier was the TIBBS trial (74), where slow-release nifedipine was compared to highly β-1 selective bisoprolol. After 1 year, event-free survival was significantly better in the β-blocker group (Figure 8-25a). Again, the potential problems of calcium blocker-induced increases in sympathetic nerve activity in younger patients were discussed (see Chapter 6).

ii) Elderly hypertensives

Without coronary heart disease

The Systolic Hypertension in Europe Trial (Syst-Eur) was a randomized, double-blind, placebo-controlled study, in 4695 elderly hypertensives, involving first-line nitrendipine with the possible addition of enalapril and hydrochlorothiazide (145). There was a significant 42% reduction in total stroke, a 44% reduction in nonfatal stroke, and a 31% reduction in fatal/nonfatal CV endpoints; total mortality remained unchanged.

In 9711 Chinese hypertensives on low-dose diuretics, felodipine was compared with randomized placebo over a 5-year period (12). Significant reductions in stroke were observed in uncomplicated hypertensives and in those older than 65 years (**Figure 8-38**), and in the latter group, there were significant reductions in all CV events and all deaths.

Two large studies compared non-dihydropyridine calcium blockers with diuretic or β-blocker therapy. The Nordic Diltiazem Study (NORDIL) (146), in 10,881 older hypertensives, compared diltiazem with diuretic or β-blocker over a 5-year period. Both interventions were the same in preventing the primary endpoint of all stroke, myocardial infarction, and other CV deaths. A similar study, but now with verapamil, the so-called Controlled Onset Verapamil Investigation of Cardiovascular End Points trial (147), arrived at the same conclusion as NORDIL.

As already noted (51), the INSIGHT study compared nifedipine GITS (is a long-acting Formulation of nifedipine) with a combination of hydrochlorothiazide and amiloride over 4 years (the second-line add-on therapy in both arms was atenolol). Both drug arms were similar in reducing CV and cerebrovascular events.

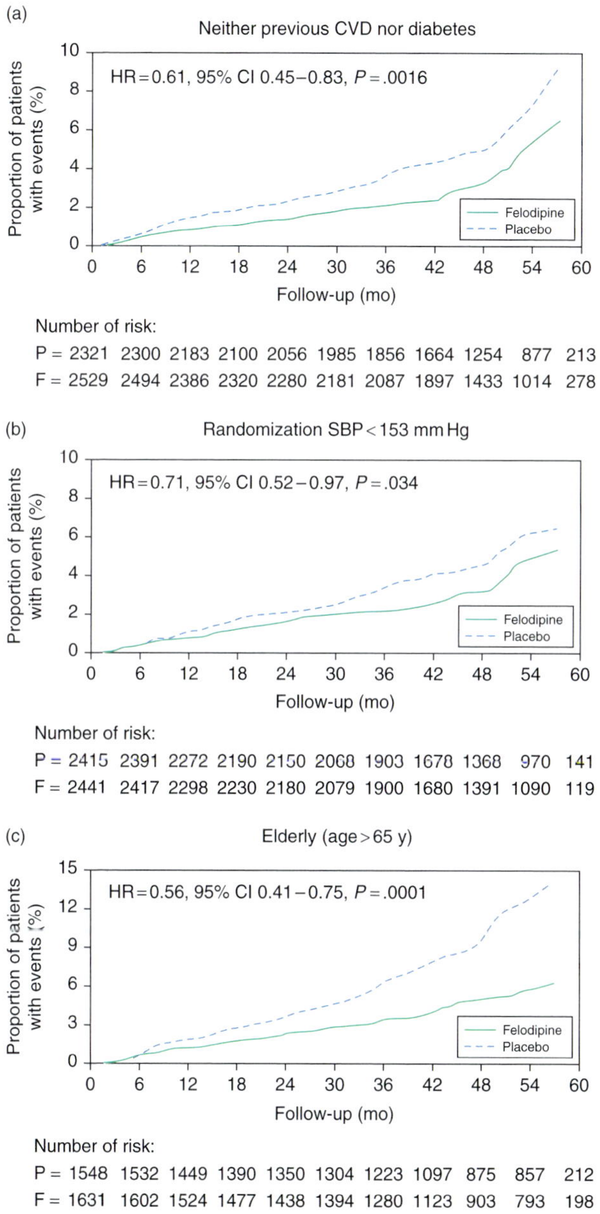

Fig. 8-38 FEVER trial: in older Chinese hypertensives, felodipine was superior to randomized placebo in improving event-free survival in various sub-groups. (From Zhang Y, Zhang X, Liu L, et al. Is a systolic blood pressure target < 140mm Hg indicated in all hypertensives? Subgroup analyses of findings from the randomised FEVER trial. *Europ Heart J* 2011;32:1500–8.)

	Amlodipine-based regimen (n=9639)		Atenolol-based regimen (n=9618)			
	Number (%)	Rate per 1000	Number (%)	Rate per 1000	Unadjusted HR (95% CI)	P
Primary endpoints						
Non-fatal myocardial infarction (including silent)+fatal CHD	429 (5%)	8.2	474 (5%)	9.1	0.90 (0.79–1.02)	0.1052
Secondary endpoints						
Non-fatal myocardial infarction (excluding silent)+fatal CHD	390 (4%)	7.4	444 (5%)	8.5	0.87 (0.76–1.00)	0.0458
Total coronary endpoint	753 (8%)	14.6	852 (9%)	16.8	0.87 (0.79–0.96)	0.0070
Total cardiovascular events and procedures	1362 (14%)	27.4	1602 (17%)	32.8	0.84 (0.78–0.90)	<0.0001
All-cause mortality	738 (8%)	13.9	820 (9%)	15.5	0.89 (0.81–0.99)	0.0247
Cardiovascular mortality	263 (3%)	4.9	342 (4%)	6.5	0.76 (0.65–0.90)	0.0010
Fatal and non-fatal stroke	327 (3%)	6.2	422 (4%)	8.1	0.77 (0.66–0.89)	0.0003
Fatal and non-fatal heart failure	134 (1%)	2.5	159 (2%)	3.0	0.84 (0.66–1.05)	0.1257
Tertiary endpoints						
Silent myocardial infarction	42 (0.4%)	0.8	33 (0.3%)	0.6	1.27 (0.80–2.00)	0.3089
Unstable angina	73 (1%)	1.4	106 (1%)	2.0	0.68 (0.51–0.92)	0.0115
Chronic stable angina	205 (2%)	3.9	208 (2%)	4.0	0.98 (0.81–1.19)	0.8323
Peripheral arterial disease	133 (1%)	2.5	202 (2%)	3.9	0.65 (0.52–0.81)	0.0001
Life-threatening arrhythmias	27 (0.3%)	0.5	25 (0.3%)	0.5	1.07 (0.62–1.85)	0.8009
Development of diabetes mellitus	567 (6%)	11.0	799 (8%)	15.9	0.70 (0.63–0.78)	<0.0001
Development of renal impairment	403 (4%)	7.7	469 (5%)	9.1	0.85 (0.75–0.97)	0.0187
Post-hoc endpoints						
Primary endpoint+coronary revascularization procedures	596 (6%)	11.5	688 (7%)	13.4	0.86 (0.77–0.96)	0.0058
Cardiovascular death+myocardial infarction+stroke	796 (8%)	15.4	937 (10%)	18.4	0.84 (0.76–0.92)	0.0003

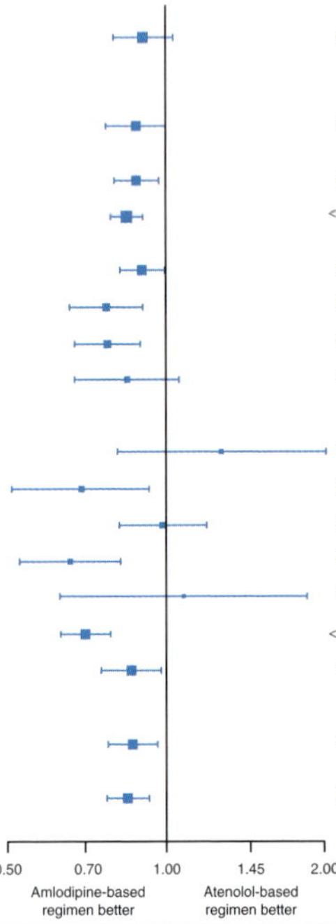

Fig. 8-39 ASCOT study: in 19, 257 elderly hypertensives, amlodipine was superior to atenolol in preventing primary, secondary, tertiary and post -hoc endpoints. (From Dahlof B, Sever P, Poulter N, et al. Prevention of cardiovascular events with an antihypertensive regimen of amlodipine adding peridopril as required versus atenolol adding bendroflumethazide as required (ASCOT-BPLA); a multicentre randomised controlled trial. *Lancet* 2005;366:895–906.)

The large ASCOT study (77) in 19,257 older hypertensives, compared amlodipine (second-line ACEI) and atenolol (second-line diuretic) and was stopped after 5.5 years of follow-up. The amlodipine-based regimen prevented more major CV events, and induced less diabetes, than the atenolol-based regimen (**Figure 8-39**). Interestingly, these advantages of amlodipine-based therapy over atenolol disappeared in those patients not randomized to atorvastatin (148)!

The large ALLHAT study (52, 55) has already been alluded to (Figure 8-19). In that study, it was clear that amlodipine was less effective than the diuretic or ACEI in preventing heart failure and subsequent hospitalization, and this applied to both systolic (reduced ejection fraction) and diastolic (normal ejection fraction) varieties of heart failure (Figure 8-20) (53). In other respects, that is, reduction in the risk of stroke, coronary heart disease, and CVD, amlodipine was similar to the comparator drugs. Though calcium blockers are less effective than diuretics and ACEIs in preventing heart failure, they are associated with less heart failure compared to randomised placebo (151)"

As already indicated (124), a recent large meta-analysis has shown that, compared to ACEIs, calcium blockers appear more effective in preventing stroke (Figure 8-35) but less effective in preventing coronary heart disease (Figure 8-35a). However, BP was slightly lower in the amlodipine arm of the studies.

The VALUE study (130), where amlodipine was compared to valsartan, has already been referred to. The calcium blocker was significantly superior in reducing the risk of myocardial infarction, and there was a strong trend in stroke reduction with amlodipine (**Figure 8-40**). Others (149, 150) have confirmed this view. Similar studies, in Japanese hypertensives, showed no difference between valsartan and amlodipine (131, 132).

With coronary artery disease

In normotensive patients with coronary artery disease amlodipine, but not enalapril, differed significantly from placebo in reducing adverse CV events (152).

As already mentioned, in the INVEST study involving elderly patients with hypertension and coronary heart disease (79), verapamil and atenolol were similar in reducing CV events (Figure 8-27), although atenolol was superior in those with a history of heart failure.

F) α-Blockers

In the ALLHAT study, 42,448 elderly hypertensive subjects were recruited, with a view to a 6-year follow-up, but the doxazosin arm of the study was stopped prematurely due to an excess of risk relating to CV events, particularly heart failure, compared to chlorthalidone (153). There was a 25% greater incidence of combined CV outcomes, and the risk of heart failure was doubled, in those randomized to doxazosin versus chlorthalidone (154)

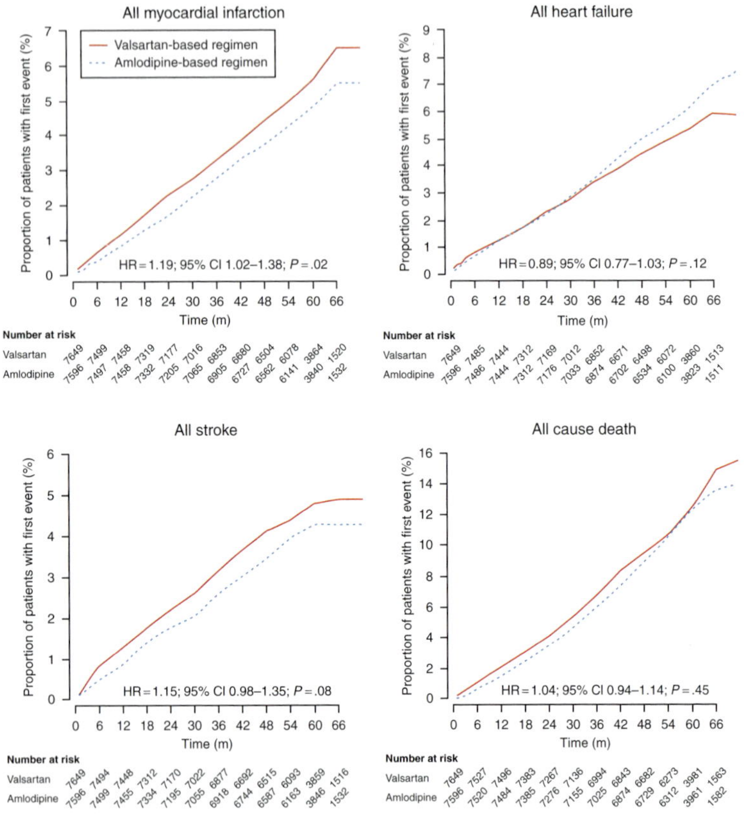

Fig. 8-40 VALUE study: in 15,245 high-risk elderly hypertensives, amlodipine was superior to valsartan in reducing the risk of stroke and MI. (From Julius S, Kjeldsen SE, Weber M, et al. Outcomes in hypertensive patients at high cardiovascular risk treated with regimens based on valsartan or amlodipine: the VALUE randomised trial. *Lancet* 2004;363:2022–31.)

G) Starting therapy with drug combinations

i) ACE/diuretic combination

The Action in Diabetes and Vascular Disease - PreterAx and DiamicroN MR Controlled Evaluation (ADVANCE) trial (155) was performed in 11,140 older hypertensives with type 2 diabetes, randomized to either placebo or a fixed-dose combination of perindopril and indapamide over a 4.3-year period. There were significant reductions in macrovascular and microvascular events (9%), CV death (18%), and all-cause death (14%) in the drug combination group; so that over 5 years, 1 death due to any cause would be averted among every 79 patients assigned to therapy. These benefits were greatest in those with renal dysfunction (156).

ii) ACE and diuretic or calcium blocker combination

The Avoiding Cardiovascular events through COMbination therapy in Patients Living with Systolic Hypertension trial (ACCOMPLISH) (157) involved 11,506 high-risk elderly hypertensives, randomized to either benazepril and amlodipine or benazepril and hydrochlorothiazide, over a 3-year period. The ACE/calcium blocker combination was clearly superior in reducing CV events (**Figure 8-41**).

iii) ACE/ARB combination

The ONTARGET study (13) has been referred to already. In that large study, in elderly mild hypertensives at high risk, randomized to ramipril, telmisartan, or the combination, however, the combination did not improve outcome, but adverse reactions such as syncope and renal dysfunction were increased.

iv) Calcium blocker plus β-blocker or ARB or diuretic

In a study of 3501 older Japanese hypertensives, patients were randomized to either calcium blocker (benidipine) and β-blocker, or ARB, or diuretic, over 3/6 years (158). All combinations were similar in preventing CV events, but prevention of stroke tended to be better on the calcium blocker/diuretic combination.

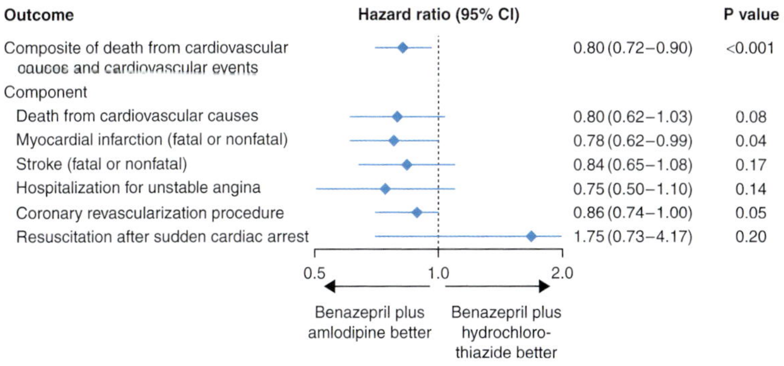

Fig. 8-41 ACCOMPLISH trial: in 11,506 high-risk elderly hypertensives, the combination of benazepril and amlodipine was superior to benazepril plus hydrochlorothiazide in reducing primary endpoints. (From Jamerson K, Weber MA, Bakris GL, et al (ACCOMPLISH trial investigators). Benazapril plus amlodipine or hydrochlorthiazide for hypertension in high-risk patients. *N Engl J Med* 2008;359:2417–28.)

v) What is the future for starting therapy with a fixed combination?

In a population-based study, involving 209,250 hypertensive patients aged 40–79 years (159), there was a clear advantage of starting with combination, versus monotherapy, in reducing CV endpoints (**Figure 8-42**).

As pointed out by Cruickshank (160), fixed-dose combinations minimize "pill burden," and drug compliance is accordingly improved, thus increasing the chance of achieving goal BP.

3. Some final thoughts

A) Patients with renal failure

Patients with chronic renal failure, even in the early phases, have high sympathetic nerve activity, as reflected in muscle, but not plasma noradrenaline or heart rate which increases as glomerular filtration rate (GFR) decreased (**Figure 8-43**). (161). High sympathetic nerve activity in chronic renal failure is a predictor of all-cause death and nonfatal CV events (162). Thus, it might have been predicted that drugs that suppress or antagonize sympathetic activity would benefit patients with renal failure in terms of prognosis. Such data are not, to date, available.

The African American Study of Kidney Disease and Hypertension study (163) in 1094 middle-aged African Americans with hypertensive renal disease addressed this issue. The aim was to compare

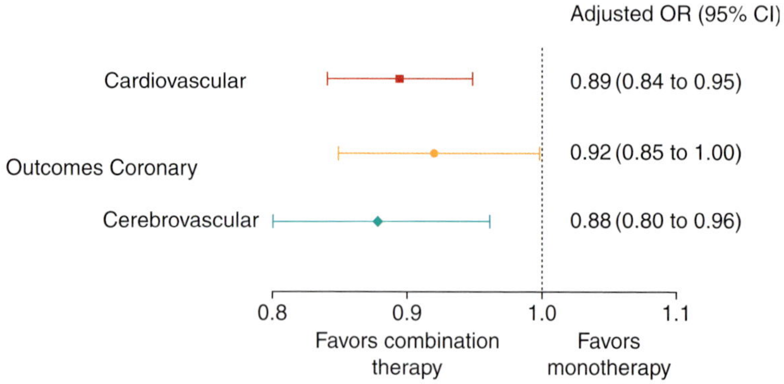

Fig. 8-42 Starting with combination therapy, compared to monotherapy, improves prognosis regarding cardiovascular, coronary, and cerebovascular outcomes. (From Corrao G, Nicotra F, Parodi A, et al. Cardiovascular protection by initial and subsequent combination of antihypertensive drugs in daily life practice. *Hypertension* 2011;58:566–72.)

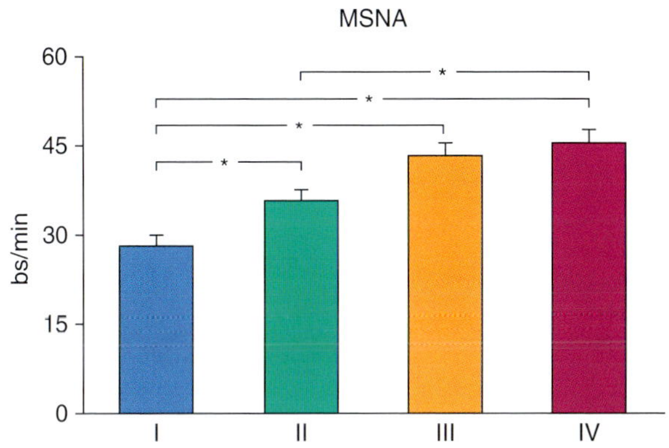

Fig. 8-43 In renal dysfunction, as GFR decreases, so muscle sympathetic nerve activity (MSNA) increases—I–IV represent quartiles of GFR. *statistical significance (From Grassi G, Quarti-Trevano F, Saravalle G, et al. Early sympathetic activation in the initial clinical stages of chronic renal failure. *Hypertension* 2011;57:846–51.)

the effects of two levels of BP control and three types of antihypertensive agent (β-blocker = metoprolol, ACEI = ramipril, and calcium blocker = amlodipine), on the decline of GFR over 3–6 years. The ACEI appeared more renoprotective, but no added benefit was observed at lower BPs. However, CV events (cardiac death, myocardial infarction, stroke, and heart failure) were not influenced by either the level of BP or the type of antihypertensive agent (164). Hyperkalemia was an occasional problem with the ACEI, decreased by diuretic therapy (165). In the 8- to 12-year follow-up cohort study, all patients were now put onto the ACEI ramipril, and the conclusion was that intensive lowering of BP did not benefit kidney disease progression unless, possibly, there was no baseline proteinuria (151).

In the RENAAL study (167), involving 1515 patients with type 2 diabetic nephropathy, patients were randomized to either placebo or the ARB losartan and followed up for 3.4 years. Losartan decreased the primary endpoint (increase in serum creatinine by 2 times, plus end-stage renal disease, plus death) by a significant 16%, but there was no effect on death rate.

In a meta-analysis of 1679 patients on dialysis (168), lowering BP by an average of 4.5/2.3 mm Hg resulted in a significant 29% reduction of both CV events and death (**Figure 8-44**), and a significant 20% reduction in all cause death. The conclusion was that renin–angiotensin system blockers, β-blockers, and calcium blockers were all suitable for use in patients on dialysis. Another meta-analysis

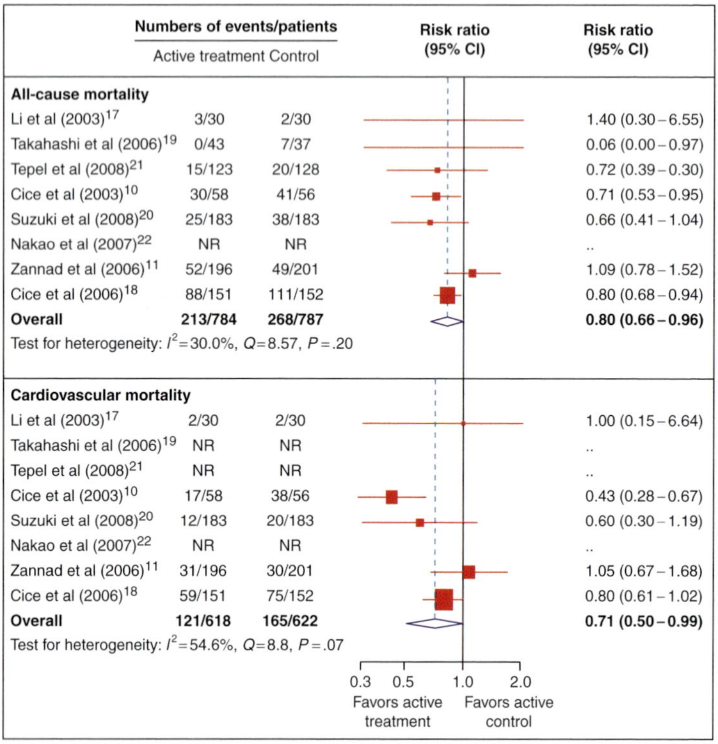

Fig. 8-44 In patients on dialysis, a treatment-induced fall of 4 5/2 3 4.5/2.3 mm Hg is linked to significant falls in all-cause and cardiovascular mortality. (From Heerspink HJ, Ninomiya T, Zoungas S, et al. Effect of lowering blood pressure on cardiovascular events and mortality in patients on dialysis: a systematic review and meta-analysis of randomised controlled trials. *Lancet* 2009;373:1009–15.)

(169) suggested that dialysis patients with high BP have the most to gain from antihypertensive therapy, with possible advantages for blockers of the renin–angiotensin system and β-blockers.

B) The age factor and β-blockers—chronological or biological age?

As indicated earlier, in young, middle-aged diastolic hypertensives, where sympathetic drive is high and β receptors are sensitized, it is clear that first-line β-blockade, versus placebo or diuretic therapy, is beneficial in terms of CV endpoint reduction (at least in nonsmokers on nonselective or only moderately β-1 selective, β-blockers) (Figure 8-23) (42, 67–69, 70); likewise, atenolol was at least as good as ACE inhibition in reducing primary endpoints (Figure 8-24) and superior in preventing all-cause death (Figure 8-25). The reverse is true in the elderly systolic hypertensive (without coronary heart disease), where β-receptors are internalized and desensitized (Table 8-4) (48, 75–77).

Tables 8.3 and 8.4 illustrate the above 8 studies in terms of mean age and pulse-pressures (P-Ps). It is tempting to conclude that hypertensive patients younger than 60 years should be suitable for first-line β-blocker, and the reverse for those older than 60 years. But what about the patient aged 60 years, or aged 59 with an imminent birthday? It all seems so arbitrary when dealing with chronological age. Would it be more sensible to deal with biological age?; aging/stiffening of the arterial system is reflected in P-P. So, would it be appropriate to conclude that a patient, whatever age, with a P-P of less than, or equal to, 65 mm Hg (reflecting relatively young arteries) should be considered for first-line β-blockade; and those with a P-P greater than 70 mm Hg should be candidates for first-line diuretic or calcium blocker: P-Ps between 66 and 69 mm Hg would require clinical judgment, for example, a resting heart rate of 90 bpm + P-P = 67 mm Hg, might be best suited to a β-blocker.

Having started a β-blocker, should it be stopped when the patient's age exceeds 60 years? The simple answer is no, the β-blocker should be continued. The classic example of this is the UKPDS study (Figure 8-24) (69), and its 20-year follow-up (Figure 8-25) (71). It is clear that, after 9–10 years of follow-up, the benefits of the β-blocker over the ACEI occur when the average age of the patients is now 65 years. Moreover, in those allocated to intensive treatment with either ACEI or β-blocker, the P-P has been reduced by 4–5 mm Hg compared to a small increase in the less-intensive treatment group (**Table 8-5**). At 20 years follow-up, when the average age of the patients is now 75 years, the advantage of β-blocker therapy over ACEI is now significant in terms of 23% fewer all-cause deaths.

C) Are drug-induced metabolic changes dangerous?

Observational studies over a 4- to 17-year period conclude that drug-induced diabetes increases the risk of a CV event to a degree intermediate between naturally occurring type 2 diabetes and those without diabetes (170, 171, 172).

TABLE 8-5 Effect of treatment with atenolol or captopril vs. less tight control of BP over 9 years, on P-P in the UK PDS study

	Age (y)		Baseline	After 9 y treatment
			56	65
P-P (mm Hg)	Less Tight BP Control		66	67
	Tight BP Control	Atenolol	66	62
		Captopril	66	61

Abbreviations: P-P, pulse pressure; BP, blood pressure.

However, randomized, controlled studies strongly suggest that drug-induced diabetes is not harmful to patients. Two studies involving ARBs versus randomized non-ARB (173) or placebo (96) over 4–5 years showed that although type 2 diabetes was less common in the ARB group, there was an excess of CV deaths.

The ALLHAT study (174) concluded that new-onset diabetes associated with chlorthalidone does not increase CVD outcomes. In that same study (175), the trends favoring chlorthalidone over lisinopril in those without the metabolic syndrome strengthened to significance in the case of heart failure and CVD prevention, in those with the metabolic syndrome (**Figure 8-45**).

Long-term, controlled studies over 14–20 years confirm that drug-induced diabetes, or increases in blood sugar, are not harmful. In the UKPDS study (54a), in spite of atenolol-induced increases in HbA1-c, after 9- to 10-year follow-up, the trends in the reduction of all 7 primary endpoints favored atenolol over captopril (Figure 8-24), and at 20 years of follow-up (55), the trends persisted, but now there was a significant 23% reduction in all-cause deaths in those originally randomized to atenolol (Figure 8-25). Perhaps, even more persuasive are the results of the mean 14.3-year follow-up of the SHEP study (176), where chlorthalidone (second-line atenolol), compared to randomized placebo, was associated with improved outcomes (Figure 8-17), particularly in those with diabetes. Strikingly, subjects who had diabetes associated with chlorthalidone therapy had no significant increase in CV events and had a better prognosis than did those with preexisting diabetes, or who developed naturally occurring diabetes while on placebo (**Figure 8-46**).

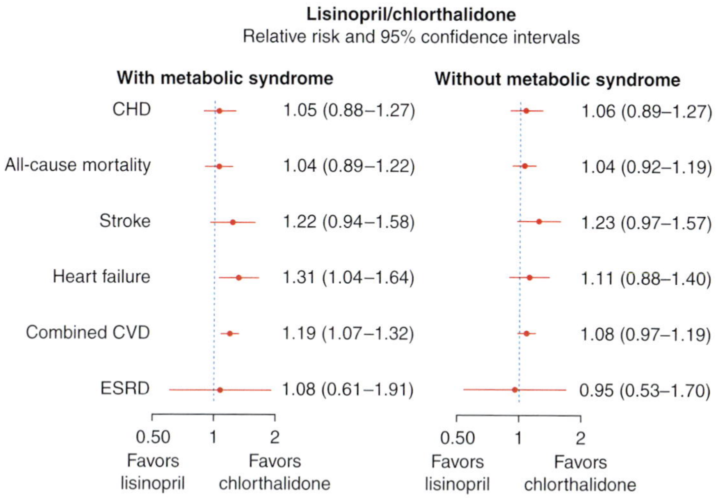

Fig. 8-45 ALLHAT, $n = 33{,}357$—chlorthalidone ± atenolol was at least equivalent to lisinopril-based therapy in reducing CV end-points in both MS and non-MS elderly hypertensives. (From Black HR, Davis B, Barzilay J, et al. Metabolic and clinical outcomes in nondiabetic individuals with the metabolic syndrome assigned to chlorthalidone, amlodipine or lisinopril as initial treatment for hyertension (ALLHAT). *Diabet Care* 2008;31:353–60.)

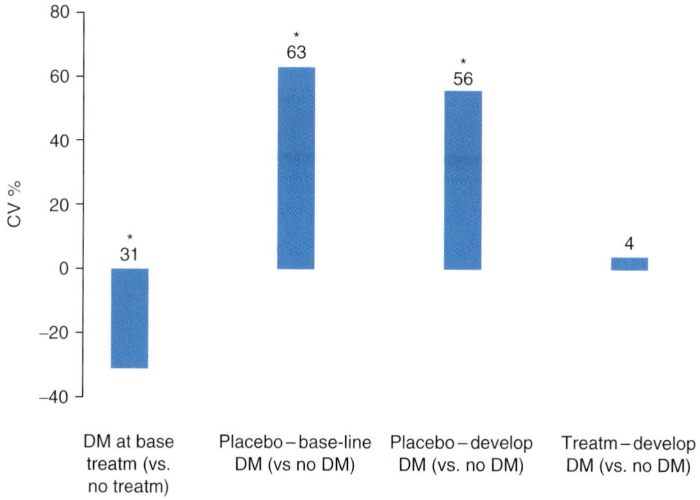

Fig. 8-46 SHEP and induced vs. natural type 2 diabetes over 14+ years—effect on CV death (%).

D) Patients' responses to risk information and the benefits of treating mild hypertension

Many patients may prefer not to take treatment for mild hypertension, if the personal risks were fully explained (177). A study in General Practice involved patients with mild hypertension and an age and sex matched group of patients with hypertension who were given a questionnaire relating to a mythical disease "SPF 2" (which actually was mild hypertension). The risk data relating to "SPF-2" were taken from the results of the MRC Mild Hypertension study (35). The questionnaire is illustrated in **Table 8-6**, and the patients' responses are given in **Table 8-7**. It is readily apparent that a patients' wish to be treated depended heavily on how the question was framed, ranging from 92% acceptance associated with "relative-risk reduction" information, to 44% acceptance associated with "personal probability of benefit" information.

The above publication certainly influenced one GP regarding her approach to treating very old hypertensives! (178).

TABLE 8-6 Risk framing questions to patients with mild hypertension in general practice

Now imagine your doctor discovered that you suffered from "SPF 2." Please tick the answer that is closest to how you would react:

1. Would you take the pills described above if they reduced your risk of having a stroke by 45%? (*risk reduction model*)
2. What if you were unlikely to have a stroke, so that it worked out that in a year you would have only a 1 in 400 chance of having a stroke, but the pills could reduce this to a 1 in 700 change? Would you take the pills? (*absolute risk reduction model*)
3. If the doctor had to treat 35 patients for 25 years in order to prevent one stroke, do you think it would be worth taking the treatment for yourself? (*number needed to teat model*)
4. If the tablets had a 3% chance of doing you good by preventing a stroke and a 97% chance of doing no good or not being needed in your case would you take them? (*personal probability of benefit from treatment model*)

From Misselbrook D, Armstrong D. Patients' responses to risk information about the benefits of treating hypertension. *Brit J Gen Pract* 2001;51:276–9.

TABLE 8-7 Responses from patients to the questionnaire in Table 8-6

Would you take treatment?	Relative risk reduction (%)	Absolute risk reduction (%)	Number needed to treat (%)	Personal probability of benefit (%)
Definitely	180 (65)	129 (47)	96 (35)	50 (18)
Maybe	75 (27)	79 (29)	92 (33)	71 (26)
Probably not	14 (5)	46 (17)	63 (23)	91 (33)
Definitely not	7 (3)	22 (8)	25 (9)	64 (23)
Proportion accepting treatment (95% confidence interval)	92% (89%–96%)	95% (70%–80%)	68% (63%–74%)	44% (38%–50%)

From Misselbrook D, Armstrong D. Patients' responses to risk information about the benefits of treating hypertension. *Brit J Gen Pract* 2001;51:276–9.

SUMMARY AND CONCLUSIONS

1. In uncomplicated hypertension, a 5–6 mm Hg reduction in DBP results in an approximate 40% reduction in stroke risk and about 15% reduction in myocardial infarction (MI); in high-risk hypertensives with diabetes, stroke reduction increases with the magnitude of BP reduction, but not so MI; lowering DBP of elderly patients with isolated systolic hypertension (ISH) may actually increase the risk of stroke and MI.
2. How far should SBP be lowered?—there is no convincing evidence to date, which suggests that treated SBP less than 140 mm Hg prevents CV events and saves lives; in high-risk electro-cardiograph (ECG-LVH) older hypertensives (LIFE study), treated SBP of less than 135 mm Hg might be associated with an increased risk of all-cause death.
3. There is a J-curve relationship between treated DBP and myocardial infarction, but not stroke, in hypertensive patients with CHD; retrospective data suggest a J-point at about 84–5 mm Hg (below which the risk of MI increases), a value supported by prospective data from the 3000 hypertensives with CHD in the

HOT study; similarly for SBP, the J-point in high-risk patients with CHD ± diabetes, or LVH, is about 130–5 mm Hg.

4. Low-sodium diets reduce BP, but there is a debate as to whether the risk of CV events will be reduced (plasma renin and noradrenaline levels are increased); only a large, prospective hard endpoint study will answer this question.
5. Diuretics—(a) In young/middle-aged hypertensives (younger than 60 years), thiazide diuretic therapy (vs. placebos) reduces stroke risk by 40%–50% but does not reduce (and may increase) the risk of MI: compared to β-blockers (nonselective or only moderately β-1 selective), diuretics are inferior in reducing the risk of MI in nonsmokers; possibly relevant is the fact that diuretics increase sympathetic nerve activity in younger patients with sensitized β-receptors; (b) in elderly systolic hypertensives (stiff vessels plus desensitized β-receptors), diuretics (vs. placebo) reduce the risk of both stroke and MI by 30%–40%; and, compared to calcium blocker or ACEI therapy, are as effective in reducing stroke and MI risk, but superior in preventing heart failure; compared to β-blockers (atenolol), diuretic therapy is superior in reducing the risk of both stroke and MI; and (c) typical diuretics, like hydrochlorothiazide, may be inferior antihypertensive agents compared to chlorthalidone or indapamide; diuretic-induced hypokalemia is associated with increases in blood sugar; diuretics reduce the risk of bone fracture.
6. β-blockers—(a) In young/middle-aged hypertensives without coronary heart disease, nonselective/poorly selective β-blockers (propranolol, oxprenolol, and metoprolol) are superior to placebo in reducing both stroke and MI in nonsmokers (but not in smokers) and are superior to diuretics in reducing MI in nonsmokers (but not in smokers); the perception that BBs do not effectively reduce stroke risk is wrong; in young/middle-aged nonsmokers, compared to placebo, propranolol reduced stroke risk by 54%, that is, the same as diuretics; the "β-blocker/smoker/adrenaline/hypertensive response" interaction can be avoided by high β-1 selectivity, for example, bisoprolol; in the one and only ACEI-β-blocker comparison (UKPDS study), atenolol was at least as good as captopril in reducing all 7 primary endpoints versus less tight control of BP (including stroke, where atenolol reduced the risk by 50% vs. less tight control of BP) after 9–10 years, and at 20-year follow-up was significantly superior in reducing all-cause death; versus calcium blockers, atenolol was equivalent to lacidipine in reducing CV events,

but, highly β-1 selective bisoprolol was significantly superior to nifedipine in reducing the hard, primary composite endpoint, in hypertensives with coronary artery disease; (b) in elderly systolic hypertensives, first-line atenolol has proved inferior in reducing hard CV endpoints to placebo, calcium blockers, and ARBs, but equal to calcium blockers if IHD was also present; second-line β-blockade, to diuretic or calcium blocker therapy, performs well in reducing hard CV endpoints; (c) the smoking/adrenaline/hypertensive interaction, metabolic disturbance, bronchospasm, weight gain, and sexual dysfunction, associated with nonselective/poorly selective BBs, can be avoided by high β-1 selectivity, for example, bisoprolol; (d) β-blockers reduce the risk of bone fracture, and also prevent, and diminish the rates of progression of, several types of cancer."

7. ACEI—(a) In young/middle-aged hypertensives, ACEIs are superior to dihydropyridine calcium blockers in preventing fatal and non-fatal MI; in obese hypertensives with type-2 diabetes (UKPDS), all 7 trends in primary end-point reduction (vs. less-tight BP control) favored atenolol versus captopril, and at 20 year follow-up the β-blocker was significantly superior in reducing all-cause death; (b) In elderly hypertensives, the ACEI was superior to placebo in reducing CV end-points; compared to diuretic and calcium blockers, ACEIs were similar in preventing CV events, but inferior to the diuretic in preventing diastolic heart failure; it is possible that ACEI are more effective than calcium blockers in preventing MI, but less effective in preventing stroke; in the elderly, compared to ARBs, ACEIs are similar in reducing the composite end-point; (c) Meta-analysis reveals that ACEIs reduce all-cause mortality by a significant 10%, compared to zero-effect of ARBs."
8. ARBs—(a) in young/middle-aged pre-hypertensives with diabetes, olmesarten was inferior to placebo in preventing CV deaths, sudden death and MI; (b) In elderly hypertensives, compared to placebo in 2 studies, the ARB was not significantly superior in reducing CV events or composite end-points; compared to atenolol, losartan was superior in preventing all CV end-points except MI; ARBs and ACEIs have similar effects in reducing composite end-points; ARBs and calcium blockers have proved similar in preventing the primary end-point; and (c) There is an ongoing debate regarding ARBs and MI prevention; certainly in young/middle-aged subjects with diabetes, ARBs increase the risk of CV events; possibly relevant is that, in younger subjects, ARBs increase sympathetic nerve

activity; (d) a meta-analysis of randomised trials shows that, unlike ACEIs, ARBs do not reduce all-cause mortality."

9. Calcium blockers—(a) In young/middle-aged subjects without coronary heart disease, calcium blockers have proved similar to atenolol, but inferior to enalapril, in reducing CV end-points; in hypertensive subjects with coronary artery disease, nifedipine was significantly inferior to highly β-1 selective bisoprolol in reducing the primary composite end-point; of possible relevance is the fact that dihydropyridine calcium blockers increase sympathetic nerve activity; (b) In elderly hypertensives without coronary heart disease, compared to placebo, calcium blockers significantly reduce CV events; compared to conventional therapy (diuretic or β-blocker), calcium blockers were similar in reducing the primary end-point; compared to diuretic therapy, calcium blockers were similar in reducing CV events, but possibly better at reducing stroke-risk, but worse in preventing heart failure; compared to atenolol, the calcium blocker amlodipine was significantly superior in preventing CV events and type-2 diabetes; compared to ACEIs, calcium blockers are similar in reducing CV events, but possibly superior in stroke-prevention, and possibly less effective in preventing MI; compared to ARBs calcium blockers may be more effective in preventing stroke and MI; (c) In elderly patients with coronary heart disease, verapamil was similar to atenolol in reducing CV events, but inferior in patients with a history of heart failure.
10. Drug-combinations—(a) Compared to placebo, in elderly patients, the fixed combination of perindopril and indapamide was superior in preventing macro-, and micro-vascular events; (b) The combination of benazepril plus amlodipine was superior to the combination of benazepril plus hydrochlorothiazide, in reducing CV events; (c) The combination of ACEI/ARB was not superior to either component alone, in reducing CV events, but did increase adverse reactions; and (d) Combinations of calcium blocker plus β-blocker, or diuretic, or ARB, were similar in preventing CV events, with a possible advantage regarding the calcium blocker/diuretic combination.
11. In patients with hypertensive renal dysfunction, intensive lowering of BP was ineffective in reducing CV events and death, and there was no difference between ACEI, β blocker and calcium blocker; in patients with diabetic nephropathy, ARB (vs. placebo) slowed progression of renal disease, but had no effect on death rate; in patients on dialysis, a modest fall in BP with renin-angiotensin system blockers, β-blockers and

calcium blockers, significantly reduced CV events and death, all being suitable agents to use.

12. First-line β-blockers are most effective in reducing CV events in younger/middle-aged patients, but not in the elderly; age may be best assessed in terms of biological age (P-P), rather than chronological age; thus a P-P of less than 65 mm Hg (denoting relatively young arteries) might be suitable for first-line β-blocker.
13. Are drug induced (diuretic or β-blocker) metabolic changes dangerous? Probably not, but there are cost-effective implications.

REFERENCES

1. MacMahon S, Neal B, Rodgers A. Blood pressure lowering for the primary and secondary prevention of coronary and cerebrovascular disease. *Schweiz Med Wochenschr* 1995;125:2479–86.
2. Blood Pressure Lowering Treatment Trialist Group. Effects of different blood-pressure-lowering regimens on major cardiovascular events. *Lancet* 2003;362:1527–35.
3. Blood Pressue Lowering Treatment Trialists' Collaboration. Effect of different regimens to lower blood pressure on major cardiovascular events in older and hunger people. *BMJ* 2008;336:1121–3.
4. Turnbull F, Woodward M, Neal B, et al. Do men and women respond differently to blood pressure-lowering treatment? *Eur Heart J* 2008;29:2669–80
5. Reboldi G, Gentile G, Angeli F, et al. Effects of intensive blood pressure reductionon myocardial infarction and stroke in diabetes. *J Hypertens* 2011;29:1253–69.
6. Thompon AM, Hu T, Eshelbrenner CL, et al. Antihypertensive treatment and secondary prevention of cardiovascular disease events among persons without hypertension. *JAMA* 2011;305:913–22.
7. Delles C. Risk factors and target organ damage: is there a special case for pre-hypertension? *J Hypertens* 2008;26:2268–70.
8. Law MR, Morris JK, Wald NJ. Use of blood pressure lowering drugs in the prevention of cardiovascular disease: meta-analysis of 142 randomised trials in the context of expectations from prospective epidemiological studies. *BMJ* 2009;338:b665. doi:10.1136/bmj. b 1665.
9. Angeli F, Reboldi G, Verdecchia P. The lower the BP the better. *Hypertension* 2010;56:182–4.
10. Somes GW, Pahor M, Shorr RI, et al. The role of diastolic blood pressure when treating isolated systolic hypertension. *Arch Int Med* 1999;159:2004–9.
11. Ogihara T, Saruta T, Rakugi H, et al. Target blood pressure for treatment of isolated systolic hypertension in the elderly. *Hypertension* 2010;56:196–202.

12. Zhang Y, Zhang X, Liu L, et al. Is a systolic blood pressure target < 140mm Hg indicated in all hypertensives? Subgroup analyses of findings from the randomised FEVER trial. *Europ Heart J* 2011;32:1500–8.
13. The ONTARGET Investigators. Telmisartan, ramipril, or both in patients at high risk for vascular events. *N Engl J Med* 2008;358:1547–59.
14. The ACCORD Study Group. Effects of intensive blood-pressure control in type 2 diabetes mellitus. *N Engl J Med* 2010;362:1575–85.
15. Anderson TW. Re-examination of some of the Framingham blood pressure data. *Lancet* 1978;2:1139–41.
16. Stewart IM. Relation of reduction in pressure to first myocardial infarction in patients receiving treatment for severe hypertension. *Lancet* 1979;1:861–5.
17. Cruickshank JM, Thorp JM, Zacharias FJ. Benefits and potential harm of lowering high blood pressure. *Lancet* 1987;1:581–4.
18. D'Agostino RB, Belanger AJ, Kannel WB, Cruickshank JM. Relation of low diastolic blood pressure to coronary heart disease death in the presence of myocardial infarction: the Framingham Study. *BMJ* 1991;303:385–9.
19. Cruickshank JM. Coronary flow reserve and the J-curve relation between diastolic blood pressure and myocardial infarction. *BMJ* 1988;297:1227–30.
20. Klocke FJ. Measurements of coronary flow reserve: defining pathophysiology versus making decisions about patient care. *Circulation* 1987;76:1183–9.
21. Protogerou AD, Safar ME, Iaria P, et al. Diastolic blood pressure and mortality in the elderly with cardiovascular disease. *Hypertension* 2007;50:172–80.
22. Strandgaard S, Haunso S. Why does antihypertensive treatment prevent stroke but not myocardial infarction? *Lancet* 1987; 2:658–60.
23. Hansson L, Zancetti A, Carruthers SG, et al. Effects of intensive blood pressure lowering and low-dose aspirin in patients with hypertension: principal results of the Hypertension Optimal Treatment (HOT) randomised trial. *Lancet* 1998;351:1755–62.
24. Cruickshank JM. Antihypertensive treatment and the J-curve. *Cardiovascular Drugs Ther* 2000;14:373–9.
25. Messerli FH, Mancia G, Conti R, et al. Dogma disputed: can aggressively lowering blood pressure in hypertensives with coronary artery disease be dangerous? *Ann Int Med* 2006;144:884–93.
26. Rothwell PM, Howard SC, Spence JD. Relationship between blood pressure and stroke risk in patients with symptomatic corotid occlusive disease. *Stroke* 2003;34:2583–92.
27. Bangalore S, Messerli FH, Wun C-C, et al. J-curve revisited: an analysis of blood pressure and cardiovascular events in the Treating to new Targets (TNT) Trial. *Eur Heart J* 2010;31:2897–908.

28. Sleight P, Redon J, Verdecchia P, et al. Prognostic value of blood pressure in patients with high vascular risk in the ongoing Telmisartan Alone and in combination with Ramipril Global End-point Trial study (ONTARGET). *J Hypertens* 2009;27:1360–9.
29. Cooper-Dehoff RM, Gong Y, Handberg EM, et al. Tight blood pressure control and cardiovascular outcomes among hypertensive patients with diabetes and coronary artery disease. *JAMA* 2010;304:61–8.
30. Dorresteijn JA, van der Graaf Y, Spiering W, et al. Relation between blood pressure nd vascular events and mortaliy in patients with manifest vascular disease. J-curve revisited. *Hypertension* 2012;59:14–21.
31. Okin PM, Hille DA, Kjeldsen SE, et al. Impact of lower achieved blood pressure on outcomes in hypertensive patients. *J Hypertens* 2012;30:802–10.
32. Robertson JI. Dietary salt and hypertension: a scientific issue or a matter of faith? *J Evaluat Clin Pract* 2003;9(1):2003.
33. Tikellis C, Pickering RJ, Tsorotes MC, et al. Activation of the renin-angiotensin system mediates the effects of dietry salt intake on atherogenesis in the apolipoprotein E knockout mouse. *Hypertension* 2012;60:98–105.
34. Cook NR, Cutler JA, Obarzanek E, et al. Long term effects of dietary sodium restriction on cardiovascular outcomes: TOHP. *BMJ* 2007;334:885–8.
35. He FJ, MacGregor GA. Salt reduction lowers cardiovascular risk: a meta-analysis of outcome trials. *Lancet* 2011;378:380–2.
36. Alderman MH. Reducing dietary sodium. The case for caution. *JAMA* 2010;303:448–9.
37. Alderman MH, Cohen H, Madhaven S. Dietary sodium intake and mortality: the National Health and Nutrition Examination Survey (NHANES I). *Lancet* 1998;351:781–5.
38. Stolarz-Skrzypek K, Kuznetsova T, Thijs L, et al. Fatal and non-fatal outcomes, incidence of hypertension, and blood pressure changes in relation to urinary sodium excretion. *JAMA* 2011;305:1777–85.
39. O'Donnel MJ, Yusuf S, Mente A, et al. Urinary sodium and potassium excretion and risk of cardiovascular disease risk. *JAMA* 2011;306:2229–38.
40. Whelton PK. Uriary sodium and cardiovascular disease risk. *JAMA* 2011;306:2262–4.
41. Report by the Management Committee. The Australian therapeutic trial in mild hypertension. *Lancet* 1980;1:1261–7.
42. Medial Research Working Party. MRC trial of treatment of mild hypertension: principal results. *BMJ* 1985;291:97–104.
43. Miall WE, Greenberg G. *Mild Hypertension–Is There Pressure to Treat?* Cambridge: Cambridge University Press; 1987, p 80.

44. Leren P, Helgeland A. Coronary heart disease and the treatment of hypertension. Some Oslo Study Data. *Am J Med* 1986;80:3–6.
45. SHEP Cooperative Research. Prevention of stroke by antihypertensive drug treatment in older persons with isolated systolic hypertension: final results of the Systolic Hypertension in the Elderly Program (SHEP). *JAMA* 1991;265:3255–64.
46. Kostis JB, Davis B, Cutler J, et al. Prevention of heart failure by antihypertensive drug treatment on older persons with isolated systolic hypertensdion. *JAMA* 1997;278:212–6.
47. Kostis JB, Cabrera J, Cheng JQ, et al. Association between chlorthalidone treatment of systolic hypertension and long-term survivial. *JAMA* 2011;306:2588–93.
48. MRC Working Party. Medical Research Council trial of hypertension in older adults: principal results. *BMJ* 1992;304:405–12.
49. Beckett NS, Peters R, Fletcher AE, et al. Treatment of hypertension in patients 80 years of age or older. *N Engl J Med* 2008;358: 1887–98.
50. Beckett N, Peters R, Tuomilehto J, et al. Immediate and late benefits of treating very elderly people with hypertension: HYVET Study. *BMJ* 2012;343:16.
51. Brown MJ, Palmer CR, Castaigne A, et al. Morbidity and mortality in patients randomised to double-blind treatment with long-acting calcium channel blocker or diuretic in the international Nifedipine GITS study: INSIGHT. *Lancet* 2000;356:366–72.
52. The ALLHAT Officers and Coordinators for the ALLHAT Collaborative Research Group. Major outcomes in high-risk hypertensive patients randomised to angiotensin-converting enzyme inhibitor or calcium channel blocker vs diuretic. *JAMA* 2002;288:2981–97.
53. Davis BR, Kostis JB, Simpson LM, et al. Heart failure with preserved and reduced left ventricular ejection fraction in the antihypertensive and lipid-lowering treatment to prevent heart attack trial. *Circulation* 2008;118:2259–67.
54. Piller LB, Baraniuk S, Simpson LM, et al. Long-term follow-up of participants with heart failure in antihypertensive and Lipid and Lowering Treatment to Prevent heart Attack Trial (ALLHAT). *Circulation* 2011;124:1811–8.
55. Wright JT, Dunn JK, Cutler JA, et al. Outcomes in hypertensive black and non-black patients treated with chlorthalidone, amlodipine and lisinopril. *JAMA* 2005;293:1595–1608.
56. Wing LM, Reid CM, Ryan P, et al. A comparison of outcomes with angiotensin converting enzyme inhibitors and diuretics for hypertension in the elderly. *N Engl J Med* 2003;348:583–92.
57. Psaty BM, Lumley T, Furberg CD, et al. Health outcomes associated with various antihypertensive therapies used first-line agents. *JAMA* 2003;289:2534–44.

58. Badarin FJ, Abuannadi MA, Lavie CJ, et al. Evidence-base diuretic therapy for improving cardiovascular prognosis in systemic hypertension. *Am J Cardiol* 2011;107:1178–84.
59. Messerli FH, Bangalore S. Half a century of hydrochlorthiazide: facts, fads, fiction and follies. *Am J Med* 2011;124:896–9.
60. Alderman MH, Pillar LB, Ford CE, et al. Clinical significance of incident hypokalemia and hyperkalemia in treated hypertensive patients in the Antihypertensive and Lipid-Lowering Treatment to Prevent Heart Attack Trial. *Hypertension* 2012;59:926–33.
61. Kotchen TA. Antihypertensive therapy-associated hypokalemia and hyperkalemia. *Hypertension* 2012;59:906–7.
62. Stears AJ, Woods SH, Watts MA, et al. A double-blind, placebo-controlled, cross-over trial comparing the effects of amiloride and hydrochlorthiazide on glucose tolerance in patients with essential hypertension. *Hypertension* 2012;59:934–42.
63. Elliott WJ. Effects of potassium sparing versus thiazide diutetics on glucose tolerance. *Hypertension* 2012;59:911–2.
64. Rouch GC, Holford TR, Guddati AK. Chlorthalidone compared with hydrochlorthiazide in reducing cardiovascular events. Systematic review and network meta-analyses. *Hypertension* 2012;59:1110–17.
65. LaCroix AZ, Wienpahl J, White LR, et al. Thiazide diuretic agents and the incidence of hip fracture. *N Engl J Med* 1990;322:286–90.
66. Schoofs MW, van der Kleft M, Hofman A, et al. Thiazide diuretics and the risk for hip fracture. *Ann Int Med* 2003;139:I 36.
67. IPPPSH Collaborative Group. Cardiovascular risk and risk factors in a randomised trial of treatment –based on the beta-blocker oxprenolol. *J Hypertens* 1985;3:379–92.
68. Wikstrand J, Warnold T, Tuomilehto J, et al. Metoprolol versus diuretics in hypertention. Morbidity results from MAPHY Study. *Hypertension* 1991;17:579–88.
69. UK Prosepective Diabetes: UKPDS 39 Study Group. Efficacy of atenolol and captopril in reducing the risk of macrovascular and microvascular complications in type-2 diabetes. *BMJ* 1998;317:713–20.
70. JM Cruickshank. *The Modern Role of Beta-Blockers in Cardiovascular Medicine.* USA Shelton, Connecticut: People's Medical Publishing House—USA; 2012.
71. Holman RR, Paul SK, Bethel MA, et al. Long-term follow-up after tight control of blood pressure in type-2 diabetes. *N Engl J Med* 2008;359:1565–76.
72. Zanchetti A, Bond G, Hennig M, et al. Calcium antagonist lacidipine slows down progression of asymptomatic carotid atherosclerosis (ELSA). *Circulation* 2002;106:2422–7.
73. Heddblad B, Wikstrand J, Janzon L, et al. Low-dose metoprolol CR/XL and fluvastatin slow progression of carotid intima thickness. *Circulation* 2001;103:1721–6.

74. von Arnim T, for TIBBS Investigators. Prognostic significance of transient ischaemic episodes: response to treatment shows improved prognosis results of the TIBBS follow-up. *J Am Coll Cardiol* 1995;25:231–8.
75. Coope J, Warrender TS. Randomised trial of treatment of hypertension in primary care (HEP). *BMJ* 1986;293:1145–51.
76. Kjeldsen SE, Dahlof B, Devereux RB, et al. Effect of losartan on cardiovascular morbidity and mortality in patients with isolated hypertension and left-ventricular hypertrophy. *JAMA* 2002;288:1491–8.
77. Dahlof B, Sever P, Poulter N, et al. Prevention of cardiovascular events with an antihypertensive regimen of amlodipine adding peridopril as required versus atenolol adding bendroflumethazide as required (ASCOT-BPLA); a multicentre randomised controlled trial. *Lancet* 2005;366:895–906.
78. JM Cruickshank. Are we misunderstanding beta-blockers? *Int J Cardiol* 2007;120:10–27.
79. Pepine CJ, Handberg EM, Cooper-Dehoff RM, et al. A calcium antagonist vs non-calcium antagonist hypertension treatment strategy for patients with coronary artery disease (INVEST). *JAMA* 2003;290:2805–16.
80. Bangalore S, Messerli FH, Cohen JD, et al. Verapamil-sustained release-based treatment strategy is equivalent to atenolol-based treatment strategy at reducing cardiovascular events in patients with prior myocardial infarction (INVEST). *Am Heart J* 2008;156:241–7.
81. Schlienger RG, Kraenzlin ME, Jick SS, et al. Use of beta-blockers and risk of fractures. *JAMA* 2004;292:1326–32.
82. Short PM, Lipworth SI, Elder DH, et al. Effect of beta-blockers in treatment of chronic obstructive pulmonary disease: a retrospective cohort study. *BMJ* 2011;342:1068.
83. Kazani S, Israel E. Treatment with beta-blockers in people with COPD. *BMJ* 2011;342:1037–8.
84. Smith C, Teitler M. Beta-bloocker selectivity at cloned human beta-1 and beta-2 adrenergic receptors. *Cardiovasc Drugs Ther* 1999;13:123–6.
85. Cryer PE, Hammond MW, Satiago JV, et al. Norepinephrine and epinephrine release and adrenergic mediation of smoking-associated hemodynamic and metabolic events. *N Engl J Med* 1976;295:573–7.
86. Hering D, Kucharska W, Kara T, et al. Smoking is associated with chronic sympathetic activation in hypertension. *Blood Pressure* 2010;19:152–5.
87. Tarnow J, Muller RK. Cardiovascular effects of low-dose epinephrine infusions in relation to the extent of pre-operative beta-blockade. *Anaesthesiology* 1991;74:1035–43.
88. Carlberg B, Samuelsson O, Lindholm LH. Atenolol in hypertension: is it a wise choice? *Lancet* 2004;364:1684–9.

89. Aronow WS. Current role of beta-blockers in the treatment of hypertension. *Experts Opin Pharmacother* 2010;11:2599–607.
90. Blackburn DF, Lamb DA, Eurich DT, et al. Atenolol as initial antihypertensive therapy: an observational study comparing first-line agents. *J Hypertens* 2007;25:1499–505.
91. Messerli FH, Grossman E, Goldbourt U. Are beta-blockers efficacious as first-line therapy for hypertension in the elderly. A systematic review. *JAMA* 1998;279:1903–7.
92. Lindholm LH, Carlberg B, Samuelsson O. Should beta-blockers remain the first choice in the treatment of primary hypertension? A meta-analysis. *Lancet* 2005;366:1545–53.
93. Opie LH. Beta-blockade should not be among several choices for initial therapy of hypertension. *J Hypertens* 2008;26:161–3.
94. Beevers DG. The end of beta-blockers for uncomplicated Hypertension? *Lancet* 2005;366:1510–12.
95. Williams B. Beta-blockers and the treatment of hypertension. *J Hypertens* 2007;25:1351–3.
96. Kaplan NM. Beta-blockers in hypertension. Adding insult to injury. *JACC* 2008;52:1490–1.
97. Cutler JA, Davis BR. Should beta-blockers and diuretics remain as first-line therapy for hypertension? *Circulation* 2008;117:2691–705.
98. Ram CV. Beta-blockers in hypertension. *Am J Cardiol* 2010;106:1819–25.
99. Kraus T, Lovibond K, Caufield M, et al. Management of hypertension: summary of NICE guidance. *BMJ* 2011;343:474–6.
100. Cruickshank JM. Don't beta-blockers still have a role in hypertension? *BMJ* 2011;343:759.
101. Williams B, Krause T, Lovibond K, et al. Authors reply. *BMJ* 2011;343:760.
102. Khan N, MacAlister FA. Re-examining the efficacy of beta-blockers for the treatment of hypertension: a meta-analysis. *Canadian MAJ* 2006;174:1737–42.
103. Kubo T, Azevedo ER, Newton GE, et al. Lack of evidence for peripheral alpha-1 adrenoceptor blockade during long-term treatment of heart failure with carvedilol. *J Am Coll Cardiol* 2001;38:1463–9.
104. Kukin ML, Kalman J, Mannino M, et al. Combined alpha-beta-blockade (doxazosin plus metoprolol) compared with beta-blockade alone in chronic heart failure. *Am J Cardiol* 1996;77:486–91.
105. Desch CE, Magorien RD, Triffon DW, et al. Development of failure. *Am J Cardiol* 1979;44:1179–82.
106. Flather MD, Shibata MC, Coats AJ, et al. Randomised trial to determine the effects of nebivolol on mortality and cardiovascular hospital admissions in elderly patients with heart failure (SENIORS). *Eur Heart J* 2005;26:215–25.
107. Schulman SP, Becker LC, Kass DA, et al. L-arginine therapy in acute myocardial infarction: the Vascular Interaction with Age in

Myocardial Infarction (VINTAGE MI) randomised clinical trial. *JAMA* 2006;295:58–64.
108. Fitzgerald PJ. Beta-blockers, norepinephrine, and cancer: an epidemiological viewpoint. *Clin Epidemiol* 2012;4:151–6.
109. Cole SW, Sood AK. Molecular pathways: beta-adrenergic signaling in cancer. *Clin Cancer Res* 2012;18:1201–6.
110. Cakir Y, Plummer HK 3rd, Titof PK, et al. Beta-adrenergic and arachidonic acid-mediated growth regulation of human breast cancer cell lines. *Int J Oncol* 2002;21:153–7.
111. Melhem-Bertrandt A, Chavez-Macgregor M, Lei X, et al. Beta-blocker use is associated with improved elapse-free survival in patients with triple-negative breast cancer. *J Clin Oncol* 2011;29:2645–52.
112. De Giorgi V, Gandini S, Grazzini M, et al. Beta-blockers: a new and emerging treatment for melanoma. *Recenti Prog Med* 2012;103: 11–16.
113. Al-Wadei HA, Al-Wadei MH, Schuller HM. Cooperative regulation of non-small cell lung carcinoma by nicotinic and beta-adrenergic receeptors: a novel target for intervention. *PLoS One* 2012;7:e29915.
114. Zhang D, Ma QY, Hu HT, et al. Beta-2 adrenergic antagonists suppress pancreatic cancer cell invasion by inhibiting CREB, NFkB and AP-1. *Cancer Biol Ther* 2010;10:19–29.
115. Perron L, Bairati I, Harel F, et al. Antihypertensive drug use and the risk of prostate cancer (Canada). *Cancer Causes Control* 2004;15:535–41.
116. Grytli HH, Fagerland MW, Fossa SD, et al. Use of beta-blockers is associated with prostate cancer-specific survival in prostate cancer patients on adrogen deprivation therapy. *Prostate* 2012;Jul 20. doi: 10. 1002/pros. 22564.
117. Estacio RO, Jeffers BW, Hiatt WR, et al. The effect of nisoldipine as compared with enalapril on cardiovascular outcomes in patients with non-insulin-dependent diabetes and hypertension. *N Engl J Med* 1998;338:645–52.
118. Hansson L, Lindholm LH, Niskanen L, et al. Effect of angiotensin-converting-enzyme inhibition compared with conventional therapy on cardiovascular morbidity and mortality in hypertension: the Captopril Prevention Project (CAPP) randomised trial. *Lancet* 1999;353:611–6.
119. The Heart Outcomes Prevention Evaluation Study Investigators. Effects of an angiotensin-converting-enzyme inhibitor, ramipril, on cardiovascular events in high risk patients. *N Engl J Med* 2000;342:145–53.
120. Heart Outcomes Prevention Evaluation (HOPE) Study Investigators. Effects of ramipril on cardiovascular and microvascular outcomes in people with diabetes mellitus: results of the HOPE Study and MICRO – HOPE Substudy. *Lancet* 2000;355:253–9.
121. HOPE/HOPE-TOO Study Investigators. Long-term effects of ramipril on cardiovascular events and on diabetes. *Circulation* 2005;112:1339–46.

122. The European trial on reduction of cardiac events with Perindopril in stable coronary artery disease investigators. Efficacy of perindopril in reduction of cardiovascular events among patients with stable coronary artery disease (EUROPA). *Lancet* 2003;362:782–8.
123. Wennberg R, Zimmermann C. The PROGRESS trial three years later: time for a balanced report of effectiveness. *BMJ* 2004;329:968–71.
124. Verdecchia P, Reboldi G, Angeli F, et al. Angiotensin-converting enzyme inhibitors and calcium channel blockers for coronary artery disease and stroke prevention. *Hypertension* 2005;46:386–92.
125. Imai E, Chan JC, Yamasaki T, et al. Effects of olmesartan on renal and cardiovascular outcomes in type-2 diabetes with overt nephropathy: a multicentre, randomised, placebo-controlled study. *Diabetologia* 2011;54:2978–86.
126. Haller H, Ito S, Izzo JL, et al. Olmesartan for the delay or prevention of microalbuminuria in type-2 diabetes. *N Engl J Med* 2011;364:907–17.
127. Staessen JA, Wang J-G, Birkenhager WH. Outcome beyond blood pressure control? *Eur Heart J* 2003;24:504–14.
128. The Telmisartan Randomised AssessmeNt study in ACEinNtolerant subjects with cardiovascular Disease (TRANSCEND) Investigators. Effects of the angiotensin receptor blocker telmisartan on cardiovascular events in high-risk patients intolerant to angiotensin-converting enzyme inhibitors: a randomised controlled trial. *Lancet* 2008;372:1174–83.
129. The NAVIGATIOR Study Group. Effect of valsartan on the incidence of diabetes and cardiovascular events. *N Engl J Med* 2010;362:1477–90.
130. Julius S, Kjeldsen SE, Weber M, et al. Outcomes in hypertensive patients at high cardiovascular risk treated with regimens based on valsartan or amlodipine: the VALUE randomised trial. *Lancet* 2004;363:2022–31.
131. Narumi H, Takano H, Shindo S, et al. Effects of valsartan and amlodipine on cardiorenal protection in Japanese hypertensive patients: the Valsartan Amlodipine Randomised Trial. *Hypertens Res* 2011;34:62–9.
132. Muramatsu T, Matsushita K, Yamaskita K, et al. Comparison between valsartan and amlodipine regarding cardiovascular morbity and mortality in hypertensive patients with gglucose intolerance. *Hypertension* 2012;59:580–6.
133. Kasanuki H, Hagiwara N, Hosoda S, et al. Angiotensin 11 receptor blocker-based vs non-angiotensin 11 receptor blocker-based therapy in patients with angiographically documented coronary artery disease and hypertension. *Eur Heart J* 2009;30:1203–12.
134. Mochizuki S, Dahlof B, Shimizu M, et al. Valsartan in Japanese population with hypertension and other cardiovascular disease (Jikei Heart Study). *Lancet* 2007;369:1431–9.
135. Yusuf S, Diener H-C, Sacco RL, et al. Telmisatan to prevent recurrent stroke and cardiovascular events. *N Engl J Med* 2008;359:1225–37.

136. Sanset EC, Bath PM, Boysen G, et al. The angiotensin-receptor blocker candesartan for treatment of acute stroke (SCAST): a randomised, placebo-controlled double-blind trial. *Lancet* 2011;377:741–50.
137. Gerc V, Buksa M, Loza V, et al. Is aliskiren superior to inhibitors of angiotensin-converting enzyme and angiotensin receptor blockers in renin-angiotensin system blockade? *Med Arch* 2009;63:343–9.
138. Reboldi G, Angeli F, Cavallini C, et al. Comparison between angiotensin-converting enzyme inhibitors and angiotensin receptor blockers on the risk of myocardial infarction, stroke and death: a meta-analysis. *J Hypertens* 2008;26:1282–9.
139. Volpe M, Tocci G, Sciaretta S, et al. Angiotensin II receptor blockers and myocardial infarction: an updated analysis of randomised clinical trials. *J Hypertens* 2009;27:941–6.
140. Verma S, Strauss M. Angiotensin receptor blockers and myocardial infarction. *BMJ* 2004;329:1248–9.
141. Stauss MH, Hall AS. Angiotensin receptor blockers may increase risk of myocardial infarction. *Circulation* 2006;114:838–54.
142. Stauss MH, Hall A. Renin-angiotensin system and cardiovascular talk. *Lancet* 2007;370:23–4.
143. Messerli FH, Bangalore S, Rushitzka F, et al. Angiotensin receptor blockers: baseline therapy in hypertension? *Eur Heart J* 2009;30:2427–30.
144. Van Varic LC, Bertrand M, Aldcerhuis KM, et al. Angiotensin-converting enzyme inhibitors reduce mortality in hypertension: a meta-analysis of randomised clinical trials of renin-angiotensin-aldosterone inhibitors involving 158,998 patients. *Eur Heart J* 2012;33:2088–97.
145. Staessen JA, Fagard R, Thijs L, et al. Randomised double-blind comparison of placebo and active treatment for older patients with isolated systolic hypertension. The Syst-Eur Trial Investigators. *Lancet* 1997;350:757–64.
146. Hansson L, Hedner T, Lund-Johansen P, et al. Randomised trial of effects of calcium antagonists compared with diuretics and beta-blockers on cardiovascular morbidity and mortality in hypertension: the Nordic Diltiazem (NORDIL) Study. *Lancet* 2000;356:359–65.
147. Black HR, Elliot WJ, Grandits G, et al. Principal results of the Controlled Onset Verapamil Investigation of Cardiovascular End Points (CONVINCE) trial. *JAMA* 2003;289:2073–82.
148. McInnes. What is the true place of blood pressure in cardiovascular risk management? *J Hypertesn* 2007;25:925–8.
149. Staessen JA, Wang J-G, Thijs L. Cardiovascular protection and blood pressure reduction: a meta-analysis. *Lancet* 2001;358:1305–15.
150. Messerli FH, Staessen JA. Safety of calcium antagonists: More ACTION. *Am J Med* 2005;118:1418–20.

151. Costanzo P, Perrone-Filardi P, Petretta M, et al. Calcium channel blockers and cardiovascular outcomes: a meta-analysis of 175, 634 patients. *J Hypertens* 2009;27:1136–51.
152. Nissen SE, Tuzcu EM, Libby P, et al. Effect of antihypertensive agents on cardiovascular events in patients with coronary artery disease and normal blood pressure. *JAMA* 2004;292:2217–26.
153. The ALLHAT Officers and coordinators. Major cardiovascular events in hypertensive patients randomised to doxazosin vs chorthalidone. *JAMA* 2000;283:1967–75.
154. Furberg CD, Psaty BM, Pahor M, et al. Clinical implications of recent findings from the Antihypertensive and Lipid-Lowering Treatment to Prevent Heart Attack Trial (ALLHAT) and other studies of hypertension. *Ann Intern Med* 2001;135:1074–8.
155. ADVANCE Collaborative Group. Effects of a fixed combination of perindopril and indapamide on macrovascular and microvascular outcomes in patients with type-2 diabetes mellitus (the ADVANCE trial): a randomised controlled trial. *Lancet* 2007;370:829–40.
156. Heerspink HJ, Ninomiya T, Perkovic V, et al. Effects of a fixed combination of perindopril and indapamide in patients with type-2 diabetes and chronic kidney disease. *Eur Heart J* 2010;31: 2888–96.
157. Jamerson K, Weber MA, Bakris GL, et al (ACCOMPLISH trial investigators). Benazapril plus amlodipine or hydrochlorthiazide for hypertension in high-risk patients. *N Engl J Med* 2008;359: 2417–28.
158. Matsuzaki M, Ogihara T, Umemoto S, et al. Prevention of cardiovascular events with calcium channel blocker-based combination thera pies in patients with hypertension a: a randomised controlled trial. *J Hypertens* 2011;29:1649–59.
159. Corrao G, Nicotra F, Parodi A, et al. Cardiovascular protection by initial and subsequent combination of antihypertensive drugs in daily life practice. *Hypertension* 2011;58:566–72.
160. Cruickshank JM. Combining beta-blockers and calcium channel blockers in the management of hypertension. *Prim Care Cardiovasc J* 2012;5(suppl 1):S13–18. Doi: 10.3132/pccj.2011.084.
161. Grassi G, Quarti-Trevano F, Saravalle G, et al. Early sympathetic activation in the initial clinical stages of chronic renal failure. *Hypertension* 2011;57:846–51.
162. Penne EL, Neumann J, Klein IH, et al. Sympathetic hyperactivity and clinical outcome in chronic kidney disease patients during standard treatment. *J Nephrol* 2009;22:208–15.
163. Wright JT, Bakris G, Green T, et al. Effect of blood pressure lowering with antihypertensive anti-hypertensive drug class on progression of hypertensive kidney disease: results from the AASK Trial. *JAMA* 2002;288:2421–31.

164. Norris K, Bourgoigne J, Gassman J, et al. Cardiovascular outcomes in the African American Study of Kidney Disease and Hypertension (AASK) Trial. *Am J Kidney Dis* 2006;48:739–51.
165. Weinberg JM, Appel LJ, Bakris G, et al. Risk of hyperkalaemia in non-diabetic patients with chronic kidney disease receiving antihypertensive therapy. *Arch Intern Med* 2009;169:1587–94.
166. Appel LJ, Wright JT, Greene T, et al. Intensive blood pressure control in hypertensive chronic kidney disease (AASK). *N Engl J Med* 2010;363:918–29.
167. Brenner BM, Cooper ME, de Zeeuw D, et al (RENAAL Investigators). Effects of losartan on renal and cardiovascular outcomes in patients with type 2 diabetes and nephropathy. *N Engl J Med* 2001;345: 861–9.
168. Heerspink HJ, Ninomiya T, Zoungas S, et al. Effect of lowering blood pressure on cardiovascular events and mortality in patients on dialysis: a systematic review and meta-analysis of randomised controlled trials. *Lancet* 2009;373:1009–15.
169. Agarwal R, Sinha AD. Cardiovascular protection with antihypertensive drugs in dialysis patients. Systematic review and meta-analysis. *Hypertension* 2009;53:860–6.
170. Verdecchia P, Reboldi G, Angeli F, et al. Adverse prognostic significance of new diabetes in treated hypertensive subjects. *Hypertension* 2004;43:963–9.
171. Aksnes TA, Kjeldsen SE, Rostrup M, et al. Impact of new diabetes mellitus on cardiac outcomes in the valsartan antihypertensive long-term use evaluation (VALUE) trial population. *Hypertension* 2007;50:467–73.
172. Dunder K, Lind L, Zethelius B, et al. Increase in blood glucose concentration during antihypertensive treatment as a predictor of myocardial infarction: a population based cohort study. *BMJ* 2003;326: 681–4.
173. Kasanuki H, Hagiwara N, Hosoda S, et al. Angiotensin II receptor blockade vs non-angiotensin receptor blocker-based therapy in patients with angiographically documated coronary artery disease and hypertension (HIJ-CREATE). *Eur Heart J* 2009;30: 1203–12.
174. ALLHAT findings revisited in the context of subsequent analysis, other trials and meta-analyses. *Arch Intern Med* 2009;169:832–42.
175. Black HR, Davis B, Barzilay J, et al. Metabolic and clinical outcomes in nondiabetic individuals with the metabolic syndrome assigned to chlorthalidone, amlodipine or lisinopril as initial treatment for hyertension (ALLHAT). *Diabet Care* 2008;31:353–60.
176. Kostis JB, Wilson AC, Freudenberger RS, et al. Long-term effect of diuretic-based therapy on fatal outcomes in subjects with isolated

systolic hypertension with and without diabetes. *Am J Cardiol* 2005;95:29–35.

177. Misselbrook D, Armstrong D. Patients' responses to risk information about the benefits of treating hypertension. *Brit J Gen Pract* 2001;51:276–9.
178. Polak L. Offer treatment as part of shared decision making. *BMJ* 2012;344:32.

Hypertension and the Heart Rate Factor

CHAPTER 9

INTRODUCTION

1. Animal kingdom

The importance of heart rate and longevity throughout the whole animal kingdom cannot be overemphasized. A study of birds and nonhibernating mammals showed a linear relationship between the resting heart rate and longevity (**Figure 9-1**) (1). The only species to fall off the predicted line for longevity was man, whose predicted life span was about 30 years. Interestingly, the average life span of a stone-age man was about 30 years! It is presumed that life span is predetermined by the basic energetics of living cells, with heart rate being a marker of metabolic rate, particularly within the heart (2). The fact that the life span of modern, westernized men and women is about 80 years is surely a mark of improved living standards and medical advances.

Certainly, in humans, increased heart rates via artificial pacing increase the myocardial oxygen consumption by 55% in normal hearts and 70% in the hearts of patients with coronary artery disease (CHD) (**Figure 9-2**) (3). Thus, in patients with CHD with high heart rates, there are 2 factors that threaten to compromise the myocardium: (1) reduced diastolic time for adequate blood supply to the myocardium and (2) increased myocardial oxygen consumption. The result is a mismatch between the oxygen demand and supply, thereby resulting in ischemia and possible angina.

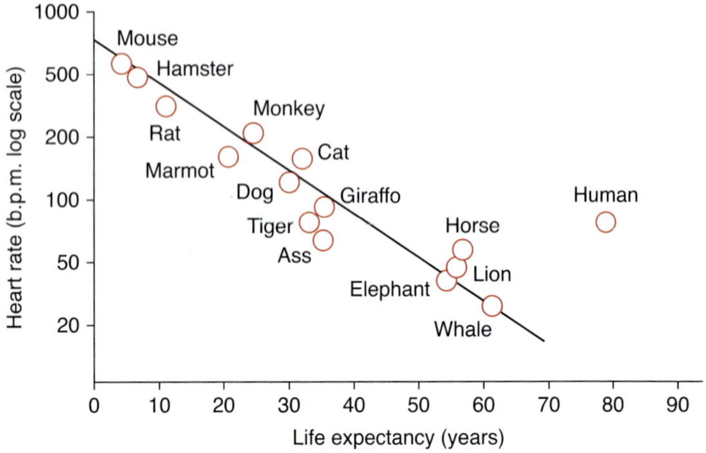

Fig. 9-1 Resting heart rate and life expectancy in mammals and man. (From Livingstone SD, Kueha LA. Similarity in the number of lifespan heart beats among non-hibernating, homeothermic animals. *Aviat, Space, Environ Med* 1979;50:1037–9.)

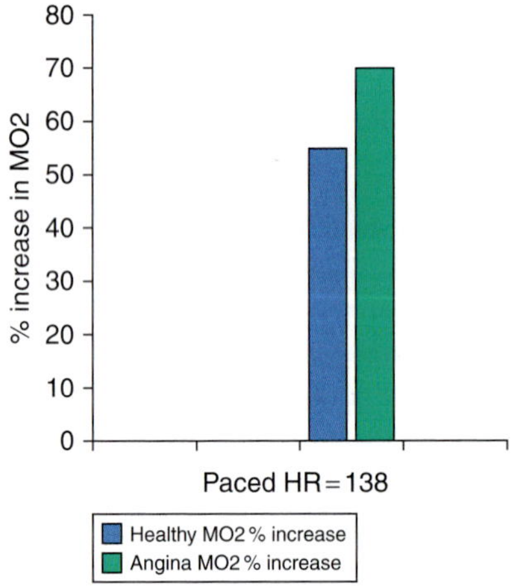

Fig. 9-2 In middle-aged men, healthy or with angina, from resting heart rate of 61 bpm, paced heart rate up to 138 bpm increased myocardial oxygen requirement (MO2) by 55%–70% (via increased coronary flow). (From Kaijser L, Berglund B. Coronary haemodynamics during isometiric handgrip and atrial pacing in patients with angina pectoris compared to healthy men. *Cardioscience* 1993;4:99–104.)

2. Heart rate as a predictor of hypertension

A high heart rate has been shown to precede arterial stiffness (4), and also the development of hypertension up to 6 years later (5). Undoubtedly, the high heart rate is a reflection of underlying

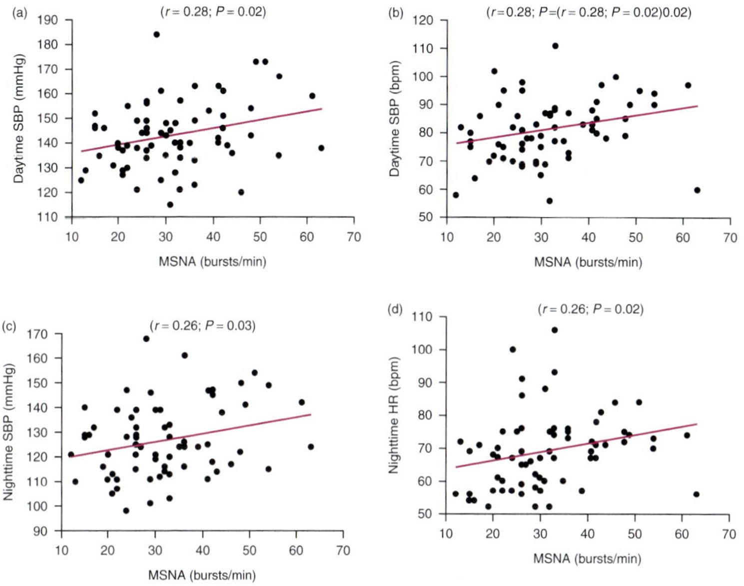

Fig. 9-3 In young/middle-aged hypertensives, high sympathetic nerve activity muscle sympathetic nerve activity (MSNA) is related to an increase in BP and heart rate. (From Hering D, Kucharska W, Kara T, et al. Resting sympathetic outflow does not predict the morning blood pressure surge in hypertension. *J Hypertens* 2011;29:2381–6.)

increased sympathetic nerve activity (6), both day and night (**Figure 9-3**) (7). Thus, high heart rates can be used as a convenient surrogate for increased sympathetic nerve activity (and/or reduced vagal tone). The relationship between the sympathetic nerve activity and the hypertension has been discussed in Chapter 4.

RESTING HEART RATE AND HEART RATE VARIABILITY AS PROGNOSTIC INDICATORS IN NONHYPERTENSIVE SUBJECTS

1. Normal population

One of the earliest studies that highlights the importance of high heart rates as a risk factor was the Chicago study, which showed a relationship between high heart rates and all-cause death and sudden coronary heart disease death (CHD) (**Figure 9-4**) (8). These results were confirmed by the Framingham Study after 30 years of follow-up (9), and applied equally to all ages, although the relationship between the

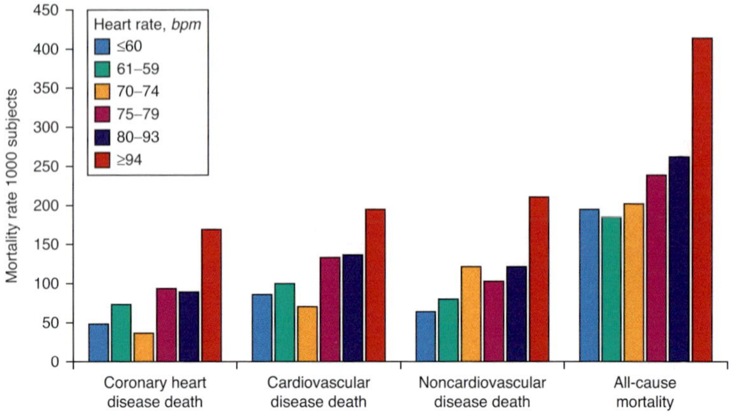

Fig. 9-4 Data from the Chicago People's Gas Company study showing the strong links between high resting heart rates and CHD, CVD, non-CVD deaths, and all-cause mortality. (From Dyer AR, et al., 1980.)

	Mean H. R,	
Age group	Male	Female
36–44	74.83	77.23
45–54	74.66	77.05
55–64	74.14	77.59
65–74	76.18	79.06
75–84	75.44	79.85

Fig. 9-5 The Framingham Study: effect of age upon resting heart rate (beats per minute) in men and women. (From Kannel WB, Kannel C, Paffenbarger RS, et al. Heart rate and cardiovascular mortality: the Framingham Study. *Am Heart J* 1987;119:1489–94.)

heart rate and the cardiovascular mortality was stronger in men than women, and the resting heart rates were higher in women than men. This study also showed that the resting heart rates remained relatively constant with increasing age in both men and women (**Figure 9-5**).

The Framingham results were confirmed by others (10–12), who also noted that there was no relationship between the resting heart rate and cancer (10).

In an 8-year follow-up of middle-aged men, a heart rate greater than 90 bpm was associated with an increased risk of cardiovascular death (13). The relationship of resting heart rate with cardiovascular and CHD deaths was more notable in men than women (14). Similarly, a change in resting heart rate over a 10-year period was significantly related to all-cause and ischemic heart disease mortality (15).

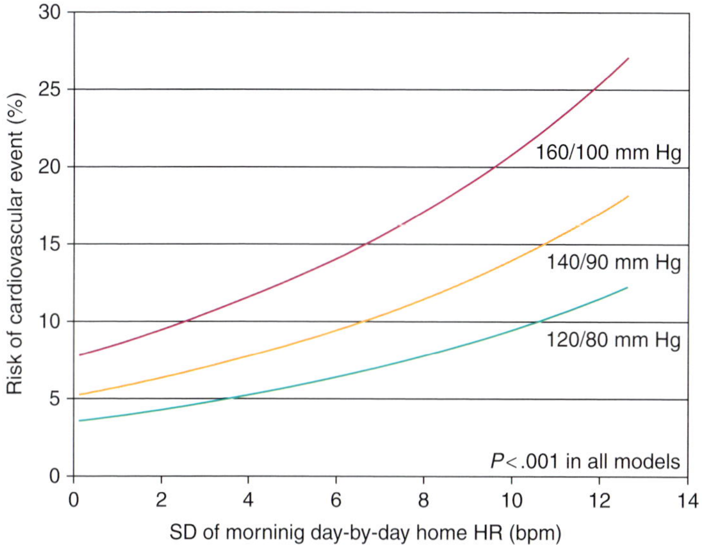

Fig. 9-5a Prognostic value of the variability standard deviation (SD) in morning home-measured heart rate. (From Johansson JK, Niiranen TJ, Puuka PJ, et al. Prognostic value of the variability in home-measured blood pressure and heart rate. The Finn-Home Study. *Hypertension* 2012;59:212–8.)

In middle-aged subjects, home-measured heart rate variability, in the morning, was a good predictor of cardiovascular events, particularly in subjects with higher blood pressures (BPs) (**Figure 9-5a**) (16).

2. Patients with stable coronary heart disease (CHD)

In 24,913 patients with suspected or proven CHD, followed up for 15 years, a high resting heart rate greater than 83 bpm was predictive of total and cardiovascular mortality, with optimal survival at heart rates less than 62 bpm (17). A similar situation pertained to patients with CHD and diabetes (**Figure 9-6**) (18).

3. Acute coronary syndromes

In 139,194 patients with non-ST segment elevation acute coronary syndromes, there was a J-shaped relationship between the resting heart rate and all-cause mortality, with heart rates less than 50 bpm being associated with increased mortality (whether or not a β-blocker was present) (**Figure 9-7**) (19).

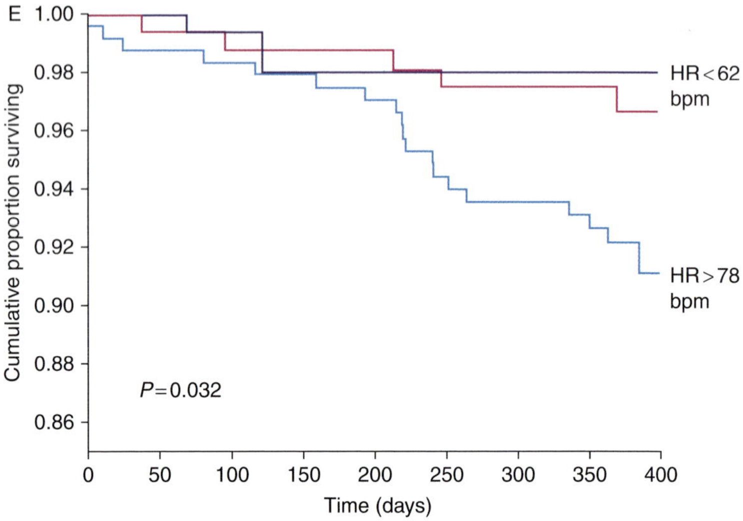

Fig. 9-6 High heart-rates are harmful in patients with stable CAD + diabetes. (From Anselmino M, Ohrvik J, Ryden L. Resting heart rate in patients with stable coronary artery disease and diabetes: a report from the Euro Heart Survey on Diabetes and the Heart. *Eur Heart J* 2010;31:3040–5.)

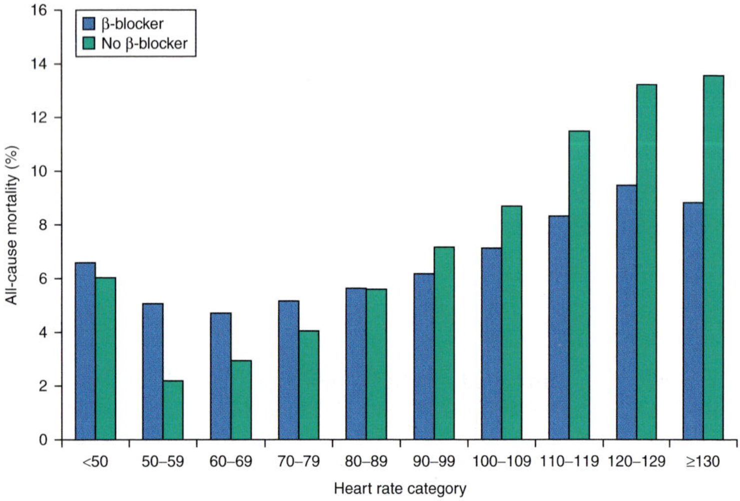

Fig. 9-7 CRUSADE: in $n = 139{,}194$ acute coronary syndrome (non-MI) cases, high and very low (<50 bpm) heart rates at presentation were linked to high all-cause mortality (in both BB and non-BB cases). (From Bangalore S, Messerli FH, Ou F-S, et al. The association of admission heart rate and in-hospital cardiovascular events in patients with non-ST-segment elevation acute coronary syndromes: CRUSADE. *Eur Heart J* 2010;31:552–60.)

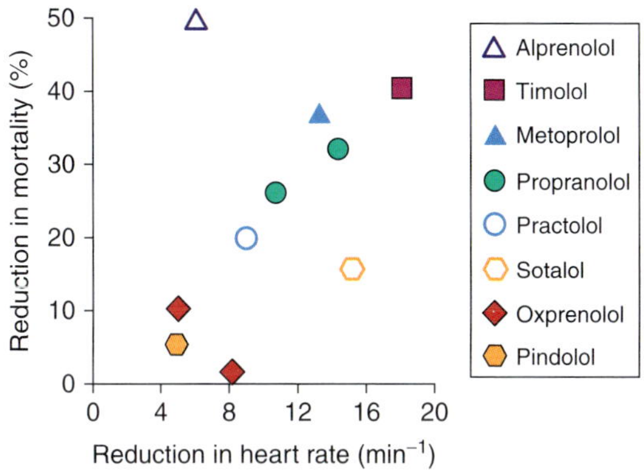

Fig. 9-7a β-Blockers and mortality in relation to reduction in heart rate in the post-MI period. (From Kjekshus J. Comments—beta-blockers: heart rate reduction a mechanism of benefit. *Eur Heart J* 1985;6(suppl A):29–30.)

4. Postmyocardial infarction

In predischarge patients with a myocardial infarction (MI), both 24-hour mean heart rate and heart rate variability were predictors of mortality over the next 2 years (20). In the postmyocardial infarction period, survival was closely related to the reduction of heart rate on β-blockers (**Figure 9-7a**) (21); notable was that β-blockers with intrinsic sympathomimetic activity (ISA), that is, pindolol and oxprenolol, were least effective in reducing both resting heart rate and mortality.

5. Patients with heart failure

In heart failure hard-endpoint studies, there is a clear relationship between change in heart rate and all-cause mortality (**Figure 9-8**) (22).

In placebo-controlled studies involving β-blockers, it is clear that β-blockers without ISA, that is bisoprolol, metoprolol, and carvedilol, lowered heart rate by 13–14 bpm and were associated with a highly significant 34%–35% reduction in all-cause mortality; whereas β-blockers with ISA, that is, xamoterol (β-1 ISA), bucindolol (β-2 ISA), and nebivolol (β-3 ISA), lowered heart rate to a lesser degree, and were associated with nonsignificant reductions (or increase in the case of xamoterol) in all-cause mortality (**Figure 9-9**) (23). A resting heart rate of 58–64 bpm is associated with the best prognosis (24).

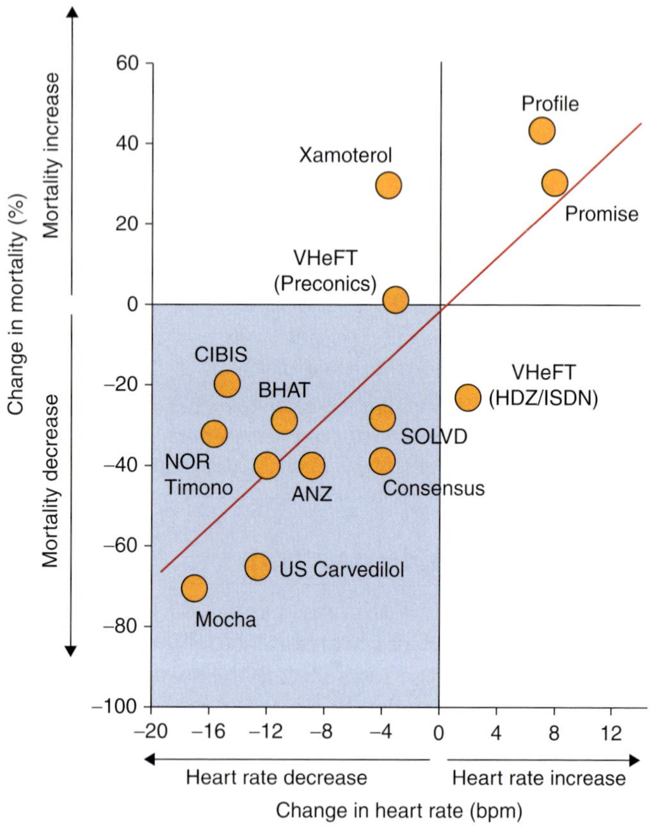

Fig. 9-8 Cardiovascular mortality in relation to changes in heart rate in chronic systolic heart failure. (From Cook S, Togni M, Schaub MC, et al. High heart rate: a cardiovascular risk factor? *Eur Heart J* 2006;27:2387–93.)

RESTING HEART RATE, OR HEART RATE VARIABILITY, AS A PROGNOSTIC INDICATOR IN PATIENTS WITH HYPERTENSION (OR PREHYPERTENSION)

1. Young/middle-aged patients with prehypertension

In 3275 middle-aged patients with prehypertension, followed up for 10 years, heart rates greater than 80 bpm were strong predictors of CHD (particularly in women) and all-cause death (25).

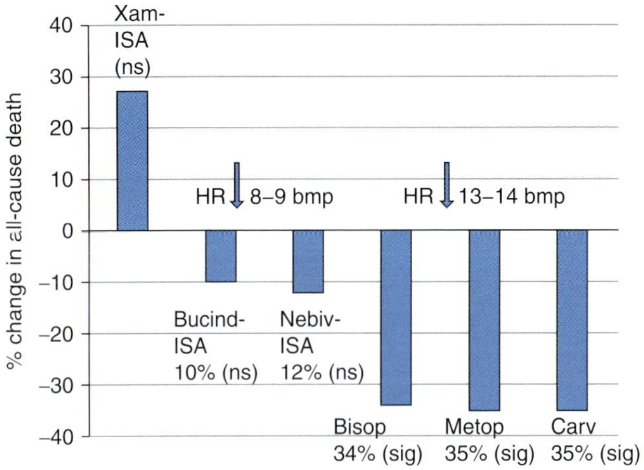

Fig. 9-9 β-Blockers and hard end-point placebo-controlled trials in heart failure; ISA reduces efficacy (all-cause death) and linked to a lesser fall in heart rate (HR). (From Cruickshank JM. *The Modern Role of Beta-Blockers in Cardiovascular Medicine*. Shelton, Connecticut: People's Medical Publishing House—USA; 2011:179.)

In middle-aged hypertensives, the Framingham Study showed that after 36-years of follow-up, high heart rates, particularly over 85 bpm, were closely linked to increased rates of all-cause death and cardiovascular and CHD events (26) in both men (**Figure 9-10**) and women (**Figure 9-11**). These findings have been confirmed by others for men, but not for women, independent of age (27).

A 17-year follow-up of middle-aged hypertensives revealed that an increase in the heart rate of 1 bpm was associated with a 1% increase in mortality, with the worst prognosis being with those whose heart rate had been increased by more than 5 bpm (28).

Undoubtedly, high heart rates in the middle-aged hypertensive are a reflection of high sympathetic nerve activity (**Figure 9-12**) (29). As discussed in Chapter 5, the study of Peng et al. in middle-aged hypertensives showed that high blood noradrenaline (NE) concentrations, independent of BP, were significantly linked to premature cardiovascular mortality (**Figure 9-13**), with increased β-receptor density and cyclic adenosine mono-phosphate (AMP) levels predicting MI, but not stroke (**Figure 9-14**).

2. Elderly hypertensive patients

High heart rates in the elderly hypertensive patients are associated with increased cardiovascular (CV) risk, but lesser than in younger

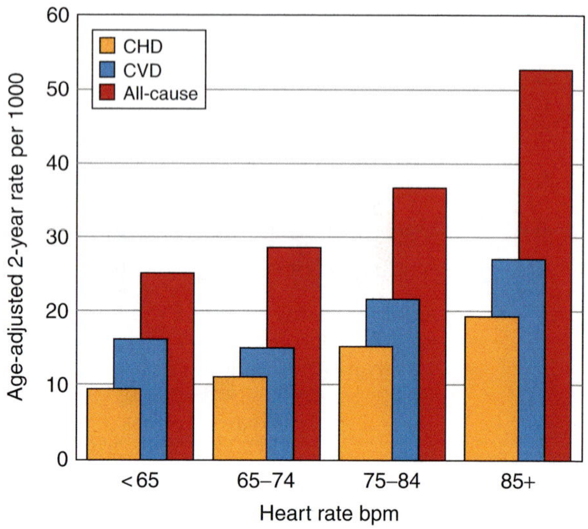

Fig. 9-10 Framingham: effect of resting heart rate on all-cause death, CHD, and CVD events in untreated male hypertensives, followed-up for 36 years. (From Gillman MW, Kannel WB, Belanger A, et al. Influence of heart rate on mortality among persons with hypertension: the Framingham Study. *Am Heart J* 1993;125:1148–54.)

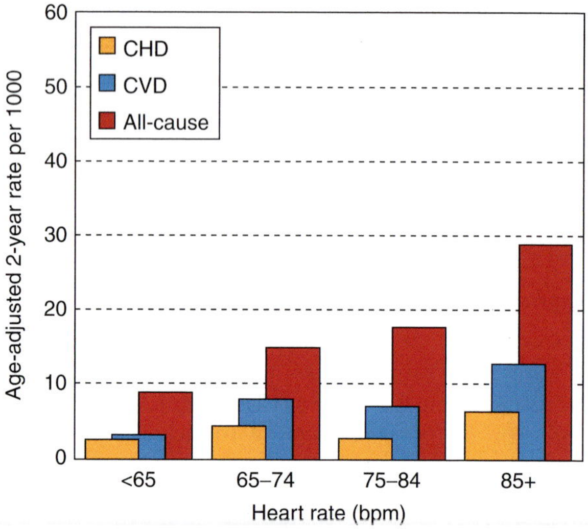

Fig. 9-11 Framingham: effect of resting heart rate on all-cause death, CHD, and CVD events in untreated female hypertensives, followed-up for 36 years. (From Gillman MW, Kannel WB, Belanger A, et al. Influence of heart rate on mortality among persons with hypertension: the Framingham Study. *Am Heart J* 1993;125:1148–54.)

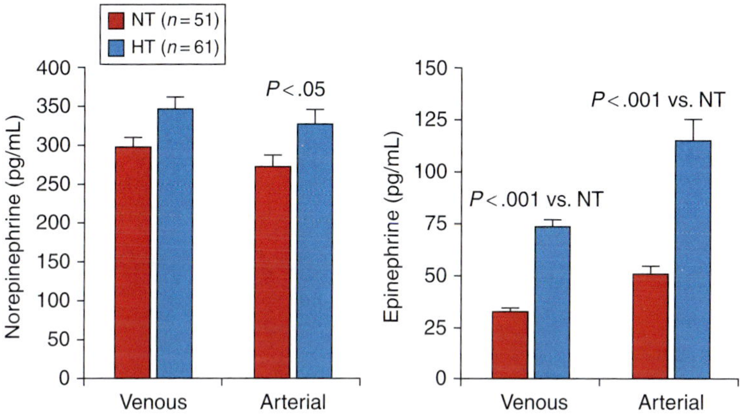

Fig. 9-12 In middle-aged male hypertensive subjects, there are significant increases in arterial NE and adrenaline. (From Trygve B et al., 2010.)

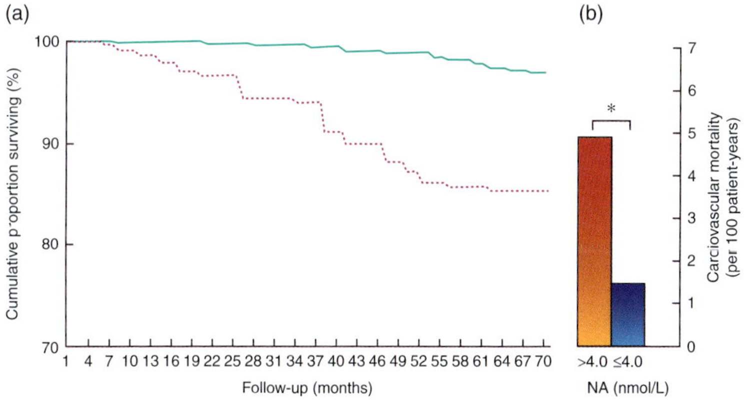

Fig. 9-13 Relationship between high (>4 nmol/L) and low (<4 nmol/L) plasma NE levels (independent of BP) and (A) survival and (B) cardiovascular mortality in middle-aged hypertensives. (From Peng Y-X et al., 2006.)

hypertensives (29). In the SYSTEUR trial (30), within the placebo (but not treated) group, the resting heart rates greater than 79 bpm predicted all-cause, cardiovascular, and noncardiovascular mortality (**Figure 9-15**). In the Systolic Hypertension in the Elderly Program (SHE) study (31), high resting heart rates also predicted an increased risk of cardiovascular death. In the INVEST study, involving elderly hypertensives with CHD, there was a mild J-shaped relationship between resting heart rate and adverse outcome incidence, with a J-point at 59 bpm (**Figure 9-16**) (32).

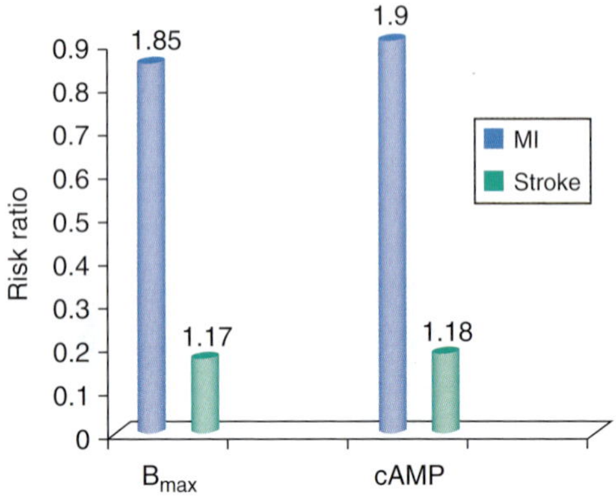

Fig. 9-14 β-receptor density (B_{max}) and cAMP levels (in lymphocytes) as predictors of MI and stroke in middle-aged hypertensives followed up for 7 years. (From Peng Y-X 2006.)

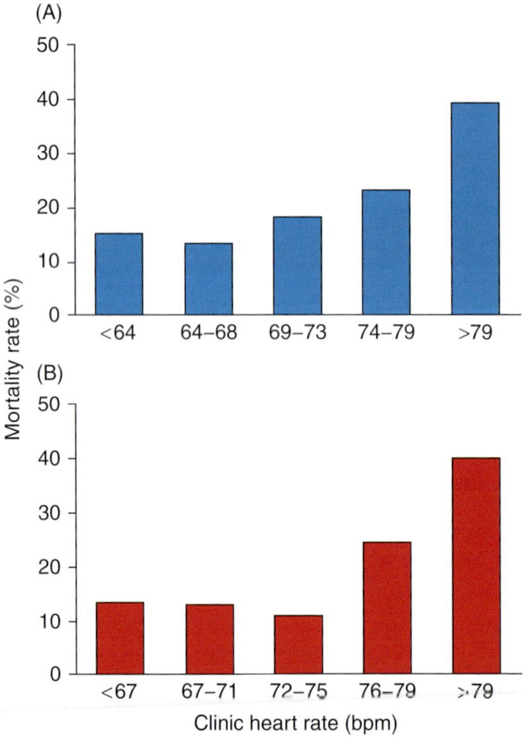

Fig. 9-15 In elderly hypertensives (SYSTEUR trial) on placebo high baseline, heart rate greater than 80 bpm were strong predictors of mortality in both (A) men and (B) women. (From Palatini P, Thijs L, Staessen JA, et al. Predictive value of clinic and ambulatory heart rate for mortality in elderly subjects with systolic hypertension. *Arch Intern Med* 2002;162:2313–21.)

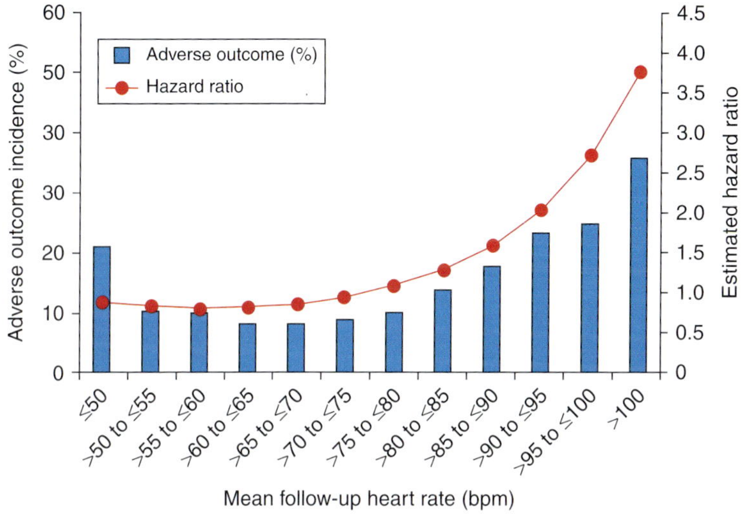

Fig. 9-16 In the INVEST trial of elderly systolic hypertensives with CHD, there was a slight J-curve relationship between follow-up resting heart rate and adverse outcomes and hazard ratio. (From Kolloch R, Legler UF, Champion A, et al. Impact of a resting heart rate on outcomes in hypertensive patients with coronary artery disease: INVEST. *Eur Heart J* 2008;29:1327–34.)

3. Heart rate and central pressures (in the elderly)

Slow paced heart rates are associated with increased central pressures (**Figure 9-17**) (34) and are linked with "timing synchronization" of the forward and backward traveling waves (35). A prolongation of the cardiac ejection phase, due to a lower heart rate, is associated with the higher augmentation of the peak SBP by the reflected wave, which is attributed to earlier systolic "timing" of the waves.

However, the ASCOT study in elderly hypertensives, comparing atenolol-based therapy with amlodipine-based therapy, revealed that the higher central pressures associated with β-blocker therapy were not due to slower heart rates but due to a greater magnitude of wave reflection (36). Hence, the magnitude of the reflected wave is less with vasodilation and is independent of heart rate.

Thus, although both atenolol and nebivolol were associated with central pressures greater than with placebo, the pressures with nebivolol (with vasodilatory β-3 ISA) were slightly lower than with atenolol (37).

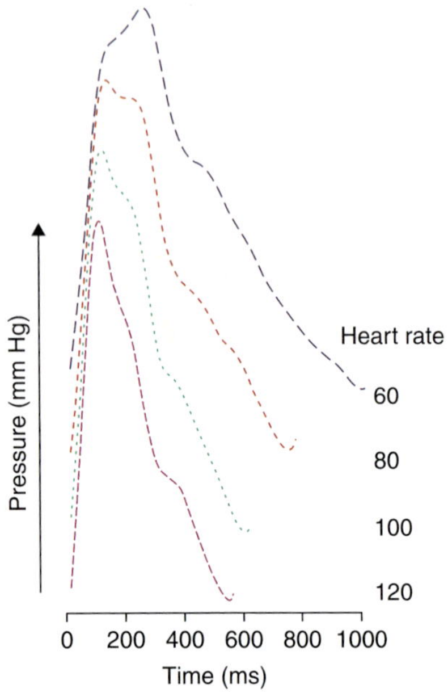

Fig. 9-17 High-paced heart rates were associated with decreased aortic pressures. (From Wilkinson IB, Mohammad NH, Tyrell S, et al. Heart rate dependency of pulse pressure amplification and arterial stiffness. *Am J Hypertens* 2002;15:24–30.)

HEART RATE AND THE VASCULAR SYSTEM

1. Vascular stiffness/compliance

Independent of BP, high heart rates were strongly related to reduced distension and increased pulse wave velocity in the carotid artery, thoracic aorta, and lower limbs of both normotensive and hypertensive subjects (38). Thus, high heart rates appear to accelerate the vascular aging process, as evidenced by increasing pulse wave velocity (**Figure 9-18**) (39). The increased load and oscillatory shear stress associated with high heart rates may impair the balance between synthesis and breakdown of collagen and elastin, thereby favoring collagen deposition and the resultant vascular stiffening (40).

2. The atheromatous process

The atheromatous process has already been addressed in Chapter 7. In brief, high heart rates and sympathetic nerve activity are involved in the atheromatous process, as well as in the development of the unstable plaque and its disruption. Areas of low endothelial shear stress, or oscillatory flow patterns, are linked to high levels of

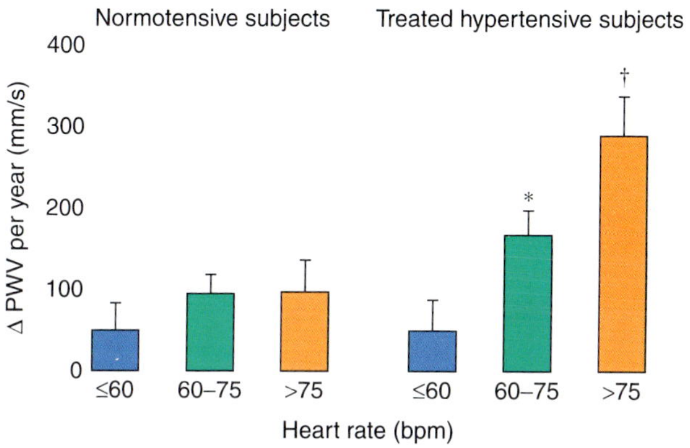

Fig. 9-18 High-resting heart rates accelerate vascular aging and speed up PWV. (From Benetos A, Adamopoulos C, Bureau J-M, et al. Determinants of accelerated progression of arterial stiffness in normotensive subjects and in treated hypertensive subjects over a 6-year period. *Circulation* 2002;105:1202–7.)

plaque formation; by contrast, laminar blood flow, associated with optimal endothelial shear stress and low heart rates, is linked to the absence of atheromatous plaque.

Coronary atheromatous plaque volume is regressed by β-blockers, partly via low heart rates. High heart rates and the absence of β-blockers are powerfully associated with the risk of plaque rupture.

IMPLICATIONS CONCERNING ANTIHYPERTENSIVE THERAPY

1. Young/middle-aged diastolic hypertension

As discussed in Chapter 4, young/middle-aged diastolic hypertension in both obese and normal-weight individuals is underpinned by increased sympathetic nerve activity. In Chapter 5, it was described how high plasma norepinephrine (noradrenaline) (NE) concentration, independent of BP, predicted premature cardiovascular events; and that high β-receptor density and cyclic AMP levels predicted MI, but not stroke. Thus, antihypertensive drugs increasing sympathetic nerve activity (and heart rate) may not be appropriate for preventing the number one killer, the MI.

High heart rates reflect increased plasma NE levels (**Figure 9-19**) (41). Which drug increases both heart rate and sympathetic nerve activity?

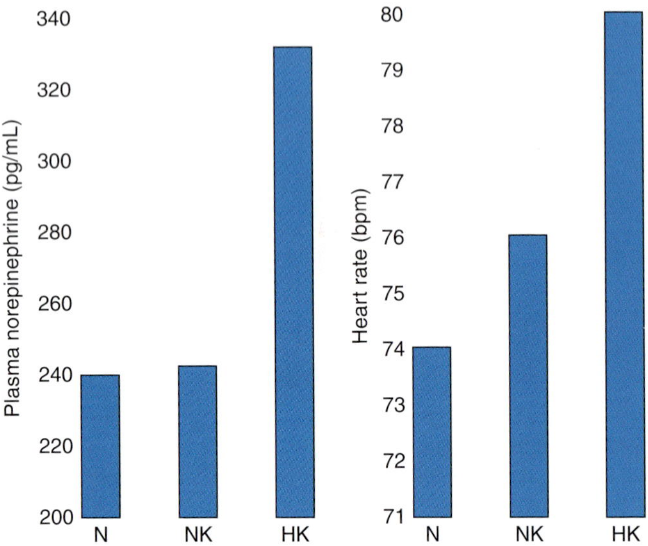

Fig. 9-19 In the Tecumseh study, resting heart rates in hyperkinetic hypertension (HK) and to a lesser extent normokinetic hypertension (NK) reflected underlying increased sympathetic nerve activity. (From Palatini P, Julius S. Association of tachycardia with morbidity and mortality: pathophysiological considerations. *J Hum Hypertens* 1997;11(1):S19–S27.)

A) Thiazide diuretics

Thiazide-type diuretics, unlike spironolactone, increase muscle sympathetic nerve activity (**Figure 9-20**) (42) and increase heart rate (43) in both low- and high-renin hypertensives (**Figure 9-21**) (44). Consequently, in both the Australian mild hypertension trial (45) and the MRC trial of mild hypertension (46), diuretic therapy was effective in reducing stroke frequency, but not the risk of MI, compared to placebo. In the Oslo study in middle-aged men, diuretic therapy actually increased the risk of MI (**Figure 9-22**) (47).

Thus, first-line diuretic therapy would be an inappropriate first-line choice in treating young/middle-aged hypertensives.

B) β-Blockers

β-Blockers lower the resting heart rate (Figure 9-21) (44). In the MRC mild hypertension study (46), the IPPPSH Study study (48), and the MAPHY Study study (49), nonselective propranolol and oxprenolol and moderately β-1 selective metoprolol reduced the risk of MI by 35%–50% versus placebo or diuretic

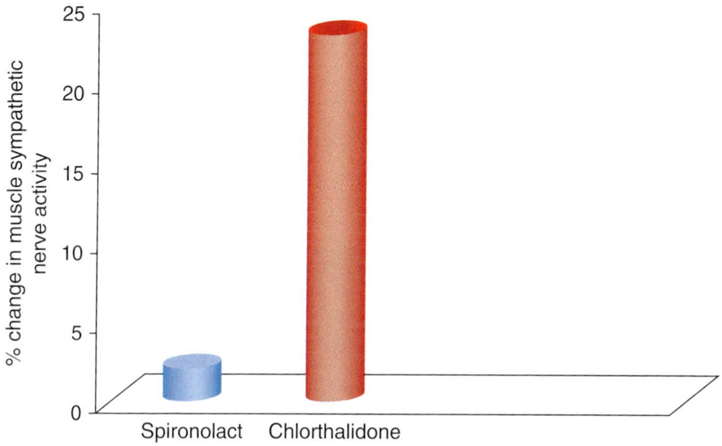

Fig. 9-20 Change in muscle sympathetic nerve activity after 3 months diuretic therapy in untreated hypertensives. (From Menon DV, Arbique D, Wang Z, et al. Differential effects of chlorthalidone vs. spironlactone on muscle sympathetic nerve activity in hypertensive patients. *J Clin Endocrinol Metab* 2009;94:1361–6.)

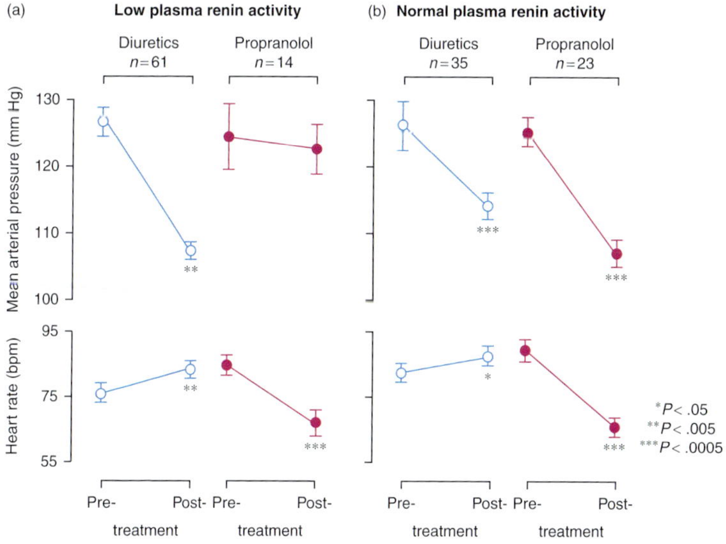

Fig. 9-21 In both low- and high-renin status hypertensive subjects, diuretic therapy increases the resting heart rate. (From Niarchos AP. Pathophysiology, diagnosis and treatment of hypertension in the elderly. *Cardiovasc Rev Rep* 1980;1:621–7.)

therapy in nonsmokers (approximately 75% of trial population) (**Figure 9-23**). The reasons for the poor results in smokers are explained in Chapter 8.

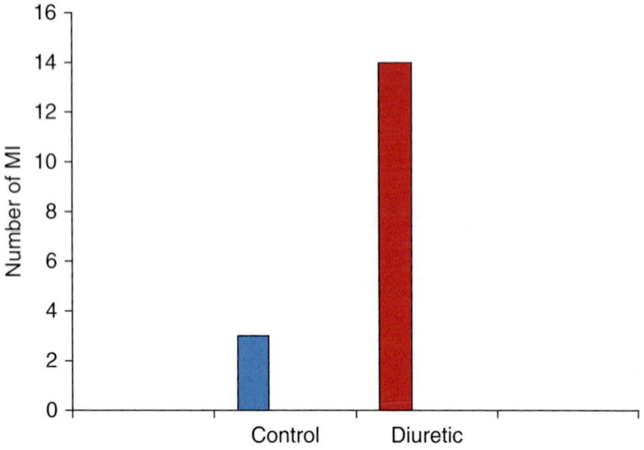

Fig. 9-22 Oslo study: 785 mildly hypertensive men, age 40–49 years, randomized to control or hydrochlorothiazide × 5.5 years; diuretics increase the risk of MI. (From Leren P, Helgeland A. Coronary heart disease and the treatment of hypertension. Some Oslo study data. *Am J Med* 1986;80:3–6.)

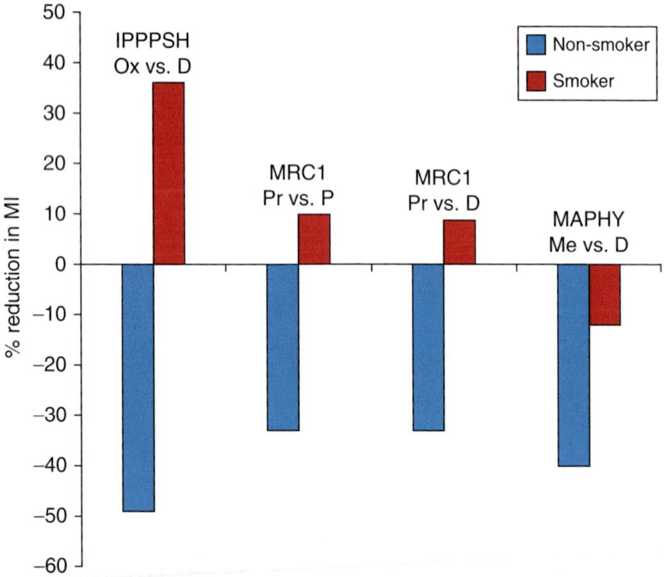

Fig. 9-23 β-Blocker/smoking interaction (MI) in young/mid-age hypertensives: the 30%–50% reduction in MI by β-blocker vs. placebo or diuretic in nonsmokers is negated in smokers. (From Cruickshank JM. *The Modern Role of Beta-Blockers in Cardiovascular Medicine*. Shelton, Connecticut: People's Medical Publishing House—USA; 2011: 179.)

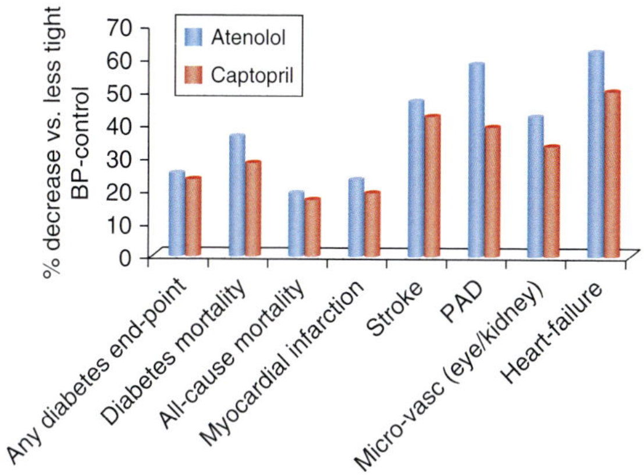

Fig. 9-24 UKPDS—the trends in reduction of all primary end-points favor atenolol vs. captopril when compared with less-tight BP control (diff = 10/5 mm Hg) over 10-year follow-up. (UK Prospective Diabetes Study Group. Efficacy of atenolol and captopril in reducing the risk of macrovascular and microvascular complications in type-2 diabetes. *BMJ* 1998;317:713–20.)

In the UKPDS study (23, 50), the ACE inhibitor captopril reduced the risk of all 7 primary endpoints (plus secondary endpoint heart failure) versus less tight control of BP, but to a lesser extent than the β-blocker atenolol (**Figure 9-24**). The reduced risk of MI on the ACE inhibitor, versus less-tight control BP, was about 20% versus 23% on atenolol. At 20-year follow-up (51), the difference in reduction of MI-risk between atenolol and captopril persisted, whereas the difference in all-cause death widened to a significant 23% reduction in favor of the β-blocker (**Figure 9-25**).

In the ELSA Study (52), comparing atenolol and lacidipine, the dihydropyridine calcium blocker, there was no difference in cardiovascular events between groups. Bisoprolol was superior to nifedipine slow release in improving event-free survival in mild hypertensives with ischemic heart disease (Figure 9-30) (23).

Thus, nonselective or moderately β-1 selective β-blockers would be a reasonable choice as first-line therapy in nonsmoking young/middle-aged diastolic hypertensives. The β-blocker/smoking hypertensive interaction can be avoided by the usage of high β-1 selectivity, for example, bisoprolol, making such a β-blocker the drug of choice for first-line treatment in young/middle-aged hypertensives (in both smokers and nonsmokers).

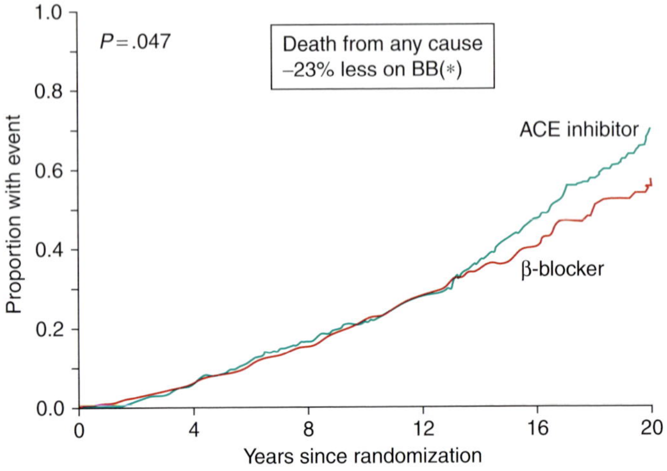

Fig. 9-25 UKPDS study: after 20-year follow-up, death from any cause was reduced by a significant 23% in those randomized to atenolol vs. captopril. (Holman RR, Paul SK, Bethel MA, et al. Long-term follow-up after tight control of blood pressure in type-2 diabetes. *N Engl J Med* 2008;359:1565–76.)

C) ACE inhibitors

Angiotensin II increases sympathetic nerve activity (54), which is reversed by ACE inhibition (which decreases angiotensin II levels), (55) but with minimal, or no change, in resting heart rate (43).

Thus, in the UKPDS study (23, 50), the ACE inhibitor reduced the risk of all 7 primary endpoints versus less tight control of BP, but to a lesser extent than the β-blocker atenolol (Figure 9-24). These differences between ACE inhibitor and atenolol persisted at 20-year follow-up, but now there was a significant 23% reduction in all-cause death in favor of the β-blocker (Figure 9-25) (51).

In the ABCD study (56), involving middle-aged diabetic hypertensives, there were significantly fewer fatal and nonfatal MIs in the enalapril, versus the calcium blocker nisoldipine, group (**Figure 9-26**).

In the Captopril Prevention Project Captopril Prevention Project (CAPP) study (57), there was no difference between captopril and conventional therapy (diuretic or β-blocker) in reducing cardiovascular mortality and morbidity.

Thus, ACE inhibitors would be a suitable choice as first-line therapy in young/middle-aged hypertensives who were intolerant of β-1 blockade.

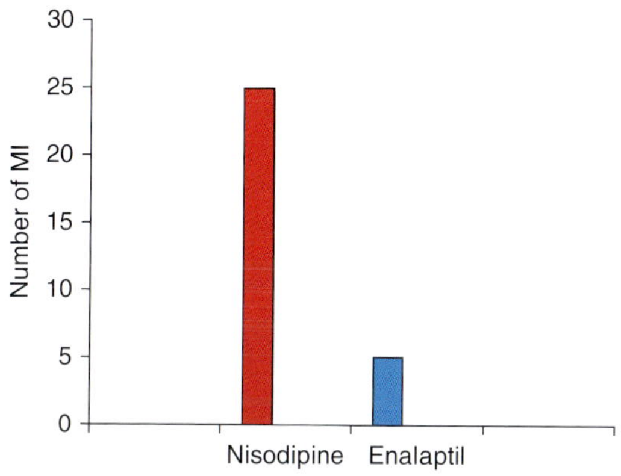

Fig. 9-26 ABCD study; in middle-aged hypertensives with diabetes randomized to enalapril or nisoldipine there was a significant increase in MI in the CB group. (From Estacio RO, Jeffers BW, Hiatt WR, et al. The effect of nisoldipine as compared with enalapril on cardiovascular outcomes in patients with non-insulin-dependent diabetes and hypertension. *N Engl J Med* 1998;338:645–52.)

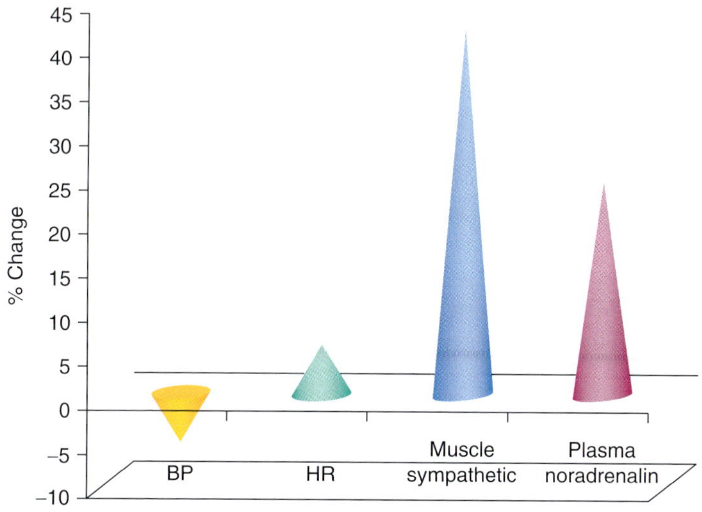

Fig. 9-27 ARBs and sympathetic nerve activity: double-blind, random, X-over, placebo-controlled study in young, hypertensive males. (From Heusser K, Vitovski J, Raasch W, et al. Elevation of sympathetic nerve activity by eprosartan inyoun male subjects. *Am J Hypertens* 2003;18:658–64.)

D) Angiotensin receptor blockers

As mentioned earlier, angiotensin II increases the sympathetic nerve activity (54). Unlike ACE inhibition, angiotensin receptor blockers (ARBs) increase the angiotensin II levels. In young hypertensives, ARBs have been noted to increase the sympathetic nerve

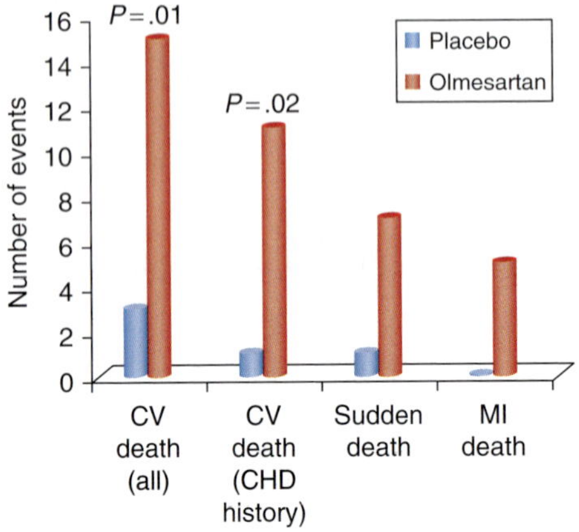

Fig. 9-28 Olmesartan vs. placebo (randomized) in 4447 DM2, mean age 57, mean BMI 31, BP 136/81, over 3.2 years: the ARB significantly increased the risk of CV endpoints and death. (From Haller H, Ito S, Izzo JL, et al. Olmesartan for the delay or prevention of microalbuminuria in type-2 diabetes. *N Engl J Med* 2011;364:907–17.)

activity (58, 59), accompanied by a small increase in heart rate (**Figure 9-27**) 60.

In patients with type 2 diabetes with overt nephropathy, olmesartan versus placebo was associated with an excess of cardiovascular deaths (58). In 4447 patients with type 2 diabetes with prehypertension, randomized to placebo or olmesartan, at 3.2-year follow-up, there was a significant increase in the cardiovascular death and also an excess of sudden death and MI in the ARB group (**Figure 9-28**) (59).

Thus, ARBs would be an inappropriate choice as first-line therapy in young/middle-aged hypertensives.

E) Dihydropyridine calcium blockers

In middle-aged hypertensives, 4 different dihydropyridine calcium blockers lowered BP to a similar extent but increased plasma NE and heart rate by varying degrees (**Figure 9-29**) (56, 61). The non-dihydropyridine verapamil does not increase the sympathetic nerve activity and reduces heart rate (62).

In the ABCD study (56), there was an excess of MI cases in patients randomized to the dihydropyridine calcium blocker, nisoldipine versus ACE inhibition (Figure 9-26). As mentioned earlier in the ELSA study (52), lacidipine and atenolol reduced cardiovascular events to a similar extent. In middle-aged mild hypertensives with CHD, slow-release nifedipine was inferior to the highly β-1 selective β-blocker bisoprolol in improving the event-free survival (**Figure 9-30**) (53).

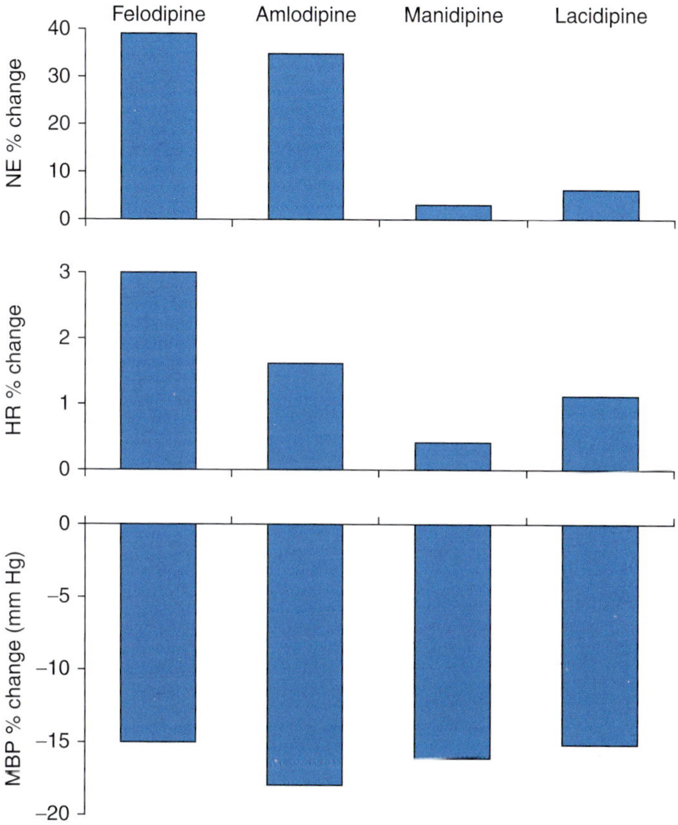

Fig. 9-29 Effect of various dihydropyridine calcium blockers on plasma NE, heart rate, and BP in middle-aged hypertensives. (From Fogari R, Zoppi A, Corradi L, et al. Effects of different dihydropyridine calcium antagonists on plasma norepinephrine in essential hypertension. *J Hypertens* 2000;18:1871–5.)

Thus, dihydropyridine calcium blockers would be an inappropriate first-line therapy for the treatment of young/middle-aged hypertensives.

2. Elderly systolic hypertensives

As discussed in Chapter 4, the Framingham Study showed clearly that elderly systolic hypertension is a quite separate condition from younger diastolic hypertension. Unlike younger diastolic hypertension, elderly systolic hypertension is a function of aging, stiff arteries. Although muscle (but not renal) sympathetic nerve activity tends to increase with age, there is an accompanying loss of β-receptor affinity/sensitivity with an associated decrease in renin/angiotensin activity.

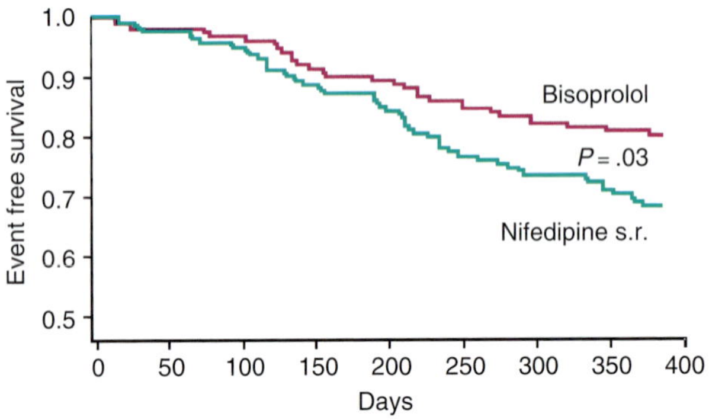

Fig. 9-30 TIBBS study: 307 CAD patients with mild hypertension; bisoprolol significantly superior to SR Nifedipine in improving event-free survival (death, MI, and hospitalization). (From Heddblad B, Wikstrand J, Janzon L, et al. Low-dose metoprolol CR/XL and fluvastatin slow progression of carotid intima thickness. *Circulation* 2001;103:1721–6.)

Accordingly, high resting heart rates in the elderly hypertensive, although still a predictor of increased CV risk (30, 31), are less potent predictors than in the younger diastolic hypertensive (29). However, with elderly systolic hypertension in the presence of CHD, high heart rates are powerful predictors of adverse outcome (Figure 9-16) (32). Interestingly, higher heart rates are associated with lower central pressures (Figure 9-17) (34); although with β-blocker-induced bradycardia, the high central pressures are linked less with low heart rates than with the greater magnitude of the reflected wave (associated with the lack of vasodilatation) (36).

A) Thiazide diuretics

The role of diuretic therapy in the treatment of the elderly systolic hypertensive is completely opposite to their role in the treatment of young/middle-aged diastolic hypertensive (where the sympathetic nerve activity is all-important).

First-line diuretic therapy has become a corner stone of treatment in the elderly. As indicated in Chapter 6, diuretics are effective in lowering central pressures, but not to a greater extent than brachial pressure.

In spite of a tendency to increase the heart rate (Figure 9-21) (44), first-line diuretic therapy has proved highly effective in reducing the risk of cardiovascular events in the elderly. In placebo-controlled studies, namely SHEP (63), MRC-elderly (64), and HYVET (65), diuretics were highly effective in reducing all-cause death, stroke, MI, and heart failure. Of particular note is the 44% reduction in the risk

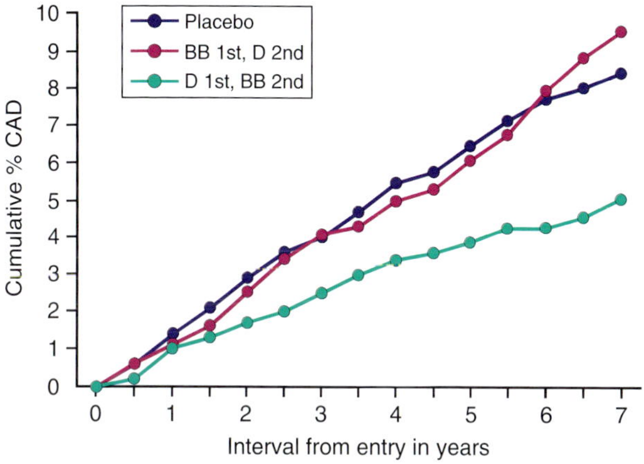

Fig. 9-31 MRC-elderly study (1992)—after 7 years follow-up only the diuretic (D) (not atenolol (BB)) significantly reduced the risk of CAD vs. placebo by 44%.

of MI in the MRC elderly study (**Figure 9-31**), a complete turnaround from the diuretic-induced increased risk of MI in the MRC study (46) and the Oslo study in younger patients (Figure 9-22) (47). Thus, it is clear that in the elderly, the risk of MI is related to central BPs, unlike in the younger hypertensive, where the risk of MI is linked to the level of the sympathetic nerve activity. In comparative studies, diuretics, particularly chlorthalidone, have fared well. In the massive ALLHAT study, the chlorthalidone was deemed the favored therapy over ACE inhibitor and calcium blocker–based therapy (66).

B) β-Blockers

Similar to diuretics, the role of β-blockers in treating elderly systolic hypertensives (without CHD) is the reverse of their role in treating young/middle-aged diastolic hypertensives. Although lowering heart rate (44), a classic β-blocker like atenolol lowers central BP in the elderly systolic hypertensive less effectively than other antihypertensive agents (67). Moreover, low heart rates have been linked to increased central pressures (Figure 9-17) (34); although when low heart rates are induced by β-blockers, the central pressures are more related to the magnitude of the reflected wave (and not heart rate), which is a function in the absence of vasodilation (36).

Accordingly, first-line β-blockade (atenolol) has performed poorly in the elderly hypertensive when compared to placebo (64), diuretics (64), ARBs (68), and calcium blockers (69).

However, in elderly systolic hypertensives with CHD, that is the INVEST study (70), atenolol was at least as effective as verapamil the (a non-dihydropyridine calcium blocker), being superior in those with a history of heart failure. In this study, there was a mild J-shaped relationship between resting heart rate and adverse outcome (Figure 9-16) (32). Heart rates on treatment were better predictors of outcome than the resting heart rates at baseline (33).

C) ACE inhibitors

ACE inhibitors do not alter the resting heart rate (43). Unlike β-blockers, first-line ACE inhibitors have fared well in the elderly, as witnessed in the HOPE study versus placebo (71). ACE inhibition was superior to hydrochlorothiazide in reducing hard endpoints in the Second Australian trial (72), but in ALLHAT (66), it was significantly inferior to chlorthalidone in preventing diastolic heart failure (see Chapter 8). In ONTARGET, ACE inhibitors and ARBs were similar in preventing the composite cardiovascular endpoint (73).

D) Angiotensin receptor blockers

The concern expressed over ARBs in young hypertensives is so less than in the elderly. Although angiotensin II levels increase with ARBs and lead to increased heart rates and sympathetic nerve activity in the young hypertensive (58, 59), interestingly in older patients (74), and those with renal failure (75), there is a fall in the sympathetic nerve activity, although not all have noted this (76).

Accordingly, the performance of ARBs in the elderly has been mixed (see Chapter 8). On balance, it appears that ARBs are relatively ineffective in reducing the risk of MI in the elderly, although effective in reducing stroke risk.

E) Calcium blockers

Although dihydropyridine calcium blockers increase the sympathetic nerve activity and heart rate (Figure 9-29) (61), causing concern relating to the excess of MIs in young hypertensives (Figure 9-26) (56, 53), this is not the case in the elderly.

In elderly systolic hypertensive patients, dihydropyridine calcium blockers have performed well in reducing cardiovascular endpoints (see Chapter 8). They are superior to the β-blocker atenolol (69); similar to diuretic therapy (66, 77), although inferior in preventing heart failure (78); more effective than ACE inhibitors in reducing stroke risk, but less effective in reducing the risk of MI (79); and more effective than ARBs in reducing the risk of MI (80).

Nondihydropine calcium blockers also confer the benefit to elderly hypertensive, but unlike dihyropyridine calcium blockers, they lower the heart rate. In the NORDIL study (81), diltiazem was similar to either diuretic or β-blocker in reducing the primary endpoint. In a similar study, Controlled Onset Verapamil Investigation of Cardiovascular End Points Controlled Investigation of Cardiovascular End Points (CONVINCE) (82), verapamil was equivalent to a β-blocker or diuretic in reducing the primary endpoint.

In elderly systolic hypertensives with CHD, INVEST study (70), verapamil was similar to atenolol in reducing the cardiovascular events, except in patients with a history of heart failure where atenolol was superior.

WHAT ABOUT SINOATRIAL NODE INHIBITORS—IVABRADINE?

Ivabradine is a sinoatrial node inhibitor that lowers the heart rate but has no effect on BP (83). It is at least as effective as a β-blocker in preventing angiotensin II-induced heart failure (84).

In patients with CHD and left ventricular systolic dysfunction (most on β-blockers), ivabradine, versus placebo, reduced the heart rate by 6 bpm, but did not reduce the primary endpoint; but in those with heart rates greater than 70 bpm, it did reduce the secondary endpoint by a significant 36% (mainly via reductions in hospital visits for fatal/nonfatal MI and coronary revascularization) (85). The drug appeared to benefit left ventricular remodeling, with increases in ejection fraction and a reduction on left ventricular systolic size (86), and heart rates of 50 bpm or less were well tolerated (87).

In patients with chronic heart failure (most on β-blockers), ivabradine versus placebo reduced the primary endpoint by a significant 18% (driven mainly by hospital admissions for worsening heart failure and deaths due to heart failure) (88). Little or no benefit accrued from treatment when baseline heart rates were less than 72–75 bpm (**Figure 9-32**) (89). Primary composite end point reduction in the ivabradine group was greatest in the group who achieved heart rates of less than 60 bpm at 28 days (**Figure 9-33**) (89).

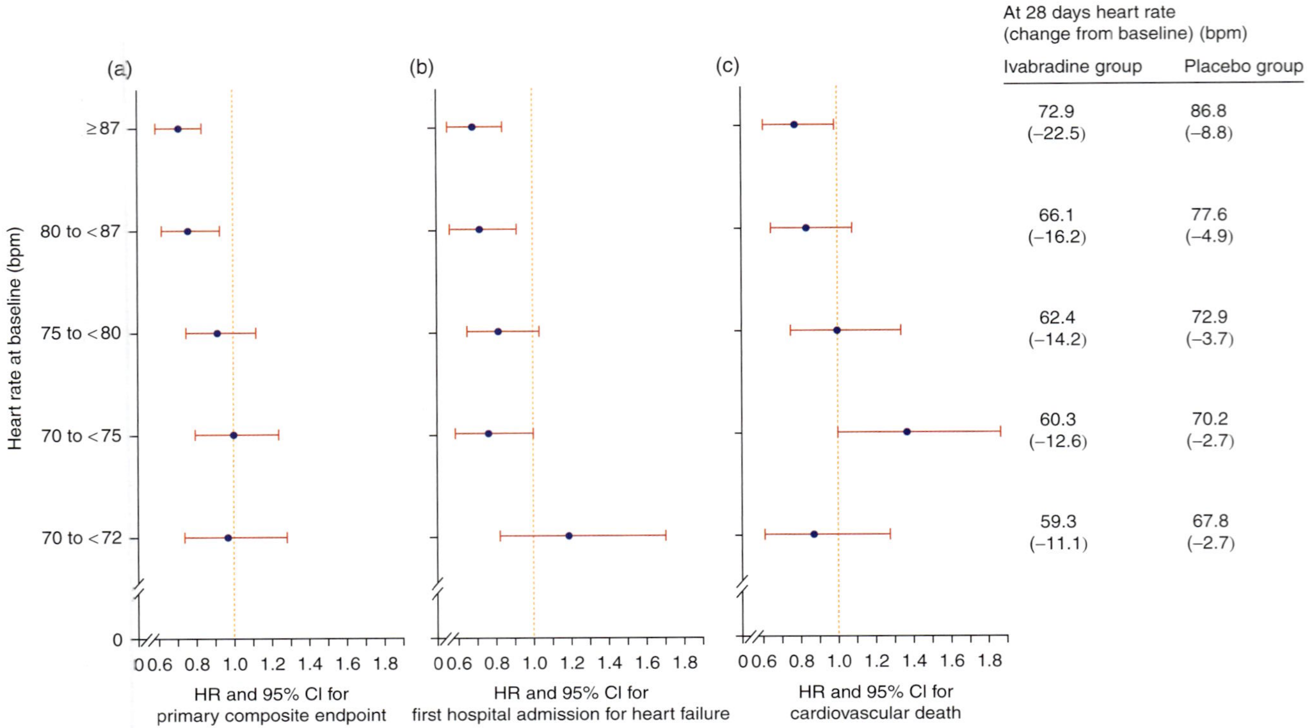

Fig. 9-32 SHIFT study in heart failure; in the placebo group, high resting heart rates were associated with poor outcomes in (A) primary composite endpoint, (B) first hospital admission, and (C) cardiovascular deaths. (From Bohm M, Swedberg K, Kamajda M, et al. Heart rate as a risk factor in chronic heart failure (SHIFT): an association between heart rate and outcomes in a randomised placebo-controlled trial. *Lancet* 2010;376:886–94.)

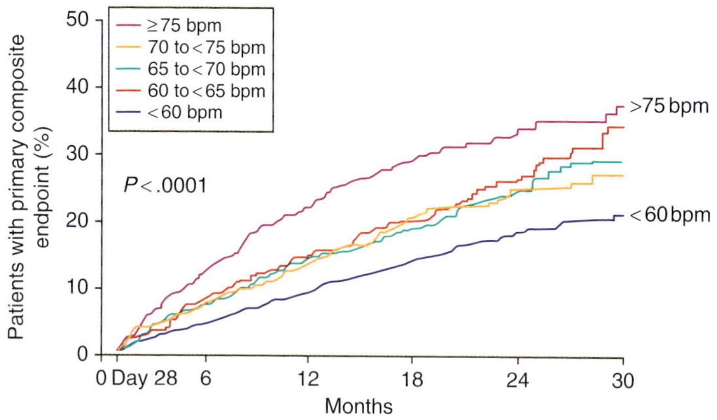

Fig. 9-33 SHIFT study in heart failure: in the ivabradine group, heart rates less than 60 bpm were associated with the best prognosis re-primary composite endpoint. (From Bohm M, Swedberg K, Kamajda M, et al. Heart rate as a risk factor in chronic heart failure (SHIFT): an association between heart rate and outcomes in a randomised placebo-controlled trial. *Lancet* 2010;376:886–94.)

The results of the Systolic Heart Failure Treatment with the I(f) Inhibitor Ivabradin Trial (SHIFT) trial have been criticized on the basis that greater than 50% of cases were on suboptimal doses of β-blockers; what would be the results if all were on optimal β-blocker dosing? (90).

Animal data indicate that ivabradine-induced reduction of heart rate (under hypercholesterolemic atherosclerotic conditions) stimulates collateral arterial growth, and possible contributing mechanisms include improved endothelial function, improved nitric oxide availability, and modulation of inflammatory cytokine gene expression (91).

There is a need for a head-to-head comparison between ivabradine and an evidence-based β-blocker (90).

HEART RATE AND THE CARDIOVASCULAR CONTINUUM

The so-called cardiovascular continuum is illustrated (**Figure 9-34**) (92). This figure is based on the original produced by Dzau and Braunwald (93). The starting point is the high-risk subject, involving possible dyslipidemia, diabetes, smoking, obesity, and hypertension. Of these risk factors, hypertension, which is number one global risk factor (see Chapter 5), is the most important.

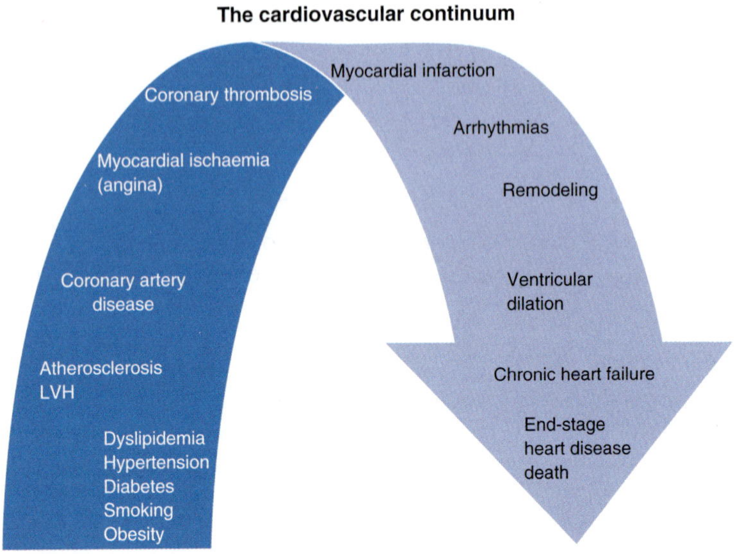

Fig. 9-34 The cardiovascular continuum. (From Zamorano JL. Heart rate management: a therapeutic goal throughout the cardiovascular continuum. *Eur Heart J* 2008;10(suppl F):F17–F21.)

1. Origin of hypertension and high heart rates

The appearance of hypertension in children and young/middle-aged adults is linked to high heart rates and increased sympathetic nerve activity (see Chapter 4).

High-risk subjects are at a risk of end organ damage.

2. End-organ damage and high heart rates

Hypertension in young/middle-aged subjects increases the risk of end organ damage. The development of left-ventricular hypertrophy (LVH), in both animals and young/middle-aged hypertension, is closely linked to increased sympathetic nerve activity and heart rate (see Chapter 7). Similarly, the development of atheroma is closely associated with the high heart rates and increased sympathetic nerve activity (see Chapter 7). In monkeys, atheromatous lesions can be largely prevented by sinoatrial node ablation. The development of atheromatous plaque is linked to disturbed blood flow patterns associated with the low endothelial shear stress, a process avoided/reversed by laminar blood flow and low heart rates (β-blocker).

3. Coronary heart disease and ischemia

As mentioned earlier, patients with CHD and high resting heart rates have an impaired prognosis (Figure 9-6) (17, 18).

4. Acute coronary syndromes

In patients with non-ST segment acute coronary syndromes, both on and off β-blockers, there was a J-shaped relationship between the resting heart rate and all-cause mortality (Figure 9-7) (19).

5. Postmyocardial infarction

In predischarge patients, a high-mean 24-hour heart rate was a strong predictor of mortality over the next 2 years (20). In the presence of β-blockers, those with the greatest reduction in heart rate had the best prognosis; β-blockers with ISA were the least cardioprotective (Figure 9-7a) (21).

6. Chronic systolic heart failure

In hard endpoint studies, slow heart rates are related to reduced all-cause mortality (Figure 9-8) (22). Thus, β-blockers without ISA, that is, bisoprolol, metoprolol, and carvedilol, are highly effective in reducing all-cause mortality, compared to β-blockers with ISA, that is xamoterol, bucindolol, and nebivolol, which are ineffective in reducing all-cause death (Figure 9-9) (23). Resting heart rates of 58–64 bpm are associate with the best prognosis (24).

7. Therapeutic implications

Beta-blockade

β-1 blockade, and to a lesser extent ACE inhibition, is effective at all stages of the cardiovascular continuum.

At stage 1, β-1 blockade (bisoprolol) is the most effective way to lower BP in the young/middle-aged hypertensive (see Chapter 6).

At stage 2, bisoprolol is at least as effective as ACE inhibition, and atenolol is more effective than diuretics, at reversing LVH in young/middle-aged hypertensives (see Chapter 7). Atheromatous plaque is regressed by β-1 blockade (see Chapter 7), via low heart rates that are linked to laminar blood flow patterns.

At stage 3, slow heart rates and β-blockers are associated with a reduced risk of atheromatous plaque rupture and ensuing acute MI (see Chapter 7).

Thus, in young/middle-aged hypertension (under-pinned by high sympathetic nerve activity), β-1 blockade reduces the risk of MI by 35%–50%, versus placebo or diuretic therapy, in nonsmokers; high β-1 selectivity avoids the β-blocker/smoking/hypertensive interaction (see Chapter 8); β-1 blockade is superior to ACE inhibition in reducing the all-cause death in the young/middle-aged hypertensive; antihypertensive agents that increase the sympathetic nerve activity and resting heart rate in young/middle-aged hypertensives, that is, diuretics, dihydropyridine calcium blockers, and ARBs, do not reduce, and may even increase, the risk of MI; in elderly systolic hypertension (a reflection of stiffening, aging of the arteries), with desensitization of β-receptors, diuretic or calcium blocker therapy is an appropriate first-line choice (but β-blockers if CAD is present).

At stage 4, in the postinfarction period, slow heart rates induced by β-blockers without ISA are associated with the reduced mortality.

At stage 5, with systolic heart failure, β-1 blockade is linked to significant reductions in resting heart rate and all-cause death, unlike β-blockers with ISA that reduce heart rate to a lesser degree and do not reduce all-cause mortality.

Sinoatrial blockade

The role of ivabradine in the cardiovascular continuum remains to be discovered, particularly as this sinoatrial node antagonist does not lower BP. Only a large, randomized comparison of ivabradine and β-1 blockade, say bisoprolol, at the various stages (including hypertension in the young/middle-aged) of the cardiovascular cycle will provide the answers.

SUMMARY AND CONCLUSIONS

1. Resting heart rate, a marker of metabolic rate, is a powerful predictor of life span within the bird and mammalian kingdoms.
2. In normal subjects, high resting heart rates (a surrogate for increased sympathetic activity) predict the development of hypertension several years later and are closely related to premature all-cause death and sudden CHD/cardiovascular death, particularly in men.

3. In normal subjects, home-measured morning heart rate variability is, particularly at higher BP levels, a predictor of cardiovascular events.
4. In patients with stable CHD, acute coronary syndromes, post-myocardial infarction period, or chronic systolic heart failure, high resting heart rates (with or without β-blockers) are associated with a poor prognosis.
5. In young/middle-aged hypertensive subjects, resting heart rates greater than 80–85 bpm are strong predictors of coronary, cardiovascular, and all-cause deaths; resting heart rates between 50–60 bpm are desirable.
6. In elderly hypertensive subjects, high resting heart rates also predict premature CV events, but less so than in young/middle-aged subjects; and, in the presence of CHD, the relationship is J-shaped (J-point at about 50 bpm).
7. In the elderly hypertensive, slow heart rates are linked to high central systolic pressures; with β-blockers, the increased central pressure is more a reflection of an increased magnitude of the reflected wave (due to the absence of vasodilatation) rather than bradycardia.
8. High resting heart rates increase vascular stiffness, encourage disturbed blood flow patterns associated with atheromatous plaque formation, and increase the risk of plaque rupture.
9. There are therapeutic implications arising from the association of high resting heart rates with a poor prognosis in young/middle-aged hypertensive subjects; underlying high sympathetic nerve activity, high β-receptor density and cyclic AMP levels, are related to an increased risk of MI (number one killer in young/middle-aged hypertensives) but not stroke.
10. In young/middle-aged hypertension, antihypertensive drugs that increase the sympathetic nerve activity and heart rate, that is thiazide-type diuretics, dihydropyridine calcium blockers, and ARBs, do not decrease (and may increase) the risk of MI; the choice remains with ACE inhibitors or β-blockers.
11. Compared with either randomized diuretics or placebo, non- or moderately β-1 selective β-blockers reduced not only heart rate but also the risk of MI by 35%–50% in nonsmokers; in smokers, where no benefit was noted, there is a 2- to 3-fold increase in adrenaline concentration, so that in the presence of β-1 plus β-2 blockade, there is unbridled α-constriction resulting in a marked increase in BP; this potentially lethal interaction can be avoided by high β-1 selectivity, for example, bisoprolol,

where maintained β-2-induced vasodilatation cancels out the α-constrictive process, thus avoiding the hypertensive response.

12. In the one and only comparison between β-blocker and ACE inhibitor, that is, UKPDS study, within the "tight-control" group, there was a randomized comparison between atenolol and captopril, and over 9 years, the trends in reduction of all 7 primary endpoints (vs. "less tight control") all favored the β-blocker; at 20-year follow-up, these trends persisted and, in the case of all-cause death, strengthened to a significant 23% reduction in those originally randomized to the β-blocker.
13. In the elderly, systolic hypertensive, with desensitized β-1 receptors and stiff, noncompliant vessels, the link between high sympathetic nerve activity and MI disappears, so that diuretic therapy, for example, is now associated with highly significant reductions in MI, as well as stroke and heart failure, whereas β-blockade (in the absence of CHD) is relatively noneffective.
14. Sinoatrial node inhibitors, for example, ivabradine, lower heart rate but do not reduce BP; their benefit in systolic heart failure (on background of β-blockers) has been observed.
15. The benefit of low heart rates has been noted throughout the cardiovascular continuum; low heart rates, via β-1 blockade, have been shown (a) to be associated with the best control of high BP in the young/middle-aged subject; (b) to be associated with the reduction of end-organ damage, for example, in reversing LVH, regressing atheromatous plaque, and decreasing the risk of plaque rupture, in middle-aged subjects; (c) to reduce the risk of MI in young/middle-aged hypertension, versus placebo and diuretics; (d) to be effective in stable and unstable ischemic heart disease; (e) to be linked to improved survival in the postmyocardial infarction period (not with β-blockers with ISA); and (f) to be linked to improved survival in chronic systolic heart failure (β-blockers with ISA lower heart rate less and do not reduce all-cause mortality).

REFERENCES

1. Livingstone SD, Kuehn LA. Similarity in the number of lifespan heart beats among non-hibernating, homeothermic animals. *Aviat Space Environ Med* 1979;50:1037–9.
2. Levine HJ. Rest heart rate and life expectancy. *J Am Coll Cardiol* 1997;30:1104–6.

3. Kaijser L, Berglund B. Coronary haemodynamics during isometiric handgrip and atrial pacing in patients with angina pectoris compared to healthy men. *Cardioscience* 1993;4:99–104.
4. Franklin SS. Arterial stiffness and hypertension. *Hypertension* 2005;45:349–51.
5. Palatini P, Dorigatti F, Zaetta V, et al. Heart rate as a predictor of development of sustained hypertension in subjects screened for stage 1 hypertension: the HARVEST Study. *J Hypertens* 2006;24:1873–80.
6. Palatini P. Role of elevated heart rate in the development of cardiovascular disease in hypertension. *Hypertension* 2011;58:745–50.
7. Hering D, Kucharska W, Kara T, et al. Resting sympathetic outflow does not predict the morning blood pressure surge in hypertension. *J Hypertens* 2011;29:2381–6.
8. Dyer AR, Persky V, Stamler J, et al. Heart rate as a prognostic factor for coronary heart disease and mortality; findings in three Chicago epidemiological studies. *Am J Epidemiol* 1980;112:736–49.
9. Kannel WB, Kannel C, Paffenbarger RS, et al. Heart rate and cardiovascular mortality: the Framingham Study. *Am Heart J* 1987;119:1489–94.
10. Mensink GB, Hoffmeister H. The relationship between resting heart rate and all-cause, cardiovascular and cancer mortality. *Eur Heart J* 1997;18:1404–10.
11. Tverdal A, Hjellvik V, Selmer R. Heart rate and mortality from cardiovascular causes: a 12 year follow-up study of 379,843 men and women aged 40–45 years. *Eur Heart J* 2008;29:2772–81.
12. Jouven X, Empana JP, Escolano S, et al. Relation of heart rate and rest and long-term (>20 years) death rate in initially healthy middle-aged men. *Am J Cardiol* 2009;103:279–83.
13. Shaper AG, Wannamethee G, Macfarlane PW, et al. Heart rate, ischaemic heart disease and sudden cardiac death in middle-aged British men. *Br Heart J* 1993;70:49–55.
14. Cooney MT, Vartiainen E, Laakitainen T, et al. Elevated resting heart rate is an independent risk factor for cardiovascular disease in healthy men and women. *Am Heart J* 2010;159:612–9.
15. Nauman J, Janszky I, Vatten LJ, et al. Temporal changes in resting heart rate and deaths from ischaemic heart disease. *JAMA* 2011;306:2579–87.
16. Johansson JK, Niiranen TJ, Puuka PJ, et al. Prognostic value of the variability in home-measured blood pressure and heart rate. The Finn-Home Study. *Hypertension* 2012;59:212–8.
17. Diaz A, Bourassa MG, Guertin M-C, et al. Long-term prognostic value of resting heart rate in patients with suspected or proven coronary artery disease. *Eur Heart J* 2005;26:967–74.
18. Anselmino M, Ohrvik J, Ryden L. Resting heart rate in patients with stable coronary artery disease and diabetes: a report from the Euro Heart Survey on Diabetes and the Heart. *Eur Heart J* 2010;31:3040–45.
19. Bangalore S, Messerli FH, Ou F-S, et al. The association of admission heart rate and in-hospital cardiovascular events in patients with

non-ST-segment elevation acute coronary syndromes: CRUSADE. *Eur Heart J* 2010;31:552–60.

20. Copie X, Hnatkova K, Staunton A, et al. Predictive power of increased heart rate versus depressed left-ventricular ejection fraction and heart rate variability for risk stratification after myocardial infarction. Results of two-year follow-up study. *J Am Coll Cardiol* 1996;27:270–6.
21. Kjekshus J. Comments—beta-blockers: heart rate reduction a mechanism of benefit. *Eur Heart J* 1985;6(suppl A):29–30.
22. Cook S, Togni M, Schaub MC, et al. High heart rate: a cardiovascular risk factor? *Eur Heart J* 2006;27:2387–93.
23. Cruickshank JM. *The Modern Role of Beta-Blockers in Cardiovascular Medicine.* Shelton, Connecticut: People's Medical Publishing House —USA; 2011:179.
24. Cullington D, Goode KM, Clark AL, et al. Heart rate achieved or beta-blocker dose in patients with chronic heart failure: which is the better target? *Eur J Heart* Fail 2012;14:737–47.
25. King DE, Everett CJ, Mainous AG, et al. Long-term prognostic value of resting heart rate in subjects with pre-hypertension. Am *J Hypertens* 2006;19:796–800.
26. Gillman MW, Kannel WB, Belanger A, et al. Influence of heart rate on mortality among persons with hypertension: the Framingham Study. Am *Heart J* 1993;125:1148–54.
27. Benetos A, Rudnicki A, Thomns F, et al. Influence of heart rate on mortality in a French population: role of age, gender and blood pressure. *Hypertension* 1999;33:44–52.
28. Paul L, Hastie CE, Li WS, et al. Resting heart rate pattern during follow-up and mortality in hypertensive patients. *Hypertension* 2010;55:567–74.
29. Thomas F, Rudnicki A, Bacri AM, et al. Cardiovascular mortality in hypertensive men according to presence of associated risk factors. *Hypertension* 2001;37:1256–61.
30. Palatini P, Thijs L, Staessen JA, et al. Predictive value of clinic and ambulatory heart rate for mortality in elderly subjects with systolic hypertension. *Arch Intern Med* 2002;162:2313–21.
31. Kostis JB, Cabrera J, Cheng JQ, et al. Association between chlorthalidone treatment of systolic hypertension and long-term survival. *JAMA* 2011;306:2588–93.
32. Kolloch R, Legler UF, Champion A, et al. Impact of a resting heart rate on outcomes in hypertensive patients with coronary artery disease: INVEST. *Eur Heart J* 2008;29:1327–34.
33. Palatini P. Is there benefit of cardiac slowing drugs in the treatment of hypertensive patients with elevated heart rate? *Eur Heart J* 2008;29:1218–20.
34. Wilkinson IB, Mohammad NH, Tyrell S, et al. Heart rate dependency of pulse pressure amplification and arterial stiffness. *Am J Hypertens* 2002;15:24–30.

35. Safar ME, Protogerou AD, Blacker J. Statins, central blood pressure and blood pressure amplification. *Circulation* 2009;119:9–12.
36. Manisty CH, Zambanini A, Parker KH, et al. Differences in the magnitude of wave reflection account for differential effects of amlodipine-versus atenolol-based regimens on central blood pressure: ASCOT Study. *Hypertension* 2009;54:724–30.
37. Dhakam Z, Yasmin, McEniery CM, et al. A comparison of atenolol and nebivolol in isolated systolic hypertension. *J Hypertens* 2008;26:351–6.
38. Cunha RS, Pannier B, Benetos A, et al. Association between high heart rate and high arterial rigidity in normotensive and hypertensive subjects. *J Hypertens* 1997;15:1423–30.
39. Benetos A, Adamopoulos C, Bureau J-M, et al. Determinants of accelerated progression of arterial stiffness in normotensive subjects and in treated hypertensive subjects over a 6-year period. *Circulation* 2002;105:1202–7.
40. Palatini P, Parati G. Persistently elevated heart rate accelerates the progression of arterial stiffness. *J Hypertens* 2010;28:653–6.
41. Palatini P, Julius S. Association of tachycardia with morbidity and mortality: pathophysiological considerations. *J Hum Hypertens* 1997;11:S19–S27.
42. Menon DV, Arbique D, Wang Z, et al. Differential effects of chlorthalidone versus spironolactone on muscle sympathetic nerve activity in hypertensive patients. *J Clin Endocrinol Metab* 2009;94:1361–6.
43. Deary AJ, Schumann AL, Murfeet H, et al. Double-blind, placebo controlled crossover comparison of 5 classes of drugs. *J Hypertens* 2002;20:771–7.
44. Niarchos AP. Pathophysiology, diagnosis and treatment of hypertension in the elderly. *Cardiovasc Rev Rep* 1980;1:621–7.
45. Report by the Management Committee. The Australian therapeutic trial in mild hypertension. *Lancet* 1980;1:1261–7.
46. Medical Research Working Party. MRC trial of treatment of mild hypertension: principal results. *BMJ* 1985;291:97–104.
47. Leren P, Helgeland A. Coronary heart disease and the treatment of hypertension. Some Oslo study data. *Am J Med* 1986;80:3–6.
48. IPPPSH Collaborative Group. Cardiovascular risk and risk factors in a randomised trial of treatment—based on the beta-blocker oxprenolol. *J Hypertens* 1985;3:379–92.
49. Wikstrand J, Warnold T, Tuomilehto J, et al. Metoprolol versus diuretics in hypertension. Morbidity results from MAPHY study. *Hypertension* 1991;17:579–88.
50. UK Prospective Diabetes Study Group. Efficacy of atenolol and captopril in reducing the risk of macrovascular and microvascular complications in type-2 diabetes. *BMJ* 1998;317:713–20.
51. Holman RR, Paul SK, Bethel MA, et al. Long-term follow-up after tight control of blood pressure in type-2 diabetes. *N Engl J Med* 2008;359:1565–76.

52. Zanchetti A, Bond G, Hennig M, et al. Calcium antagonist lacidipine slows down progression of asymptomatic carotid atherosclerosis (ELSA). *Circulation* 2002;106:2422–7.
53. von Arnim T; for TIBBS Investigators. Prognostic significance of transient ischaemic episodes: response to treatment shows improved prognosis results of the TIBBS follow-up. *J Am Coll Cardiol* 1995;25:231–8.
54. Grassi G. Renin-angiotensin-sympathetic crosstalks in hypertension: reappraising the relevance of peripheral interactions. *J Hypertens* 2001;19:1713–6.
55. Miyajima E, Shigemasa T, Yamada Y, et al. Angiotensin II blunts, while angiotensin-converting enzyme inhibitor augments, reflex sympathetic inhibition in humans. *Clin Exp Pharmacol Physiol* 1999;26:797–802.
56. Estacio RO, Jeffers BW, Hiatt WR, et al. The effect of nisoldipine as compared with enalapril on cardiovascular outcomes in patients with non-insulin-dependent diabetes and hypertension. *N Engl J Med* 1998;338:645–52.
57. Hansson L, Lindholm LH, Niskanen L, et al. Effect of angiotensin-converting-enzyme inhibition compared with conventional therapy on cardiovascular morbidity and mortality in hypertension: the Captopril Prevention Project (CAPP) randomised trial. *Lancet* 1999;353:611–6.
58. Imai E, Chan JC, Yamasaki T, et al. Effects of olmesartan on renal and cardiovascular outcomes in type-2 diabetes with overt nephropathy: a multicentre, randomised, placebo-controlled study. *Diabetologia* 2011;54:2978–86.
59. Haller H, Ito S, Izzo JL, et al. Olmesartan for the delay or prevention of microalbuminuria in type-2 diabetes. *N Engl J Med* 2011;364:907–17.
60. Heusser K, Vitovski J, Raasch W, et al. Elevation of sympathetic nerve activity by eprosartan inyoun male subjects. *AM J Hypertens* 2003;18:658–64.
61. Fogari R, Zoppi A, Corradi L, et al. Effects of different dihydropyridine calcium antagonists on plasma norepinephrine in essential hypertension. *J Hypertens* 2000;18:1871–5.
62. Binggeli C, Corti R, Sudano I, et al. Effects of chronic calcium channel blockade on sympathetic nerve activity on hypertension. *Hypertension* 2002;39:892–6.
63. SHEP Cooperative Research. Prevention of stroke by antihypertensive drug treatment in older persons with isolated systolic hypertension: final results of the Systolic Hypertension in the Elderly Program (SHEP). *JAMA* 1991;265:3255–64.
64. MRC Working Party. Medical Research Council trial of hypertension in older adults: principal results. *BMJ* 1992;304:405–12.
65. Beckett NS, Peters R, Fletcher AE, et al. Treatment of hypertension in patients 80 years of age or older. *N Engl J Med* 2008;358:1887–98.

66. The ALLHAT Officers and Coordinators for the ALLHAT Collaborative Research Group. Major outcomes in high-risk hypertensive patients randomised to angiotensin-converting enzyme inhibitor or calcium channel blocker vs diuretic. *JAMA* 2002;288:2981–97.
67. Morgan T, Lauri J, Bertram D, et al. Effect of different antihypertensive drug classes on central aortic pressure. *Am J Hypertens* 2004;17:118–23.
68. Kjeldsen SE, Dahlof B, Devereux RB, et al. Effect of losartan on cardiovascular morbidity and mortality in patients with isolated hypertension and left-ventricular hypertrophy. *JAMA* 2002;288:1491–8.
69. Dahlof B, Sever P, Poulter N, et al. Prevention of cardiovascular events with an antihypertensive regimen of amlodipine adding peridopril as required versus atenolol adding bendroflumethiazide as required (ASCOT-BPLA); a multicentre randomised controlled trial. *Lancet* 2005;366:895–906.
70. Pepine CJ, Handberg EM, Cooper-Dehoff RM, et al. A calcium antagonist vs non-calcium antagonist hypertension treatment strategy for patients with coronary artery disease (INVEST). *JAMA* 2003;290:2805–16.
71. The Heart Outcomes Prevention Evaluation Study Investigators. Effects of an angiotensin-converting-enzyme inhibitor, ramipril, on cardiovascular events in high risk patients. *N Engl J Med* 2000;342: 145–53.
72. Wing LM, Reid CM, Ryan P, et al. A comparison of outcomes with angiotensin converting enzyme inhibitors and diuretics for hypertension in the elderly. *N Engl J Med* 2003;348:583–92.
73. The ONTARGET Investigators. Telmisartan, ramipril, or both in patients at high risk for vascular events. *N Engl J Med* 2008;358: 1547–59.
74. Bechir M, Enseleit F, Chenevard R, et al. Effect of Losartan on muscle sympathetic activity and baroceptor function in systemic hypertension. *Am J Cardiol* 2005;95:129–31.
75. Goodfriend TL, Elliot ME, Catt KJ. Angiotensin receptors and their antagonists. *N Engl J Med* 1996;334:1649–54.
76. Ligtenberg G, Blankestijn PJ, Oey PL, et al. Reduction of sympathetic hyperactivity by enalapril in patients with chronic renal failure. *N Engl J Med* 1999;340:1321–8.
77. Brown MJ, Palmer CR, Castaigne A, et al. Morbidity and mortality in patients randomised to double-blind treatment with long-acting calcium channel blocker or diuretic in the international Nifedipine GITS study: INSIGHT. *Lancet* 2000;356:366–72.
78. Davis BR, Kostis JB, Simpson LM, et al. Heart failure with preserved and reduced left ventricular ejection fraction in the antihypertensive and lipid-lowering treatment to prevent heart attack trial. *Circulation* 2008;118:2259–67.

79. Verdecchia P, Reboldi G, Angeli F, et al. Angiotensin-converting enzyme inhibitors and calcium channel blockers for coronary artery disease and stroke prevention. *Hypertension* 2005;46:386–92.
80. Brege E. Should high blood pressure be lowered in the acute stroke? *J Hypertens* 2011;29:1478–9.
81. Hansson L, Hedner T, Lund-Johansen P, et al. Randomised trial of effects of calcium antagonists compared with diuretics and beta-blockers on cardiovascular morbidity and mortality in hypertension: the Nordic Diltiazem (NORDIL) study. *Lancet* 2000;356:359–65.
82. Black HR, Elliot WJ, Grandits G, et al. Principal results of the Controlled Onset Verapamil Investigation of Cardiovascular End Points (CONVINCE) trial. *JAMA* 2003;289:2073–82.
83. Palatini P, Benetos A, Julius S. Impact of heart rate on clinical outcomes in hypertension. *Drugs* 2006;66:133–44.
84. Becher PM, Lindner D, Miteva K, et al. Role of heart rate reduction in the prevention of experimental heart failure. *Hypertension* 2012;59:949–57.
85. Fox K, Ford I, Steg PG, et al. Ivabradine for patients with stable coronary artery disease and left ventricular systolic dysfunction (BEAUTIFUL). *Lancet* 2008;372:807–16.
86. Ceconi C, Freedman SB, Tardiff JC, et al. Effect of heart rate reduction by ivabradine on left ventricular remodelling in the echocardiographic substudy of BEAUTIFUL. *Intern J Cardiol* 2011;146:408–14.
87. Tendera M, Talajic M, Robertson M, et al. Safety of Ivabradine in patients with coronary artery disease and left ventricular systolic dysfunction (BEAUTIFUL). *Am J Cardiol* 2011;107:805–11.
88. Swedberg K, Komajda M, Borer JS, et al. Ivabradine and outcomes in chronic heart failure (SHIFT). *Lancet* 2010;376:875–85.
89. Bohm M, Swedberg K, Kamajda M, et al. Heart rate as a risk factor in chronic heart failure (SHIFT): an association between heart rate and outcomes in a randomised placebo-controlled trial. *Lancet* 2010;376:886–94.
90. Teerlink JR. Ivabradine in heart failure—no paradigm SHIFT yet. *Lancet* 2010;376:847–9.
91. Schirmer SH, DEgan A, Baumhakel M, et al. Heart rate reduction by If-channel inhibition with ivabradine restores collateral artery growth in hypercholesterolemic atherosclerosis. *Eur Heart J* 2012;33:1223–31.
92. Zamorano JL. Heart rate management: a therapeutic goal throughout the cardiovascular continuum. *Eur Heart J* 2008;10(suppl F):F17–F21.
93. Dzau V, Braunwald E. Resolved and unresolved issues in the prevention and treatment of coronary heart disease: a workshop concensus statement. *Am Heart J* 1991;121:1244–61.

The UK, European, and US Guidelines Regarding the Treatment of Essential Hypertension

CHAPTER 10

The first thing that strikes the reader of the UK, European, and US guidelines regarding the treatment of hypertension, is the massive disparity in the advice given. Maybe this is not so surprising if one accepts the view that about 50% of guideline recommendations arise from judgement or experience, rather than from the evidence-based data (1). In the United States and Canada, possible financial conflicts among guideline panel members have been highlighted as worrying features (2). What is needed is a change of culture in which serving 2 masters becomes socially unacceptable as smoking a cigarette! (3).

THE UK—NATIONAL INSTITUTE FOR HEALTH AND CLINICAL EXCELLENCE (NICE)

1. History of NICE committee guidelines

The 2004 British Hypertension Society guidelines for hypertension (4) sensibly incorporated the so-called AB/CD rule (**Figure 10-1**) (5). This rule reflects the fact that hypertension can be broadly classified into "high renin" and "low renin" hypertension. Thus, "high renin" hypertensives are best treated first line with the inhibitors of the renin–angiotensin system, that is, angiotensin converting-enzyme (ACE) inhibitors (A) or β-blockers (B), and "low renin" hypertensives are best

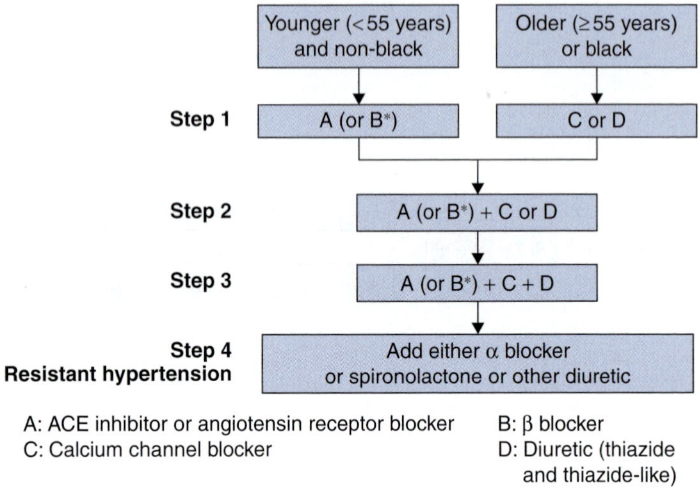

Fig. 10-1 Recommendations for combining blood pressure lowering drugs (AB/CD rule). (From Brown MJ, Cruickshank JK, Dominiczak AF, et al. Executive Committee British Hypertensive Society. Better blood pressure control: how to combine drugs. *J Hum Hypertens* 2003;17:81–6.)

treated first line with drugs that do not inhibit the renin–angiotensin system, that is, calcium blockers (C) or diuretics (D). Young/middle-aged diastolic hypertensives (younger than 55 years), and white, tend to have higher renin concentrations than older, or black, subjects. If 2 drugs are required, logical combinations are (A or B) plus (C or D).

The above guidelines were updated in 2006 (6), but now β-blockers were no longer recommended as the first-line therapy for the young/middle-aged hypertensives (**Figure 10-2**). For such patients, an Angiotensin converting enzyme inhibitor (ACEI) or an angiotensin receptor blocker (ARB) was the recommended first-line therapy for uncomplicated hypertension.

The main stated reasons for the omission of β-blockers as first-line drugs for uncomplicated hypertension were (i) reduced efficacy in preventing the risk of stroke, (ii) a tendency to precipitate diabetes mellitus, and (iii) they are accordingly the least cost-effective choice for the treatment of hypertension (7).

Then came the most recent 2011 NICE Committee guidelines (8), which demoted diuretics as first-line therapy for the treatment of hypertension (**Figure 10-3**). If a diuretic has to be given, then it should be either low-dose chlorthalidone or low-dose indapamide, in preference to a conventional thiazide diuretic such as

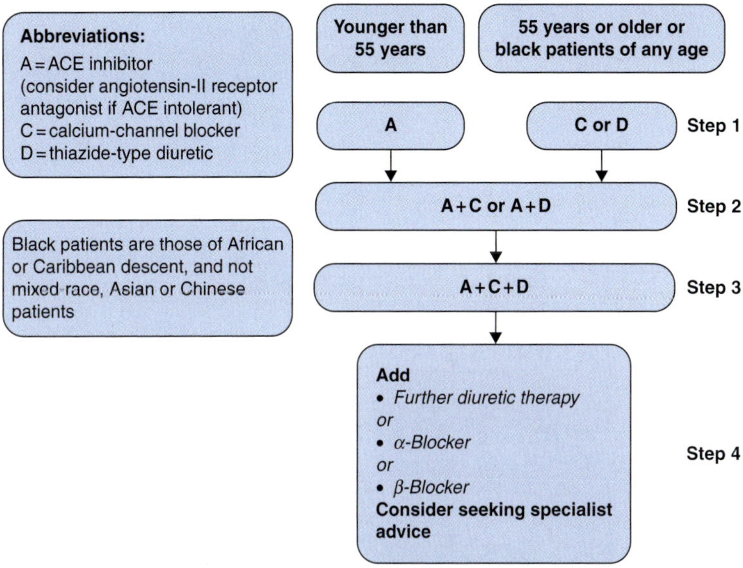

Fig. 10-2 Choosing drugs for patients newly diagnosed with hypertension. (From National Institute for Health and Clinical Excellence. Hypertension: management of hypertension in adults in primary care (Clinical guidelines 34) 2006. www.nice.org.uk/CG034.)

hydrochlorothiazide or bendroflumethiazide. In addition, ambulatory blood pressure (BP) monitoring was recommended as a cost-effective way of confirming the diagnosis of hypertension.

2. Cost-effectiveness aspects of treating hypertension

A) How to measure?

As indicated in Chapter 5 (ref 1, Figure 5-1), hypertension is the number one risk factor for premature death, heart attack, stroke, and heart failure around the world. Most of this burden is in low-/middle-income countries, as well as in people with prehypertension (ref 2, Chapter 5). Although risk associated with hypertension continues down to SBP of 115 mm Hg, the clinical and cost effects of treating prehypertension (SBP of 130–140 mm Hg) are unknown; adequately powered trials are required to assess cost effectiveness.

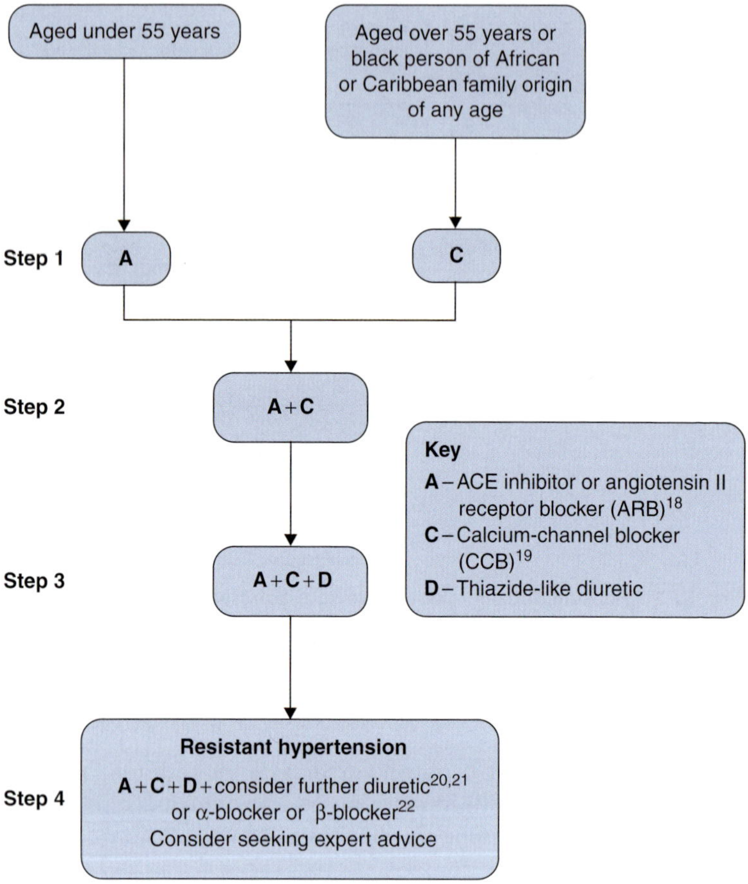

Fig. 10-3 Choosing drugs for the treatment of newly diagnosed hypertension. (From NICE guidelines 2011.)

In assessing cost effectiveness of treating hypertension, many factors have to be taken into account, including health care costs, non-health care costs, and the cost of drug therapy (**Table 10-1**) (9). Assuming 100% compliance in taking drug therapy, even taking drug costs into account, it is highly cost effective to treat hypertension (**Table 10-2**). Observing from a Health Service perspective, a useful way of expressing cost effectiveness is the disability-adjusted life years (DALY), which takes into account the avoidable events such as heart and stroke events, and deaths and disability-adjusted life years (**Table 10-3**) (10).

TABLE 10-1 The global cost of treating hypertension

Health care costs	Non-health care costs	Contributors to the cost of drug therapy
Hypertension-related visits	Informal care	Price of drug
Clinical and laboratory evaluation	Productivity loss	Clinical and laboratory costs
Consultations		Compliance
Hospitalization		Persistence
Cardiovascular complications		
Drug therapy		

From Ambrosioni E, Borghi C. Pharmacoeconomic and cost-benefit aspects. In: Mancia G, Grassi G, Kjeldsen SE, editors. Manual of hypertension of the European Society of Hypertension. Informa UK Ltd; 2008. p. 316–20.

TABLE 10-2 Annual expenditure for acute MI, heart failure, and stroke with a hypertension prevalence of 36% of the population in Italy

	Current situation	If 100% patients treated
Drugs	2.84	6.08
Costs for NHS of CV events	16.30	10.24
Total costs	19.14	16.32
Savings 2.82 billions £/yr!		

Abbreviations: CV, cardiovascular; NHS, National Health System.
From Ambrosioni E, Borghi C. Pharmacoeconomic and cost-benefit aspects. In: Mancia G, Grassi G, Kjeldsen SE, editors. Manual of hypertension of the European Society of Hypertension. Informa UK Ltd; 2008. p. 316–20.

B) Most cost-effective measures

So, what are the most cost-effective measures regarding hypertension? Clearly, being sure of the diagnosis is important. Thus, abolishing "white-coat" hypertension is essential; hence, the usage of ambulatory BP monitoring is highly cost effective (11).

Lifestyle changes, thereby cutting out drug-costs, are an attractive proposition, for example, weight loss, exercise, reduction of

TABLE 10-3 Assessing avoidable burden of CV Disease: how the DALY is derived

Outcome	Comment
• Deaths and avoidable deaths	Avoidable deaths are the difference in deaths from interventions compared to current situation
• YLLs; nondiscounted and discounted	Difference between the age at the "avoidable death" and the expected life of someone of that age in England—we used a cutoff age of 100 years. Nondiscounted calculated simply by multiplying the number of deaths in each age year by the LE, using 100 years as cutoff. We used the WHO formula to obtain the discounted LE and then applied this to the deaths (both IHD/stroke and other deaths)
• YLDs; nondiscounted and discounted	This is total number of people with a history of IHD and a history of stroke for each of the 5 years, multiplied by the disability weights and the life expectancy for each age. We used the survival estimates to calculate YLD. For people who survived a CVD event, the estimate for the duration of time lived with disability was from the time of the event to the 10-year cutoff for the model (i.e., of a person had a stroke in year 8 of the model and survived beyond 10 years, and the duration of disability was2 years
• DALYs nondiscounted and discounted	The sum of YLLs and YLDs, with and without discounting at 3.5% rate

Abbreviations: CVD, cardiovascular disease; DALYs, disability-adjusted life years; IHD, ischemic heart disease; LE, life expectancy; YLDs, years lived with a disability; YLLs, years of life lost.

From Dodhia H, Phillips K, Zannou M-I, et al. Modeling the impact of available cardiovascular disease burden and costs of interventions to lower SBP in the England population. *J Hypertens* 2012;30:217–26.

excessive alcohol, and dietary aspects. However, compliance with such an approach is problematical (12). Reducing the amount of salt in the diet is attractive (10), particularly at a governmental/food-industry level (13). This approach assumes that lowering BP by such a method will save lives. As pointed out in Chapter 6, low-sodium diets lower BP, but increase the renin/sympathetic nervous activity; thus, stroke prevention is likely, but what about myocardial infarction (MI)? Clearly, a major outcome study is required.

It is thus evident that antihypertensive drug therapy is cost effective (14). However, there is a problem of noncompliance with drug therapy, which is clearly not cost effective (15). In the setting of finite health care resources, antihypertensive drugs that might increase the risk of heart failure or diabetes will be less attractive (16). Thus, all things being considered, a drug which does not induce metabolic changes will be preferable to one that does (17). Similarly, the perception that a particular drug was less effective in reducing the risk of stroke (7) would make it an unattractive choice and non-cost effective. Thus, older non-, or poorly, selective β-blockers and diuretics have come out badly when assessed in these cost-effective terms (**Figure 10-4**) (18).

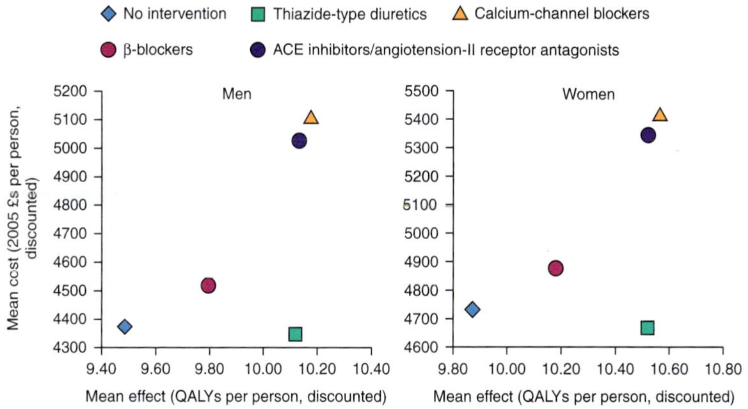

Fig. 10-4 Cost-effectiveness of treating hypertension with different types of drugs; data expressed as UK sterling per quality quality-adjusted life year (QALY) for each treatment versus no intervention: β-blockers are the least cost-effective treatment. (From Williams B. Beta-blockers and the treatment of hypertension. *J Hypertens* 2007;25:1351–3.)

3. Major criticisms of the 2011 NICE guidelines

A) The β-blocker issue

In response to the NICE 2011 guidelines (8), Cruickshank wrote a letter to the BMJ (19) as follows:

"Sir

In the summary NICE guidance on the management of hypertension (1), the advice on the first-line treatment of younger/middle-aged hypertensives with either an ACE inhibitor or ARB, with no mention of beta-blockade, is worrying.

There has been only one randomised, hard-endpoint comparison between ACE-inhibitors and beta-blockers ie UKPDS study (2). After 9–10 years follow-up the trends in the reduction of all 7 primary endpoints favoured atenolol. After 20 years the earlier trends persisted, and for all-cause death strengthened to a significant 23% reduction (3). So how could an ACE inhibitor be favoured over a beta-blocker? Is a brief increase in HbA1-c (plus cost implications) to be considered more important than a life-saving quality? Besides, high beta-1 selectivity (bisoprolol) not only avoids metabolic disturbance but is the most effective way to lower blood pressure in young-middle-aged hypertensives (4).

The apparent disappointing results of other beta-blocker studies in middle-aged hypertensives i.e. MRC, IPPPSH and MAPHY, was due to an important smoking-interaction (4). In non-smokers beta-blockers reduced the risk myocardial infarction by 30-45% versus placebo or diuretic (4). This benefit was totally cancelled out in the smokers due to the marked hypertensive reaction occurring with non/poorly-selective beta-blockers in the presence of smoking-induced increases in adrenaline (4). This dangerous interaction can be avoided by high beta-1 selectivity (4).

ARBs may increase the risk of myocardial infarction, a concern underlined by the results of a recent study in middle-aged type-2 diabetics with pre-hypertension (5). The number of deaths from cardiovascular causes was higher in the ARB, than in the placebo, group (13 vs. 3, $p = 0.01$), owing primarily to more cases of fatal myocardial infarction (5 vs. 0) and sudden cardiac deaths (7 v 1) in the ARB group.

Is it too late for the NICE guidance group to modify their recommendations?

References

1. Krause T, Lovibond K, Caufield M, McCormack T, Williams B. Managment of hypertension: summary of NICE guidance. *BMJ* 2011;343: d 4891.

2. UK Prospective Diabetes Study Group. Efficacy of atenolol and captopril in reducing risk of macrovascular and microvascular complications in type 2 diabetes: UKPDS 39. *BMJ* 1998;317:713–9.
3. Holman RR, Paul SK, Bethel MA, Neil HA, Matthews DR. Long-term follow-up after tight control of blood pressure in type-2 diabetes. *N Eng JM* 2008;359:1565–76
4. Cruickshank JM. *The Modern Role of Beta-Blockers in Cardiovascular Medicine.* People's Medical Publishing House, USA Shelton, Connecticut, 20
5. Haller H, Sadayoshi I, Izzo JL, Januszewicz A, Katayama S, Menne J etal. Olmesartan for the delay or prevention of microalbuminuria in type-2 diabetes. *N Engl J Med* 2011;364:907–17."

The NICE reply (20) was:

"In response to Cruickshank, the 2006 NICE hypertension guideline recommended that β blockers are not preferred treatment for hypertension unless there is a compelling indication for them beyond the need to lower blood pressure.[2] In the new guideline they were the least cost effective treatment option. Furthermore, similar conclusions have been reached in other independent analysis.[3 4] Cruickshank's assertion that more selective β blockers may be better than older generation β blockers at reducing cardiovascular risk in people with hypertension cannot be substantiated by referring to evidence from clinical outcome trials with these drugs in people with hypertension.

Bryan Williams professor of medicine, Department of Cardiovascular Sciences, University of Leicester and Leicester NIHR Cardiovascular Biomedical Research unit, Glenfield Hospital, Leicester LE2 7UK bw17@le.ac.uk

Taryn Krause senior project manager, research fellow

Kate Lovibond senior health economist, National Clinical Guideline Centre Acute and Chronic Conditions, Royal College of Physicians, London NW14LE, UK

Mark Caulfield professor of clinical pharmacology, William Harvey Research Institute, Barts and the London School of Medicine, and NIHR Cardiovascular Biomedical Research Unit, Queen Mary University of London, London EC1M 6BQ, UK

Terry McCormack general practitioner, Whitby Group Practice, Spring Vale Medical Centre, Whitby YO21 1SD, UK, On behalf of the Guideline Development Group

Competing interests: A full list of competing interest is available at www.bmj.com/content/343/bmj/d4891.full.

A correction is published at www.bmj.com/content/343/bmj.d6255.full and a fuller version of this letter is available at www.bmj.com/content/343/bmj.d4891/reply#bmj-el-271066.

1. Lovibond K, Jowett S, Barton P, Caulfield M, Heneghan C, Hobbs R, et al. Cost-effectiveness of options for the diagnosis of high blood pressure in primary care: a modelling study. *Lancet* 2011;378:1219–30.
2. National #Collaborating Centre for Chronic Conditions. Hypertension: management in adults in primary care: pharmacological update. (Pharmacological update of CG 18.) Royal College of Physicians, 2006.
3. Wiysonge C, Bradley H, Myose B et al. Beta-blockers for hypertension. *Cochrane Database Syst Rev* 2007;1:CD002003.
4. Bangalore S, Messerli FH, Kostis JB, Pepine CJ. Cardiovascular protection using beta-blockers: a critical review of the evidence. *J Am Coll Cardiol* 2007;50:563–72.

Cite this as: BMJ 2011;343:d6506."

Remarkable in the NICE reply above are the following points:

1. The quoting of 2 supportive meta-analyses, neither of which took the age, or smoking, factors into account.
2. The simple restatement that β-blockers are not cost effective clearly reflected the 2006–2007 position (6, 7), which preceded the 20-year follow-up of the UKPDS study published in 2008 (21), which indicated that the group initially randomized to atenolol displayed a significant 23% reduction in all-cause death compared to those randomized to the ACE inhibitor captopril (**Figure 10-5**). One is left to conclude that the significant 23% excess deaths in the ACE inhibitor group are cost effective!
3. One of the main reason for labeling β-blockers as non-cost effective, that is, lack of efficacy in stroke reduction (7), is untenable when taking the original UKPDS study (in obese, middle-aged, diabetics, diastolic hypertensives) results into account (**Figure 10-6**) (22); where compared to "less tight control" of BP, atenolol reduced stroke risk by 50%, an effect even greater than with the ACE inhibitor. Also, in the MRC mild hypertension study in middle-aged diastolic hypertensives, propranolol reduced the risk of stroke by over 50%, versus placebo, in nonsmokers (Figure 10-16) (23). The NICE opinion on β-blockers and stroke relates only to elderly systolic hypertensives, where β-blockers are not recommended as the first-line therapy.
4. By ignoring the nonselective/moderately selective β-blocker-smoking interaction, the NICE committee appear to be quite unaware of the fact that compared to randomized placebo or diuretic therapy, there was a massive reduction of about 30%–45% in the

risk of MI in those randomized to β-blockers in the non-smoking group (75% of total) (**Figure 10-7**) (24) (no other drug can compare with this β-blocker effect on the number one killer, MI, in young/middle-aged diastolic hypertension).

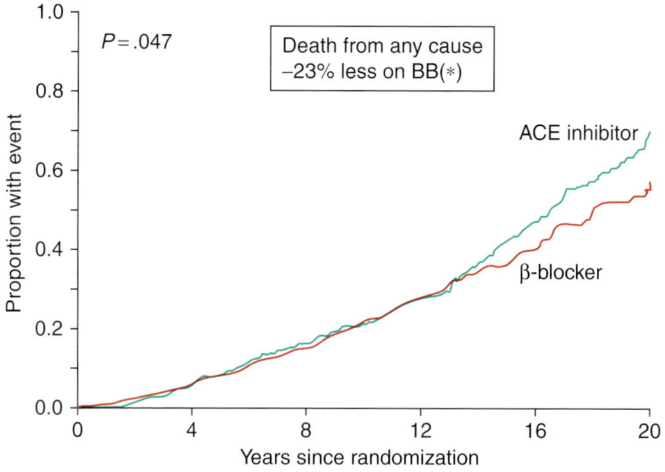

Fig. 10-5 UKPDS study: after 20-year follow-up, death from any cause was reduced by a significant 23% in those randomized to atenolol versus captopril. (From Holman RR, Paul SK, Bethel MA, et al. Long-term follow-up after tight control of blood pressure in type-2 diabetes. *N Engl J Med* 2008;359:1565–76.)

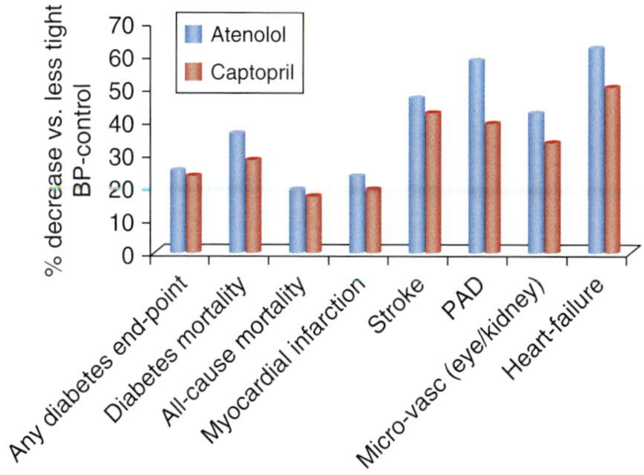

Fig. 10-6 UKPDS—the trends in reduction of all primary endpoints favor atenolol versus captopril when compared with less tight BP control (diff = 10/5 mm Hg) over 10-year follow-up. (From UK Prospective Diabetes Study Group. Efficacy of atenolol and captopril in reducing the risk of macrovascular and micro-vascular complications in type 2 diabetes; UKPDS 39. *BMJ* 1998;317: 713–20.)

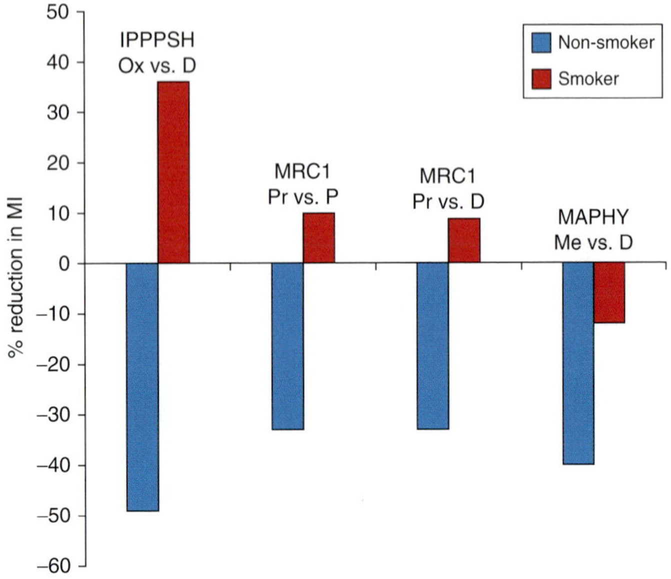

Fig. 10-7 β-Blocker/smoking interaction (MI) in young/mid-age hypertensives: the 30%–50% reduction in MI by β-blocker versus placebo or diuretic in non-smokers is negated in smokers. (From Cruickshank JM. *The Modern Role of Beta-Blockers in Cardiovascular Medicine*. Shelton, Connecticut: People's Medical Publishing House; 2011.)

5. The fact that the metabolic/blood sugar/smoking-interaction problems with nonselective/moderately selective β-blockers could be avoided by highly β-1 selective bisoprolol was dismissed by the NICE Committee based on that there were no hard endpoint data in hypertension with bisoprolol. In fact, the NICE group is wrong, as in mild hypertensives with coronary artery disease, who were randomized to either bisoprolol or nifedipine, there was a significant increase in the event-free survival in those randomized to bisoprolol (**Figure 10-8**) (25). It is also counterintuitive that a highly β-1 selective β-blocker like bisoprolol, which intervenes significantly at numerous stages in the cardiovascular (CV) continuum (**Figure 10-9**) (26), would not be highly effective in reducing hard endpoints in uncomplicated diastolic hypertension (24), as (a) it is the most effective antihypertensive agent in the young/middle-aged, (b) it is at least as effective as ACE-inhibitors in reversing LVH in middle-aged hypertensives, (c) as just mentioned, it is superior to nifedipine in improving the event-free survival in middle-aged mild-hypertensives with CAD, (d) in high-risk ischemic patients undergoing noncardiac surgery, it significantly improved postoperative survival when

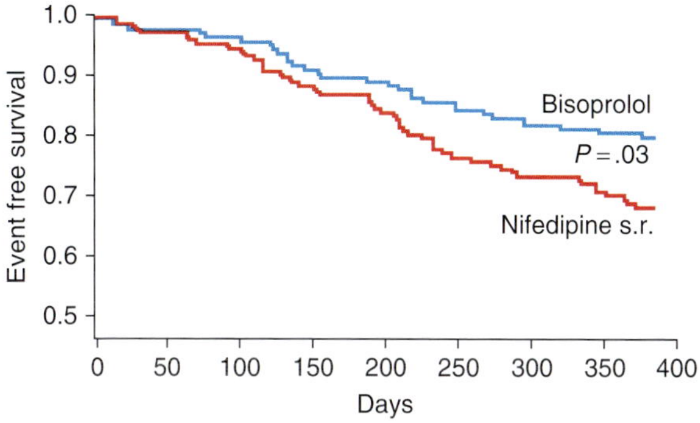

Fig. 10-8 TIBBS study: 307 CAD patients with mild hypertension; bisoprolol is significantly superior to SR nifedipine in improving event-free survival (Death, M.I. Hospitalization). (From von Armin T, for the TIBBS Investigators. Prognostic significance of transient ischaemic episodes: response to treatment shows improved prognosis. *J Am Coll Cardio* 1996;28:20–4.)

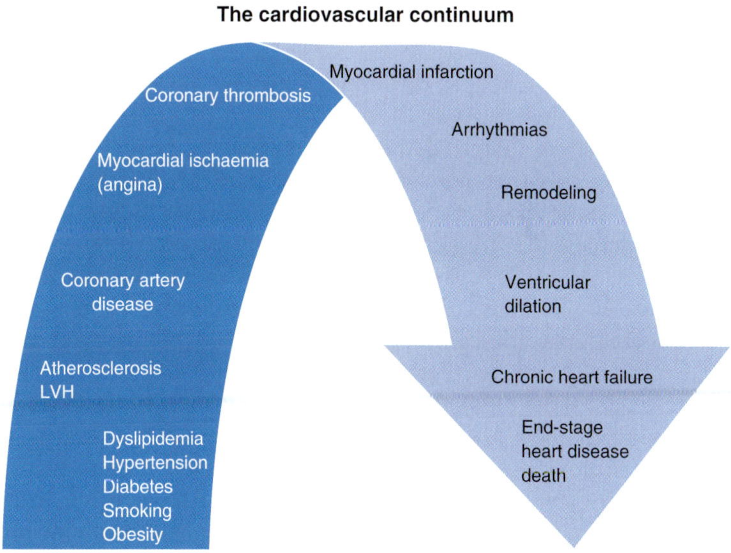

Fig. 10-9 The CV continuum. (From Zamorano JL. Heart rate management: a therapeutic goal throughout the cardiovascular continuum. *Eur Heart J* 2008;10(suppl F):F17–F21.)

prescribed 2- to 3-week preoperation, (e) in systolic heart failure, bisoprolol reduced all-cause death by a significant 34% versus placebo, and (f) in systolic heart failure, it is superior to an ACEI in reducing the risk of sudden death.

Others have also criticized the NICE 2011 guidelines (27). Sofat et al. made several points: (1) In the ASCOT study, the apparent inferiority of atenolol versus amlodipine was due to a lesser fall in BP, (2) many meta-analyses condemning β-blockers are flawed, (3) the massive Blood Pressure Treatment Trialist Collaboration concluded that all classes of drugs were broadly equivalent with respect to protection from serious CV events, (4) Law and colleagues found β-blockers to have a specific action over and above their BP lowering the effects in preventing a reoccurrence in the first few years of a coronary heart disease event; they stated that it seemed counterintuitive that β-blockers should be an unfavored treatment before a patient had a coronary event, but a preferred option immediately afterward, and (5) the small β-blocker-induced increases in blood sugar could take a subject with a blood level just below 7.0 mml/L into an arbitrary diabetic range, thereby giving a false impression that β-blockers commonly induce type 2 diabetes; such small blood sugar changes would be unlikely to be associated with an increased risk of stroke.

B) The angiotensin receptor blocker issue

The 2011 NICE guidelines recommend for the young/middle-aged hypertensive, either an ACEI or an ARB.

As presented in Chapter 8, there is great concern about ARBs and the possibility that they may increase the risk of MI. Unlike ACEIs, ARBs increase the concentration of angiotensin II as well as (in younger subjects) increase the sympathetic nerve activity (**Figure 10-10**). Meta-analyses have suggested that, unlike ACEIs, ARBs increase the risk of MI (**Figure 10-11**). This concern was amply justified by the results of 2 randomized, placebo-controlled studies in young/middle-aged subjects with type 2 diabetes (**Figure 10-12**) (28, 29).

These data were highlighted in the author's letter in the BMJ in response to the new NICE guidelines (see earlier) (19). The NICE guideline authors' response to Cruickshank's points on ARBs was—"nothing"! In spite of these damning data on ARBs in young/middle-aged subjects, the NICE guideline committee still recommends these drugs as first-line agents for the young/middle-aged hypertensive! Clearly (see above results, 20-year follow-up of the UKPDS study), excess deaths are cost effective!

C) The diuretic issue

Two publications, in particular, were critical of the new NICE guidelines, which omitted diuretics as the first-line therapy (30, 31). The criticisms in these articles are important (and surprising) in that all three authors have close associations with British Hypertension Society guideline committees.

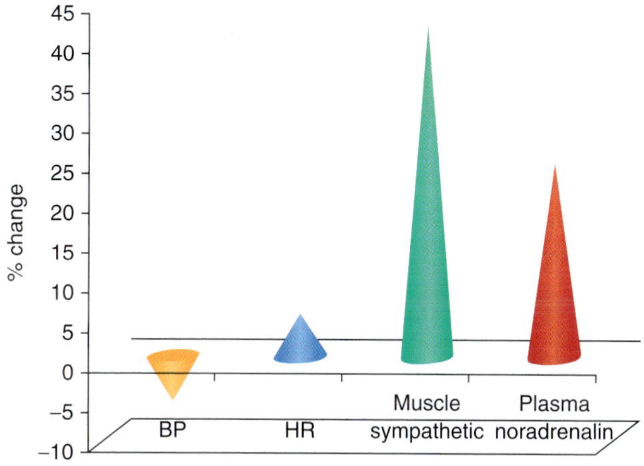

Fig. 10-10 ARBs and sympathetic nerve activity; double-blind, random, X-over, placebo-controlled study in young, hypertensive males. (Heusser K, Vitovski J, Raasch W, et al. Elevation of sympathetic nerve activity by eprosartan inyoun male subjects. *AM J Hypertens* 2003;18:658-64.)

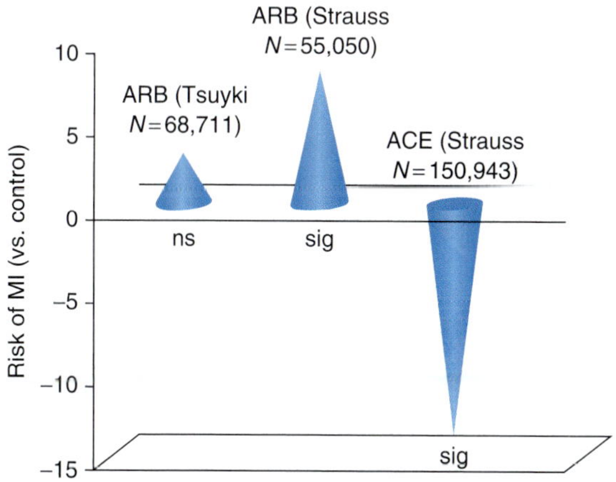

Fig. 10-11 Relative risk of MI in meta-analyses of ARB and ACE-inhibitors. (From Stauss MH, Hall AS. Angiotensin receptor blockers may increase risk of myocardial infarction. *Circulation* 2006;114:838–54.)

Brown (30) points out that NICE differs from all other international guidelines by dropping diuretics from the first-line therapy. Other salient points are as follows:

a. Low-renin hypertension (predominant in the elderly) was closely associated with sodium retention, thus particularly suitable for diuretic therapy.
b. Resistant hypertension is commonly due to the iatrogenic underdosing of diuretics

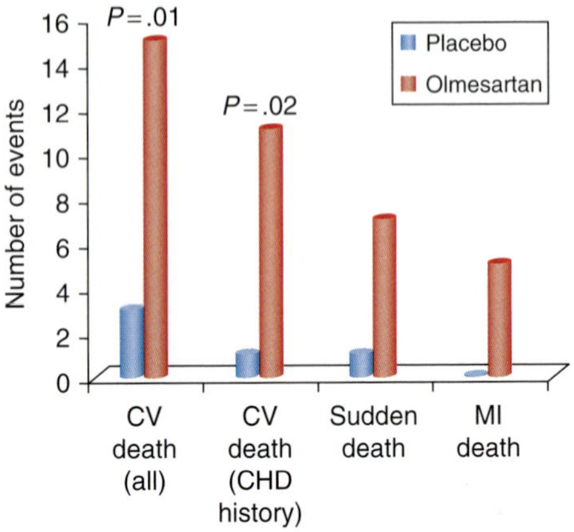

Fig. 10-12 Olmesartan versus placebo (randomized) in 4447 DM2, mean age 57, mean BMI 31, BP 136/81, over 3.2 years: the ARB significantly increased the risk of CV endpoints and death. (From Haller H, Ito S, Izzo JL, et al. Olmesartan for the delay or prevention of microalbuminuria in type-2 diabetes. *N Engl J Med* 2011;364:907–17.)

c. The tendency for diuretics to induce diabetes may be linked to the loss of potassium (see Chapter 8, Figure 8.22a), a fault corrected by the use of potassium-sparing diuretics such as amiloride (**Figure 10-13**).
d. The combination of hydrochlorothiazide and amiloride (co-amilozide), compared to placebo or atenolol, in the MRC elderly study (32), reduced coronary events by a remarkable 44% (**Figure 10-14**); thus, "pending further research," co-amilozide should be the first-line recommendation for patients aged >55 years as an alternative to CCBs.
e. The demotion of diuretics by NICE rests largely on the assumption that calcium blockers reduce the BP variability more effectively than other drugs, yet BP variability has never been tested prospectively; noteworthy is the fact that in the largest prospective, randomized hard endpoint study ever done, that is, Antihypertensive and Lipid-lowering Treatment to Prevent heart Attack Trial (ALLHAT) (33), first-line diuretic therapy was the preferred treatment over ACEIs and calcium blockers.

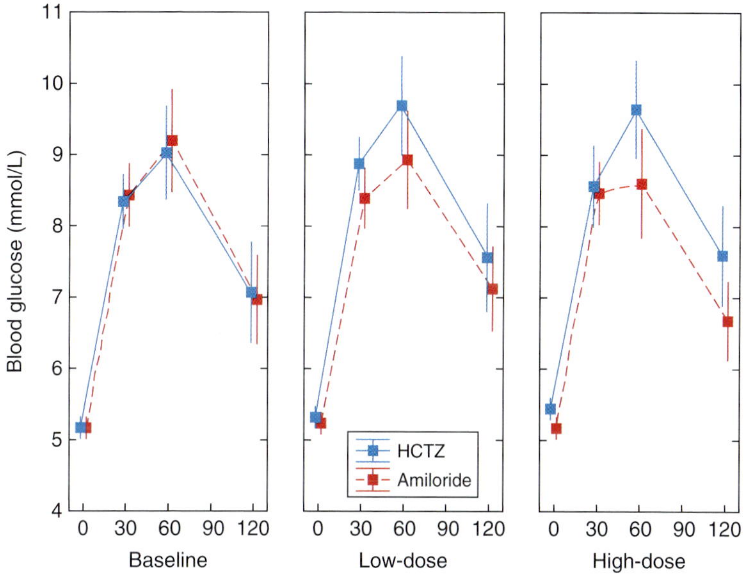

Fig. 10-13 Hydrochlorothiazide, but not amiloride, impairs glucose tolerance. (From Brown MJ. The choice of diuretic in hypertension: saving the baby from the bathwater. *Heart* 2011;97:1547–51.)

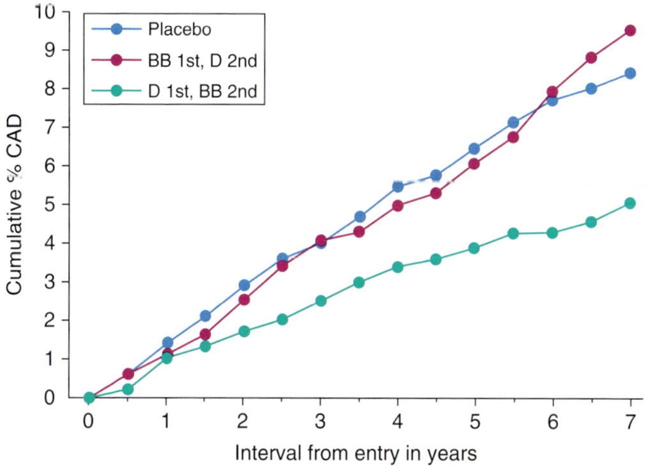

Fig. 10-14 MRC-elderly study (1992)—after 7-year follow-up only the diuretic (not atenolol) significantly reduced the risk of CAD versus placebo by 44%.

THE US, JNC 7, GUIDELINES

The recommendation was that for uncomplicated hypertension, a thiazide diuretic should be used in most cases, either alone or combined with drugs from other classes.

1. Major criticisms of the JNC-7 guidelines

Surprisingly, the Joint National Committee-7 (JNC-7) guidelines (34) did not take age into account with respect to recommended pharmacological treatment. The US Framingham group (35) showed clearly that diastolic hypertension developed mainly in the young/middle-aged and was linked to a high BMI; in contrast, systolic hypertension developed mainly in the elderly and was a function of aging and stiffening of the arteries. As discussed in Chapter 4, young/middle-aged diastolic hypertension is linked to high plasma renin levels, high sympathetic nerve activity, and sensitized β-receptors. In contrast, elderly systolic hypertension is linked to low plasma renin activity, desensitized β-receptors and salt retention—a situation ideal for diuretic therapy.

Certainly, in elderly systolic hypertensives hard endpoint studies, first-line diuretic therapy has performed exceedingly well, as witnessed in the MRC Elderly study (Figure 10-14) (32), the ALLHAT study (33), and the SHEP study (38). These studies were described in Chapter 8.

However, as indicated in Chapter 8, in randomized, hard endpoint studies in young/middle-aged hypertensives, first-line diuretics have not performed well in terms of preventing the number one killer, MI. In the Australian Mild Hypertension study (36), compared to randomized placebo, diuretic therapy showed a significant 45% fall in stroke risk, but no effect on fatal and nonfatal MI (**Figure 10-15**). A similar result was observed in the large MRC trial of mild hypertension (**Figure 10-16**) (23), where diuretic therapy was highly effective in reducing stroke risk in both smokers and nonsmokers, but had no effect at all in reducing the risk of MI (in contrast to propranolol that reduced MI risk by 33% in nonsmokers). Finally, in the Oslo study (37) involving middle-aged men, diuretics versus randomized nontreatment, diuretic therapy was associated with a significant increase in the risk of MI (**Figure 10-17**). As indicated earlier (Figure 10-7) (24), in the MRC, IPPPSH, and MAPPHY studies, and in nonsmokers, the risk of MI was 30%–45% less in those allocated to either propranolol, oxprenolol, or metoprolol, versus diuretic or placebo therapy.

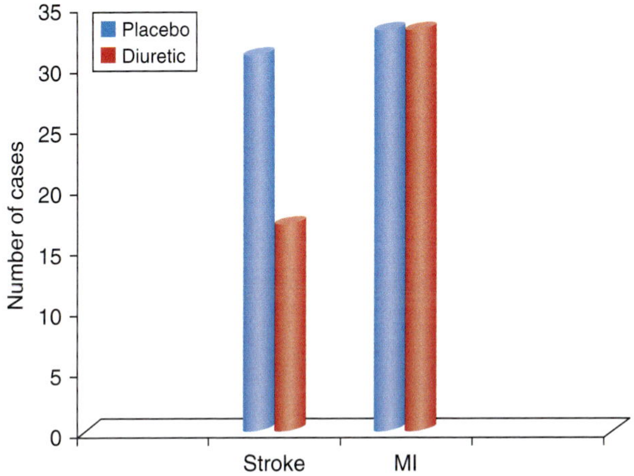

Fig. 10-15 Australian Mild Hypertension study—diuretic versus placebo in 3427 hypertensives (mean age 50 y): diuretics prevent stroke but not MI. (From Report by the Management Committee. The Australian therapeutic trial in mild hypertension. *Lancet* 1980;1:1261–7.)

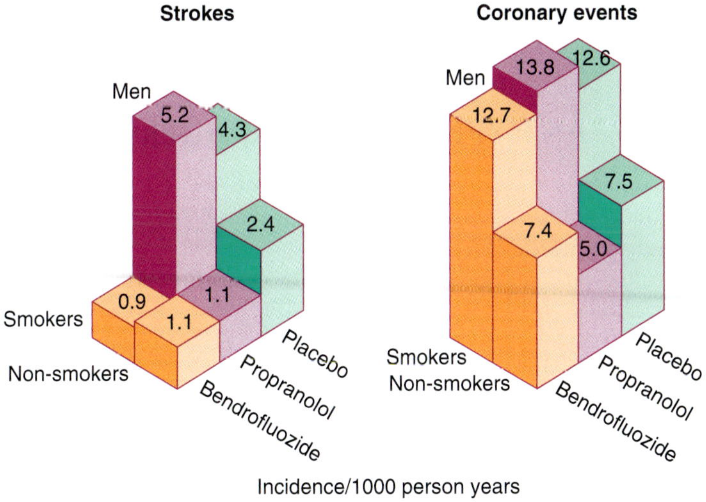

Fig. 10-16 MRC mild hypertension study (1985); diuretics reduce stroke but not coronary events.

As discussed in Chapter 6, thiazide-type diuretics increase the sympathetic nerve activity, and this is likely the reason why diuretics reduce the stroke risk (related to level of BP), but not the risk of MI

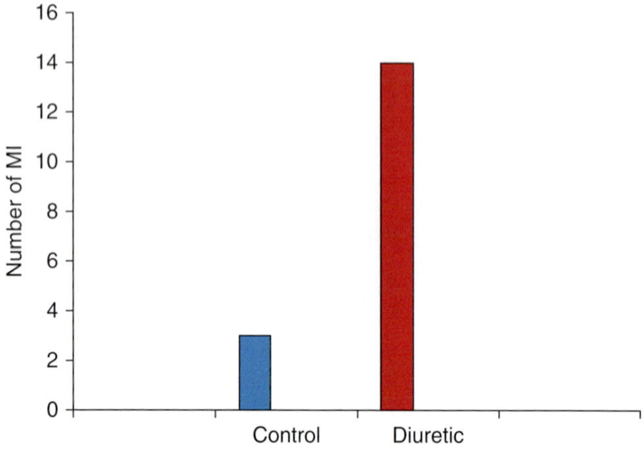

Fig. 10-17 Oslo study; 785 mildly hypertensive men, age 40–49 years, randomized to control or hydrochlorothiazide dosed for 5.5 years; diuretics increase the risk of MI. (From Leren P, Helgeland A. Coronary heart disease and the treatment of hypertension. Some Oslo study data. *Am J Med* 1986;80:3–6.)

(related to the level of sympathetic nerve activity (see Chapter 5)), in young/middle-aged patients with sensitized β-receptors.

EUROPEAN HYPERTENSION GUIDELINES

Compared to the UK NICE Committee and the US JNC-7 guidelines, the 2009 European guidelines appear to be relatively sensible and well balanced (38).

The key points regarding the choice of antihypertensive drugs are as follows:

i. Diuretics, ACE-I, calcium blockers, ARBs, and β-blockers do not differ significantly in their overall ability to reduce BP.
ii. All drug classes are similar in their ability to reduce the risk of CV events, even in the elderly or diabetics.
iii. CV protection depends on BP lowering *per se*, regardless of how it is achieved.
iv. The traditional ranking of drugs into first, second, third, and subsequent choice has little scientific and practical justifications and should be avoided.
v. The combination of β-blockers and diuretics should be avoided, particularly in patients with the metabolic syndrome (due to risk of diabetes) (39).

1. Criticism of the European guidelines

i. All antihypertensive drugs are not similar in their ability to lower BP and prevent CV events. This would have been apparent had age been taken into account.

As indicated by the Framingham Group (35), diastolic hypertension develops mainly in young/middle-aged and is linked to obesity; in contrast, systolic hypertension develops mainly in the elderly and is a function of aging and stiffening of the arteries. As discussed in Chapter 4, young/middle-aged diastolic hypertension is underpinned by high sympathetic nerve activity in the presence of sensitized β-receptors. Accordingly, β-blockade (bisoprolol) was the most effective way to lower 24-hour BP in young/middle-aged hypertensive (**Figure 10-18**) (40).

Thus, in high-risk, middle-aged, diastolic hypertensives, β-blockers have performed well, versus ACEIs (Figures 10-5 and 10-6) (22, 24), and versus placebo and diuretics (Figure 10-7) (24), in preventing MI. Agents that increase the sympathetic nerve activity, that is, diuretics, dihydropyridine calcium blockers, and ARBs (see Chapter 6) do not reduce (and might increase) the risk of MI in young/middle-aged subjects (see Chapter 8).

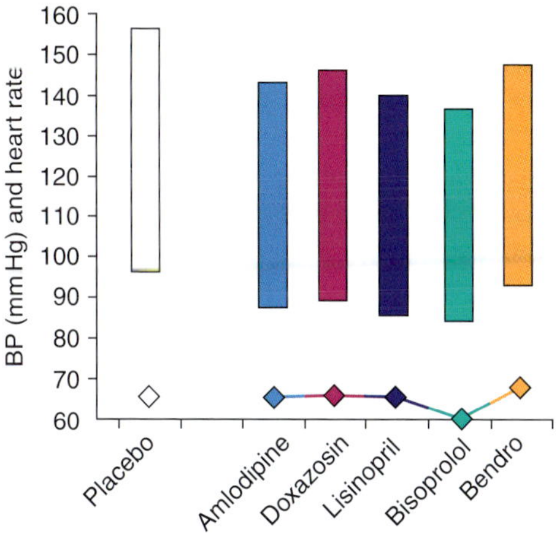

Fig. 10-18 In 34 young/middle-age (28–55 years) hypertensives, bisoprolol 5 mg was more effective than amlodipine 5 mg, doxazosin 104 mg, bendrofluazide 2.5 mg, and lisinopril 2.5–10 mg (double-blind, crossover, 1 month each). (From Deary AJ, Schumann AL, Murfeet H, et al. Double-blind, placebo controlled crossover comparison of 5 classes of drugs. *J Hypertens* 2002;20:771–7.)

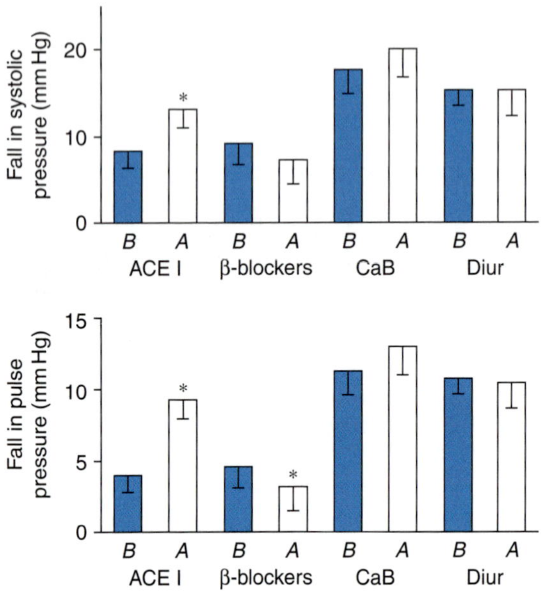

Fig. 10-19 Under randomized, double-blind, crossover conditions, in elderly systolic hypertensives the β-blocker atenolol was the least effective in reducing central (*A*) aortic and (*B*) brachial pressures. (From Morgan T, Lauri J, Bertram D, et al. Effect of different antihypertensive drug classes on central aortic pressure. Am *J Hypertens* 2004;17:118–23.)

In contrast, in the elderly, β-blockade (atenolol) was relatively ineffective in reducing the central pressures (**Figure 10-19**) (41). Accordingly, in hard endpoint studies involving the elderly hypertensive (**Table 10-4**) (32, 44–46), first-line atenolol did not perform well, versus placebo, ARBs, calcium blockers, and diuretics. Only when there was an accompanying coronary artery disease, as in the INVEST study, was first-line atenolol similar to calcium blockade (46).

ii. Cardiovascular (CV) protection does not depend on lowering BP *per se*, regardless of how it is achieved. As mentioned earlier, in the young/middle-aged diastolic hypertensives, agents that effectively lower BP, but increase the sympathetic nerve activity, that is diuretics, dihydropyridine calcium blockers, and ARBs (Chapter 6), while reducing the stroke risk, they do not reduce (and might increase) the risk of MI (Chapter 8). In contrast, β-blockers and ACE inhibitors do reduce the risk of MI (Figure 10-6) (22). Nonselective/poorly selective β-blockers, compared to randomized placebo or diuretic therapy, reduce the risk of MI by 30%–45% in nonsmokers (Figure 10-7) (24). The β-blocker/smoking/high adrenaline/hypertensive interaction

TABLE 10-4 First-line β-blockers (atenolol) perform poorly in elderly hypertension (wide pulse-pressure)

Trial	β-Blocker	Mean age (years)	Initial BP (mm Hg)	Pulse-pressure (mm Hg)	Result
MRC elderly	Atenolol (vs. placebo vs diuretic)	70	185/91	94	Only first-line diuretics differed from placebo in stroke prevention; diuretic superior to first-line atenolol in reducing coronary events
HEP	Atenolol (vs. non-treatment)	69	196/99	97	Significant reduction in stroke but no effect on coronary events by atenolol
LIFE	Atenolol (vs. losartan)	67	174/98	76	Losartan superior to atenolol in reducing cardiovascular mortality and non-fatal and fatal stroke
ASOCT	Atenolol ± diuretic (vs. amlodipine ± perindopril)	63	164/94	70	Amlodipine ± perindopril was superior to atenolol ± diuretic in reducing all-cause mortality and all coronary and stroke end-points

From Cruickshank JM. Are we misunderstanding beta-blockers? *Int J Cardiol* 2007;120:10–27.

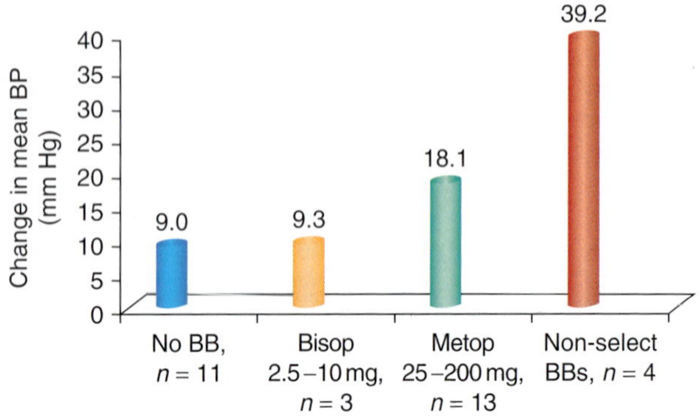

Fig. 10-19a Peri-operative interaction between adrenaline and β-blockers: hypertensive blockers: response with nonselective/poorly selective BBs. (From Tarnow J, Muller RK. Cardiovascular effects of low-dose epinephrine infusions in relation to the extent of pre-operative beta-blockade. Anaesthesiology 1991;74:1035–43.)

can be avoided by high β-1 selectivity, that is, bisoprolol (**Figure 10.19a**, see Chapter 8) (19, 24).

iii. Traditional ranking of drugs does have merit. As indicated earlier, in the young/middle-aged diastolic hypertensive (underpinned by high sympathetic nerve activity and sensitized β-receptors), β-1 blockade is highly effective in reducing the risk of MI, whereas drugs such as diuretics, dihydropyridine calcium blockers, and ARBs do not. By contrast, in the elderly systolic hypertensive (associated with aging/stiff arteries), first-line atenolol has not performed well in reducing CV events, versus placebo, diuretics, calcium blockers, and ARB, unless coronary artery disease is also present.

iv. The combination of β-blockers and diuretics should not be avoided. Such a combination has performed exceedingly powerfully in the elderly hypertensive, particularly in patients with the metabolic syndrome.

As described in Chapter 8, in the MRC elderly study (Figure 10-14) (32), the ALLHAT (33) and the SHEP studies (38), first-line diuretics/second-line β-blockers performed extremely well in reducing fatal and nonfatal CV events. In the ALLHAT study, the diuretic/β-blocker combination was especially effective, versus ACEI, α-blocker, and calcium blocker, in preventing heart failure (47) (**Figure 10-20**).

Of particular interest was that in the ALLHAT study (48), nondiabetic individuals with the metabolic syndrome survived particularly well (in terms of less heart failure and fewer CV events) on the diuretic/β-blocker combination, especially versus ACEI therapy (**Figure 10-21**). Thus, the group of patients whom the European

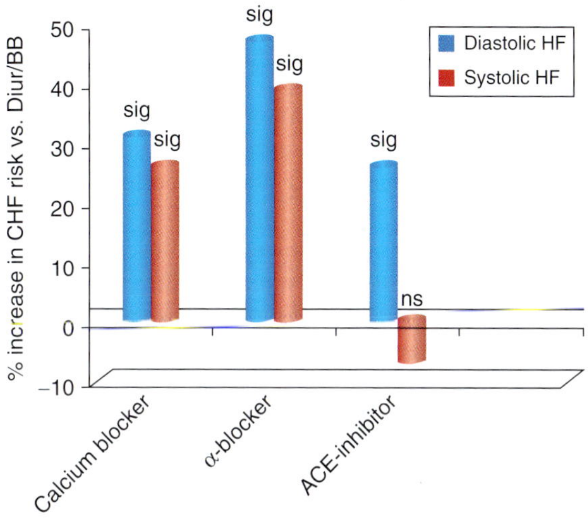

Fig. 10-20 Superiority of Diur/BB combination in the prevention of systolic and diastolic CHF versus calcium blocker and α-blocker, and diastolic CHF versus ACEI, in elderly hypertension. (From Davis BR, Kostis JR, Simpson LM et al. Heart failure with preserved and reduced left ventricular ejection fraction in the antihypertensive and lipid-lowering treatment to prevent heart attack trial. *Circulation* 2008;118:2259–67.)

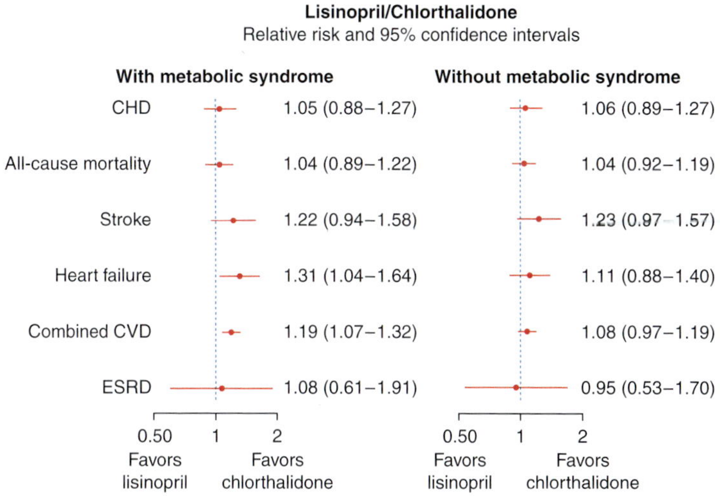

Fig. 10-21 ALLHAT, $n = 33\,357$—chlorthalidone ± atenolol was at least equivalent to lisinopril-based therapy in reducing CV endpoints in both MS and non-MS elderly hypertensives. (From Black HR, Davis B, Barzilay J, et al. Metabolic and clinical outcomes in nondiabetic individuals with the metabolic syndrome assigned to chlorthalidone, amlodipine or lisinopril as initial treatment for hypertension. *Diabetes Care* 2008;31:353–60.)

Guidelines advise not to receive the diuretic/β-blocker combination is the very important group who will benefit the most.

Another important factor in favor of a diuretic/β-blocker combination in the elderly hypertensive is that both diuretic (49) and β-blocker (50) reduce the risk of bone fracture, with a 30% reduction in fracture risk with the combination of diuretic and β-blocker (50).

Finally, metabolic disturbance with diuretics can be avoided by the use of potassium sparing diuretics like amiloride (Figure 10-13) (30). Regarding β-blocker-induced metabolic disturbance, this can be avoided by the use of highly β-1 selective bisoprolol (24).

SUMMARY AND CONCLUSIONS

1. Guidance on the treatment of hypertension from 3 leading guideline groups such as UK NICE Committee, the US JNC-7, and European guidelines varies markedly; NICE has demoted β-blockers and diuretics as the first-line therapy for uncomplicated hypertension, recommending ACE/ARB as the first-line therapy for the young/middle-aged hypertensives and calcium blockers as first-line for the elderly hypertensives; US JNC-7 guidelines recommends first-line diuretics for all hypertensives; and European guidelines recommends all classes of antihypertensive agents for all hypertensives, thus confusion reigns.
2. The NICE recommendations are based on cost-effectiveness calculations, which highlight the metabolic disturbance caused by thiazide-type diuretics and nonselective (or moderately selective) β-blockers, and the notion that β-blockers are ineffective at reducing the risk of stroke; and calcium blockers are favored due to their ability to reduce SBP variability.
3. Critics of the NICE position on diuretics point out that (a) potassium sparing diuretics, for example, co-amilozide, avoid metabolic disturbance and are linked to a remarkable 44% reduction in the risk of MI in the elderly (MRC elderly study), (b) the importance of reduced BP variability with calcium blockers has not been tested prospectively, and (c) in the largest ever hard endpoint study, that is ALLHAT, diuretic therapy was favored over calcium blocker and ACEI therapy.
4. Critics of the NICE β-blocker position point out that (a) in nonsmoking (75% of population) young/middle-aged diastolic hypertensives, nonselective (or poorly selective) β-blockers

reduce the risk of MI (number one killer), versus placebo or diuretics, by a sizable 30%–45%; (b) in the only β-blocker/ACEI comparison (UKPDS study, in high-risk, middle-aged, diabetic, diastolic hypertensives), the reduction in all 7 primary endpoints, versus "less tight control of BP," favored the β-blocker, and at 20-year follow-up, there was a significant 23% reduction in all-cause death in those randomized to the β-blocker; clearly, excess deaths are cost effective!; (c) in the UKPDS study, there was a 50% reduction in stroke risk in those randomized to β-blocker, versus less tight control of BP (similar to the 50+% reduction in stroke risk by propranolol, versus placebo, in nonsmokers in the MRC mild hypertension study in middle-aged diastolic hypertensives); the NICE position on β-blockers and stroke risk is relevant only to elderly systolic hypertensives; and (d) the most effective way to lower 24-hour BP in young/middle-aged, diastolic hypertensives is via high β-1 selectivity, that is, bisoprolol (which also avoids metabolic disturbance).

5. Critics of the NICE ARB position point out that (a) meta-analyses indicate that ARBs may not reduce (and may increase) the risk of MI, (b) in the only 2 hard endpoint studies involving ARBs in young/middle-aged subjects, the ARB increased the risk of CV events versus placebo; as with the ACEI/β-blocker issue, excess deaths are clearly cost effective!, and (c) ARBs, like diuretics and dihydropyridine calcium blockers, increase the sympathetic nerve activity, and with it the risk of MI, in young/middle-aged diastolic hypertensives.
6. The US JNC-7 recommendations that diuretics should be present in all prescriptions for the treatment of hypertension, are based on meta-analyses that do not take age into account; most hard end point diuretic studies have been in elderly systolic hypertensives, where first-line diuretics perform extremely well.
7. Critics of JNC-7 point out that (a) in the 3 randomized, hard-endpoint studies in young/middle-aged diastolic hypertensives, first-line diuretic therapy was highly effective in reducing the stroke risk, versus placebo, but did not reduce (and may increase) the risk of MI and (b) thiazide-type diuretics, like ARBs and dihydropyridine calcium blockers, increase the sympathetic nerve activity, and with it the risk of MI, in young/middle-aged diastolic hypertensive (with already raised sympathetic nerve activity and sensitized β-receptors).
8. The European guidelines state that (a) all drug classes reduce BP to a similar extent, (b) all drug classes reduce the risk of CV events to a similar extent, (c) CV protection is purely

dependent on achieved treated BP, (d) ranking of first-line therapy is inappropriate, and (e) the combination of diuretics and β-blockers should be avoided.

9. Critics of the European guidelines point out that (a) had age been taken into account, it would be apparent that the β-1 blockade is the most effective way to lower BP in the young/middle-aged, but is relatively ineffective at reducing central pressures in the elderly; (b) diastolic hypertension in young/middle-aged is underpinned by high sympathetic nerve activity and sensitized β-receptors, thus β-1 blockade is effective in reducing the risk of both MI and stroke (nonselective/poorly selective β-blockers are effective only in nonsmokers; the smoking hypertensive interaction can be avoided by high β-1 selectivity, i.e., bisoprolol); (c) drugs that increase the sympathetic nerve activity in young/middle-aged diastolic hypertensives, that is, diuretics, dihydropyridine calcium blockers, and ARBs, reduce the stroke risk, but not risk of MI; (d) in the elderly systolic hypertensive, first-line β-blockade compares poorly versus diuretics or calcium blockers, regarding the reduction of CV risk; (e) diuretic/β-blocker combinations have been highly effective in reducing the risk of stroke and MI in the elderly, and may be preferred to ACEI, or calcium blocker, therapy; (f) metabolic disturbance associated with diuretic/β-blocker combination therapy can be avoided by the use of potassium-sparing diuretic therapy combined with highly β-1 selective β-blockade; (g) elderly patients with the metabolic syndrome benefit (in terms of CV event, and heart failure, reduction) as least as well as patients without the syndrome, from a diuretic/β-blocker combination; and (h) the diuretic/β-blocker combination is highly effective in reducing the risk of bone fracture in the elderly.

REFERENCES

1. Alpert JS. A review of clinical guidelines with some thoughts about their utility and appropriate use. *Am J Med* 2010;123:573–6.
2. Neuman J, Korenstein D, Ross JS, et al. Prevalence of financial conflicts of interest among guideline panel members in Canada and United States: cross sectional study. *BMJ* 2011;342:d5621.
3. Gale EA. Conflicts of interest in guideline panel members. *BMJ* 2011;343:d5728; doi:10.1136/bmj.d5728.
4. Williams B, Poulter NR, Brown MJ, et al. British Hypertension Society guidelines for hypertension management 2004 (BHS-IV): summary. *BMJ* 2004;328:634–40.

5. Brown MJ, Cruickshank JK, Dominiczak AF, et al.; Executive Committee British Hypertensive Society. Better blood pressure control: how to combine drugs. *J Hum Hypertens* 2003;17:81–6.
6. National Institute for Health and Clinical Excellence. Hypertension: management of hypertension in adults in primary care (Clinical guidelines 34) 2006. www.nice.org.uk/CG034
7. Williams B. The obese hypertensive. The weight of evidence against beta-blockers. *Circulation* 2007;115:1973–4.
8. Krause T, Lovibond K, Caufield M, et al. Management of hypertension: summary of NICE guidance. *BMJ* 2011;343:d4891; doi:10.1136/bmj:d4891.
9. Ambrosioni E, Borghi C. Pharmacoeconomic and cost-benefit aspects. In: Mancia G, Grassi G, Kjeldsen SE, editors. *Manual of hypertension of the European Society of Hypertension*. Informa UK Ltd; 2008. p. 316–20.
10. Dodhia H, Phillips K, Zannou M-I, et al. Modelling the impact of available cardiovascular disease burden and costs of interventions to lower SBP in the England population. *J Hypertens* 2012;30:217–26.
11. Lovibond K, Jowett S, Barton P, et al. Cost-effectiveness options for the diagnosis of high blood pressure in primary care: a modelling study. *Lancet* 2011;378:1219–30.
12. Mancia G, De Backer G, Dominiczak A, et al. The task force for the management of arterial hypertension of the European Society of Hypertension, The task force for the management of arterial hypertension of the European Society of Cardiology. The Task Force for the management of arterial hypertension of the European Society of Hypertension (ESH) and the European Society of Cardiology 2007 Guidelines for the management of arterial hypertension. *Eur Heart J* 2007;28:1462–536.
13. Murray CI, Lauer JA, Hutubessy RC, et al. Effectiveness and cost of interventions to lower systolic blood pressure and cholesterol: global and regional analysis on reduction of cardiovascular disease risk. *Lancet* 2003;361:717–25.
14. Stason WB. Hypertension: a policy perspective, 1976–2008. *J Am Soc Hypertens* 2009;3:113–8.
15. Muszbek N, Brixner D, Benedict A, et al. The economic consequences of non-compliance in cardiovascular disease and related conditions: a literature review. *Int J Clin Pract* 2008;62:328–35.
16. Klarenbach SW, McAllister FA, Johansen H, et al. Identification of factors driving differences in cost effectiveness of first-line pharmacological therapy for uncomplicated hypertension. *Can J Cardiol* 2010;26:e158–e163.
17. Grimm C, Kobenein J, Wiosna W, et al. New-onset diabetes and antihypertensive treatment. *GMS Health Technol Assess* 2010;6:Doc 03.
18. Williams B. Beta-blockers and the treatment of hypertension. *J Hypertens* 2007;25:1351–3.

19. Cruickshank JM. Don't beta-blockers still have a role in hypertension? *BMJ* 2011;343:d6495.
20. Williams B, Krause T, Lovibond K, et al. Authors' reply. *BMJ* 2011;343:d6501.
21. Holman RR, Paul SK, Bethel MA, et al. Long-term follow-up after tight control of blood pressure in type-2 diabetes. *N Engl J Med* 2008;359:1565–76.
22. UK Prospective Diabetes Study Group. Efficacy of atenolol and captopril in reducing the risk of macrovascular and micro-vascular complications in type 2 diabetes; UKPDS 39. *BMJ* 1998;317:713–20.
23. Medical Research Working Party. MRC trial of treatment of mild hypertension: principal results. *BMJ* 1985;291:97–104.
24. Cruickshank JM. *The Modern Role of Beta-Blockers in Cardiovascular Medicine*. Shelton, Connecticut: People's Medical Publishing House; 2011.
25. von Armin T; for the TIBBS Investigators. Prognostic significance of transient ischaemic episodes: response to treatment shows improved prognosis. *J Am Coll Cardiol* 1996;28:20–4.
26. Zamorano JL. Heart rate management: a therapeutic goal throughout the cardiovascular continuum. *Eur Heart J* 2008;10(suppl F):F17–F21.
27. Sofat R, Casas JP, Grosso A, et al. Could we simplify NICE guidance on choosing anti-hypertensive drugs? *BMJ* 2012;343:d8078.
28. Imai E, Chan JC, Yamasaki T, et al. Effects of olmesartan on renal and cardiovascular outcomes in type-2 diabetes with overt nephropathy: a multicentre, randomised, placebo-controlled study. *Diabetologia* 2011;54:2978–86.
29. Haller H, Ito S, Izzo JL, et al. Olmesartan for the delay or prevention of microalbuminuria in type-2 diabetes. *N Engl J Med* 2011;364:907–17.
30. Brown MJ. The choice of diuretic in hypertension: saving the baby from the bathwater. *Heart* 2011;97:1547–51.
31. Brown M, Cruickshank K, MacDonald T. Navigating the shoals in hypertension discovery and guidance. *BMJ* 2012;344:23–6.
32. MRC Working Party. Medical Research Council trial of hypertension in older adults: principal results. *BMJ* 1992;304:405–12.
33. The ALLHAT Officers and Coordinators for the ALLHAT Collaborative Research Group. Major outcomes in high-risk hypertensive patients randomised to angiotensin-converting enzyme inhibitor or calcium channel blocker vs diuretic: the Antihypertensive and Lipid-lowering Treatment to Prevent heart Attack Trial (ALLHAT). *JAMA* 2002;288:2981–97.
34. Chobanian AV, Bakris GL, Black HR, et al. Seventh report of the Joint National Committee on prevention, detection, evaluation, and treatment of high blood pressure. *Hypertension* 2003;42:1206–52.
35. Franklin SS, Pio JR, Wong ND, et al. Predictors of new-onset diastolic and systolic hypertension. The Framingham Heart Study. *Circulation* 2005;111:1121–7.

36. Report by the Management Committee. The Australian therapeutic trial in mild hypertension. *Lancet* 1980;1:1261–7.
37. Leren P, Helgeland A. Coronary heart disease and the treatment of hypertension. Some Oslo study data. *Am J Med* 1986;80:3–6.
38. Mancia G, Laurent S, Agabiti-Rosei E, et al. Reappraisal of European guidelines on hypertension management: a European Society of Hypertension Task Force document. *J Hypertens* 2009;27:2121–58.
39. Redon J, Cifkova R, Laurent S, et al. The metabolic syndrome in hypertension: European society of hypertension position statement. *J Hypertens* 2008;26:1891–1900.
40. Deary AJ, Schumann AL, Murfeet H, et al. Double-blind, placebo controlled crossover comparison of 5 classes of drugs. *J Hypertens* 2002;20:771–7.
41. Morgan T, Lauri J, Bertram D, et al. Effect of different antihypertensive drug classes on central aortic pressure. *Am J Hypertens* 2004;17:118–23.
42. Coope J, Warrender TS. Randomised trial of treatment of hypertension in primary care (HEP). *BMJ* 1986;293:1145–51.
43. Kjeldsen SE, Dahlof B, Devereux RB, et al. Effect of losartan on cardiovascular morbidity and mortality in patients with isolated hypertension and left-ventricular hypertrophy. *JAMA* 2002;288:1491–8.
44. Dahlof B, Sever P, Poulter N, et al. Prevention of cardiovascular events with an antihypertensive regimen of amlodipine adding peridopril as required versus atenolol adding bendroflumethazide as required (ASCOT-BPLA); a multicentre randomised controlled trial. *Lancet* 2005;366:895–906.
45. Cruickshank JM. Are we misunderstanding beta blockers? *Int J Cardiol* 2007;120:10–27.
46. Pepine CJ, Handberg EM, Cooper-Dehoff RM, et al. A calcium antagonist vs non-calcium antagonist hypertension treatment strategy for patients with coronary artery disease (INVEST). *JAMA* 2003;290:2805–16.
47. Davis BR, Kostis JR, Simpson LM, et al. Heart failure with preserved and reduced left ventricular ejection fraction in the antihypertensive and lipid-lowering treatment to prevent heart attack trial. *Circulation* 2008;118:2259–67.
48. Black HR, Davis B, Barzilay J, et al. Metabolic and clinical outcomes in nondiabetic individuals with the metabolic syndrome assigned to chlorthalidone, amlodipine or lisinopril as initial treatment for hypertension. *Diabetes Care* 2008;31:353–60.
49. LaCroix AZ, Wienpahl J, White LR, et al. Thiazide diuretic agents and the incidence of hip fracture. *N Engl J Med* 1990;322:286–90.
50. Schlienger RG, Kraenzlin ME, Jick SS, et al. Use of beta-blockers and risk of fractures. *JAMA* 2004;292:1326–32.

Index

H

Y